THE YANG TÀIJÍ
24-STEP SHORT FORM

by the same author

Tàijí Jiàn 32-Posture Sword Form
James Drewe
ISBN 978 1 84819 011 5

of related interest

Tàijíquán
Li Deyin
Foreword by Siu-Fong Evans
ISBN 978 1 84819 004 7

What is 'Tai Chi'?
Peter A. Gilligan
ISBN 978 1 84819 024 5

Chen
Living Taijiquan in the Classical Style
Master Jan Silberstorff
Translated by Michael Vorwerk
ISBN 978 1 84819 021 4

Alchemy of Pushing Hands
Oleg Tcherne
ISBN 978 1 84819 022 1

JAMES DREWE

THE YANG TÀIJÍ 24-STEP SHORT FORM

A STEP-BY-STEP GUIDE FOR ALL LEVELS

SINGING
DRAGON

London and Philadelphia

Extracts from the BCCMA Competition Manual reprinted with kind permission from the BCCMA

First published in 2011
by Singing Dragon
an imprint of Jessica Kingsley Publishers
116 Pentonville Road
London N1 9JB, UK
and
400 Market Street, Suite 400
Philadelphia, PA 19106, USA

www.singing-dragon.com

Copyright © James Drewe 2011
Illustrations copyright © Damian Johnston 2011

All rights reserved. No part of this publication may be reproduced in any material form (including photocopying or storing it in any medium by electronic means and whether or not transiently or incidentally to some other use of this publication) without the written permission of the copyright owner except in accordance with the provisions of the Copyright, Designs and Patents Act 1988 or under the terms of a licence issued by the Copyright Licensing Agency Ltd, Saffron House, 6–10 Kirby Street, London EC1N 8TS. Applications for the copyright owner's written permission to reproduce any part of this publication should be addressed to the publisher.

Warning: The doing of an unauthorised act in relation to a copyright work may result in both a civil claim for damages and criminal prosecution.

Library of Congress Cataloging in Publication Data
A CIP catalog record for this book is available from the Library of Congress

British Library Cataloguing in Publication Data
A CIP catalogue record for this book is available from the British Library

ISBN 978 1 84819 041 2

Printed and bound in the United States by
Thomson-Shore, Inc.

Outer expression can *lead* to inner experience, but it can never substitute for it. Yet when inner experience leads to outer expression, the circle is complete – and this is the purpose of Life, and the function of the World, and of the entire Universe as well.

Neale Donald Walsh

Acknowledgements

I would like to thank several people for their help in writing this book: Richard Watson for his support and for originally introducing me to and teaching me the Yang Tàijí 24-Step Short Form; Simon Watson for his many discussions with me on the subject and for modelling for the photographs; Professor Li Deyin for teaching me the 24-Step Form; Beryl Tollady for teaching me the Alexander Technique over many years; Master Huang Ping for showing me yet another perspective of the Form; many of my students for their loyalty and for asking me questions about the Form, forcing me to seek the answers; and my wife Georgina for supporting my enthusiasm for tàijí and for doing the first editorial check.

Photography: Simon Butcher, Zebu Design.

Anatomical drawings: Damian Johnston.

Photographs of Simon Watson, Longfei Taijiquan Association.

Contents

1.	Introduction	13
	Brief history	14
	What is a tàijí form or routine?	15
	Ways of performing tàijí	15
	Why do tàijí?	16
	Traditional and modern tàijí	17
2.	Warm-Up Exercises	19
	1. Bouncing – arms forwards and backwards	19
	2. Turning to left and right	21
	3. Arms drop and swing	22
3.	Posture	25
	The balance points on the feet	25
	Body alignment	26
	Tàijí and posture	27
4.	Grounding	28
	Preparation	28
	The feet	29
	The knees	29
	The hips, the pelvis and the waist	30
	The shoulders	30
	The hands and arms	30
	Freeing the neck	31
	Keeping the neck free in tàijí	33
	The jaw	33
	The crown	34

	Standing up out of the feet	34
	Qì 气 (氣 traditional)	35
5.	Relaxation and Release	37
	The mind	37
	The body	37
	Tàijí for health	40
	Tàijí for self-defence	40
6.	The Hands and the Hand Positions	42
	The open palm	42
	The fist	43
	The crane's beak	43
7.	The Arms and Shoulders	44
	Moving the arms	44
8.	The Knees	46
	Looking after the knees	46
9.	Stances (步形 Bùxíng)	48
	1. Open Stance (standing with feet apart)	48
	2. Horse Stance	49
	3. Bow Stance	49
	4. Empty Stance	50
	5. T-Stance	51
	6. One-legged Stance	52
	7. Crouch Stance (like a servant)	52
10.	Footwork Techniques (步法 Bùfǎ)	54
	Forwards step	54
	Backwards step	54
	Withdrawing step	54
	Swing step	55
	Grinding step	55
	Turning-in step	55

11. The Process of Stepping	56
1. How to step	56
2. Problems in stepping	58
3. Finding the right stepping distance	59
4. Stepping to push	59
12. Breathing in the Form	60
Abdominal breathing exercise	61
13. Definitions	62
The centre, centre-turn and the centreline of the body	62
Sitting back	63
Holding the ball	63
Tucking under/Coccyx/Tailbone/Pelvic tilt/	
Pull in lower abdominal muscles	63
Slipping the (rear) heel	64
Screwdriver turn of the hand	64
The clock system of defining directions	65
The Kuà 胯	66
The hypothenar eminence	67
Key to foot patterns	67
Note on pronunciation of Chinese words	68
Yang Tàijí 24-Step Form with music	68
14. Structure of the Standardized Yang Tàijí 24-Step Short Form	70
Section 1 (3 movements)	70
Section 2 (3 movements)	70
Section 3 (2 movements)	71
Section 4 (3 movements)	71
Section 5 (4 movements)	71
Section 6 (2 movements)	72
Section 7 (3 movements)	72
Section 8 (4 movements)	72

15. Description of the Yang Tàijí 24-Step Short Form ... 73
    Ready Position ... 74

    Section 1 (3 movements) ... 76
        1. Commencing Form ... 76
        2. Parting the Wild Horse's Mane (Left and Right) ... 81
        3. Stork Spreads its Wings ... 99

    Section 2 (3 movements) ... 105
        4. Brush Knee and Twist Step (Left and Right) ... 105
        5. Play the Pipa ... 124
        6. Curve Back Arms (Left and Right) ... 129

    Section 3 (2 movements) ... 141
        7. Grasp the Bird's Tail (Left Style) ... 141
        8. Grasp the Bird's Tail (Right Style) ... 159

    Section 4 (3 movements) ... 170
        9. Single Whip ... 170
        10. Cloud Hands ... 180
        11. Single Whip ... 192

    Section 5 (4 movements) ... 195
        12. High Pat on Horse ... 195
        13. Kick with Right Heel ... 200
        14. Strike (Opponent's) Ears with Both Fists ... 211
        15. Turn and Kick with Left Heel ... 215

    Section 6 (2 movements) ... 222
        16. Push Down and Stand on One Leg (Left Style) ... 222
        17. Push Down and Stand on One Leg (Right Style) ... 234

    Section 7 (3 movements) ... 249
        18. Jade Lady Weaves Shuttles ... 249
        19. Needle at Sea Bottom ... 260
        20. Flash Arms ... 266

    Section 8 (4 movements) ... 270
        21. Turn, Deflect Downwards, Parry and Punch ... 270
        22. Apparent Close-Up ... 279
        23. Cross Hands ... 284
        24. Closing Form ... 288

16. Easy Reference ... 293
    Ready Position ... 293

    Section 1 (3 movements) ... 294
        1. Commencing Form ... 294
        2. Parting the Wild Horse's Mane (Left and Right) ... 295
        3. Stork Spreads its Wings ... 296

Section 2 (3 movements)	296
4. Brush Knee and Twist Step (Left and Right)	296
5. Play the Pipa	298
6. Curve Back Arms (Left and Right)	298
Section 3 (2 movements)	300
7. Grasp the Bird's Tail (Left Style)	300
8. Grasp the Bird's Tail (Right Style)	301
Section 4 (3 movements)	302
9. Single Whip	302
10. Cloud Hands	302
11. Single Whip	304
Section 5 (4 movements)	305
12. High Pat on Horse	305
13. Kick with Right Heel	305
14. Strike (Opponent's) Ears with Both Fists	306
15. Turn and Kick with Left Heel	306
Section 6 (2 movements)	307
16. Push Down and Stand on One Leg (Left Style)	307
17. Push Down and Stand on One Leg (Right Style)	308
Section 7 (3 movements)	309
18. Jade Lady Weaves Shuttles	309
19. Needle at Sea Bottom	310
20. Flash Arms	310
Section 8 (4 movements)	311
21. Turn, Deflect Downwards, Parry and Punch	311
22. Apparent Close-Up	312
23. Cross Hands	312
24. Closing Form	313
17. Beyond the Basics	**314**
General points on the Form	314
Connecting the body in tàijí	321
Yin and Yang in the Form	332
The centre	334
18. Open (Kâi 开) and Close (Hé 合)	**341**
How to close the centre	342
Exercise in 'opening' and 'closing' the arms	343
Function of closing the centre	344
Opening and closing the limbs	345
Péng energy	345

The Bows of the Arms, Legs and Back	347
Testing moves	352
Educated relaxation	354
Intention (Yĭ)	354
Fā jìn	355
The Yang Tàijí 24-Step Short Form music: Breakdown of beats per movement	361
The Yang Tàijí 24-Step Short Form in competition	364
19. Footprint of the Form	369
Key to foot patterns	369
ABOUT THE AUTHOR	381
FURTHER READING	382

1

Introduction

Understanding the Absolute by practising in the Relative.

I first began to learn the Chinese Martial Arts in 1975 and took to them instantly. It was particularly appealing that the movements used *all* of me and nothing else; it was completely self-contained. After all, there *is* nothing other than you, is there? Everything else is either a projection or a reflection of you…and tàijí has all of it, it's the Universe and simultaneously your *own* universe constantly fluctuating and changing, expanding and contracting, breathing in and out from its core… But I didn't think all of this at the time; I just knew that there was something about it that appealed to me.

So for me, tàijí is about understanding myself, the world (the 'Relative') that I live in, and my relationship to that Relative world so that I can understand how the entire Universe (the 'Absolute') functions – after all, if everything is a microcosm, I think I stand a chance of getting there! But I know that this isn't everyone's reason for doing the art, and in the section on p.16 entitled 'Why do tàijí?' I have mentioned other reasons that I know people take it up.

As I wrote the descriptive text of the book, I became more and more aware that our language was inadequate for describing the *feeling* behind the movements, particularly when it came to describing the 'open' and 'close' feelings that are at the heart of the idea of the body working from the core.

I've done my best with it, but am conscious of the shortcomings of some of the detailed descriptions of the movements (thus the 'Notes' at the end of each movement). Throughout the text I have repeated a considerable amount, but to have a complete text, it would require endless amounts of repetition – the same material being mentioned for almost every movement, as the principles of tàijí repeat continuously.

Therefore, to a certain extent, the reader will need to apply the principles mentioned in some movements to other movements.

I've chosen the Yang Tàijí 24-Step Short Form not because it was the first form that I learnt (it wasn't, it was the fourth), but because it is currently the most practised form. But it really doesn't matter which form you practise, the principles remain constant in any set of tàijí movements.

BRIEF HISTORY

The Yang Tàijí 24-Step Short Form was created by the National Physical, Cultural and Sports Committee of the People's Republic of China in 1956.

It was formed from the movements of the Traditional Long Form, which is sometimes known as the Original Long Form, the 108, 105, 103, 85 or 81 posture forms (the reason for the different numbering is that the postures are counted in different ways).

The Original 108 can take two or more years for a beginner to become familiar with the shape of the movements alone, and takes anything from 15–25 minutes to perform. In addition to this, there is a great deal of repetition in the movements, and students can find the structure of the Form both confusing and difficult to remember. For many it is hard to devote the time and maintain the momentum to learn the entire set of movements, and it was felt that a shorter form would be beneficial to encourage the growth of the Yang Tàijí.

The 24-Step Short Form was therefore constructed to make tàijí more accessible to a wider range of people. It is not a daunting task for the younger student to learn it, it is not too tiring for the older student, and, for those who have busy lives and time constraints, practising it is easier and more realistic. The 24-Step Form is referred to as a 'standardized' routine because it is performed in the same way globally, unlike the traditional 108-Step Form, which is performed in as many different ways as there are instructions.

The Form is constructed entirely of movements taken from the Traditional Yang Style Form (see also 'Traditional and modern tàijí' on p.17) but also included are some movements that in the Traditional Form are only performed on one side (i.e. in left or right style). So, for example, Grasp the Bird's Tail, instead of only being performed in right style as in the Traditional Form, is also performed in left style, and the same is true for Push Down and Stand on One Leg.

The Form is also designed so that the movements increase in complexity from start to finish. In the footwork, apart from Form 1, the next eight forms use only Bow, Empty and 'T' Stances, and it is only after this that the range of foot movement increases. This is generally true for the hand movements as well; they are more complicated in the last two-thirds of the Form, especially in conjunction with the more complex foot patterns.

WHAT IS A TÀIJÍ FORM OR ROUTINE?

A form or routine is a series or pattern of movements using Chinese Martial Arts techniques. These techniques can be kicks, pushes, punches, strikes, throws, wrist or arm locks, deflections, defensive blocks, etc. that have been combined into a series of continuous movement, where one 'application' flows smoothly into another, sometimes with connective movements, sometimes not.

WAYS OF PERFORMING TÀIJÍ

It isn't necessary to practise tàijí as though you were an athlete; it can be done in many ways, and for many different purposes, and no one method is better than another because, *however* you do it, you will always get something out of it, even though it may not be obvious at the time.

- There are days when you want to put your all into it, low postures – a real physical workout that leaves you sweating, and your muscles aching.
- It can be done almost completely standing up with straight legs, simply running through the arm and body movements to get the coordination and the feel of the movements. This way is good just for the memory of the movements, but it is also good if you have very little space because the steps will be smaller.
- It can be done as 'shadow boxing', feeling the martial applications of every movement you make.
- It can be done as a *Yìquán* exercise[1] where you feel the contractions and expansions of your joints working against each other – like magnets, sometimes attracting, and sometimes repelling each other.
- You can do it very lightly and rapidly so that it only takes a few minutes.

---

1 Please see www.yiquan.org.uk/art-pom2 for Karel Koskuba's description of Yìquán.

- You can do it focusing on a particular aspect, for example the 'open/close' of the body, the way that the centre moves, your balance, your breathing, the way in which you place the foot when taking a step, where you place your eyes, how you hold the tàijí hand, how you release your neck, how relaxed you are…and so on.
- You can do it slowly so that it takes 15 or more minutes.

It's not really important *how* you do it because the next time you come to do it, it won't be the same – it never is, that's the great thing about it. You'll be focusing on something else, you'll be more relaxed or less relaxed than the last time; you'll notice something else about it that you haven't noticed before, and occasionally you'll have one of those moments of epiphany when you think 'Oh! Of course, *that's* why you do that!', and ten minutes later it will seem so obvious that you cannot think why you hadn't seen it before!

WHY DO TÀIJÍ?

Tàijí is a very adaptable art, and there are many and various reasons for learning it.

- It doesn't involve any equipment. It's your own personal gym – great for exercise, such as stretching and toning muscles and loosening the body.
- It's good for your general health.
- It's good for coordination.
- It's good for balance.
- It's good for flexibility.
- It teaches relaxation and calmness.
- It is very gentle exercise, but at the same time can be as demanding as you want it to be.
- It is sometimes known as a 'moving meditation', bringing focus, improving concentration, and clearing the mind.
- It builds confidence in your body.
- It develops the sensitivity of your body and awareness of your relationship to your surroundings.
- It connects mind, body and spirit.

- Many people like the weapons aspect of it (sword, stick, staff, fan, etc.).
- It is good for both men and women equally.
- It is excellent for the elderly.
- It helps you to meet other like-minded people – a social activity.
- It is a very effective martial art, which, because it is practised slowly, provides a non-aggressive learning approach to martial arts.
- It achieves balance of the left and right side of the brain (analytical/intuitive, etc.).

…and many other reasons…

I know that in tàijí we talk a lot about working from the 'centre', but the more I do tàijí the more that I feel as though we are learning to work from the heart.

If your body is a reflection of the entire world, or even of the entire cosmos, this means that by working with your body you are learning to understand how the world itself functions, how life 'works'. The more that you observe about yourself and the way in which your body connects and operates, and the more that you compare this to the way in which the world operates, the more similarities you find and the more you understand.

It seems to me that in working from the dāntián – the abdominal energy centre, we are learning the mechanics of the way in which the world functions. But when you start to use partner work, you simultaneously work from the energy centre of the heart, for tàijí is also about 'feeling', or perhaps a better word is 'sensing'.

The 'heart' doesn't really refer to the organ of the heart, but it does relate to that area in the chest, sometimes called the middle dāntián. It is a metaphorical heart that connects your feeling/sensing abilities to the world and is said to be the bridge between the mind and the soul – the bridge between thinking and feeling/sensing.

TRADITIONAL AND MODERN TÀIJÍ

Although the Yang 24-Step Form has now been classified as a 'traditional' form, as it is over 50 years old, it is still really a 'modern' form in the scheme of things.

Much of the beginning of my tàijí career was taken up in learning one of the older and more 'traditional' Yang forms, the 108-Step, sometimes known as the 'Original Long Form'. All of us who were learning at this time agreed that this was the peak of tàijí perfection – we were learning from a genuine tàijí master… it couldn't get any better. This was especially true for one or two friends of mine who had been learning with another teacher for whom they had lost all respect; they felt that they had wasted five years in his school. Twenty or so years later, I came across one of those friends with whom I had lost contact. He was now with a different teacher. 'Ah,' he said to me, 'Now I've really found the *true* tàijí.'

The 'true tàijí' lies in you, not in some master or other. I've seen a few 'masters' over the years, and yes, I'm sure that some of them are very good. Others have a wealth of knowledge but aren't really interested in passing it on, some just want your money, some have called themselves 'master', some want to display their skills, and some want to be set up on a pedestal and admired. And then there are those who are great teachers; they are the ones who are very generous with all that they know, who will devote time to correcting you patiently, and who have the foresight to push you in your learning neither too hard nor too fast.

There are some tàijí teachers who view the 'modern' forms as being second-rate, a watered-down version of 'the true tàijíquán'; they feel that the heart of tàijí has been lost in the modern forms, and that these same forms are often displays of great gymnastic skill, with little of what might be termed 'internal skill'. Having studied something of both, I cannot agree with this view; the underlying principles of tàijí are the same whether traditional or modern.

The twenty-first-century beginner, desiring quicker results, is undoubtedly more impatient than the nineteenth or twentieth-century beginner, and the endless repetitive teaching methods of the traditional schools don't suit most people nowadays – a shame, because as a foundation in the art it is probably much better. The modern student requires explanations, whereas in actual fact the answers appear when you've repeated a movement enough times and the question answers itself. (Many of my contemporaries who know me and who are reading this will undoubtedly be amused at this, as they know me to be the greatest question-asker of them all!) My only defence is that I am constantly asked questions by my students and often need definitive answers but, even as I write this, I know that actually the answers appear when you *feel* the movement correctly – obviously more practice is necessary!

2

Warm-Up Exercises

Most tàijí classes begin with some warm-ups that are aimed at loosening the joints of the body to avoid damage during the class.

The three warm-ups described below work on a variety of levels. I have used them for many years, and find that they loosen up the parts of the body most likely to be strained, particularly when the students coming to the classes have been sitting at desks for most of the day. But these exercises also work at a different level; they teach how the movements should come from the centre of the body.

1. BOUNCING – ARMS FORWARDS AND BACKWARDS

Basic

Place the feet a shoulder's width apart.

Allow the knees to bend and the body to 'bounce' lightly and not too slowly. Think of the 'bounces' as being in twos or pairs.

Do this for a while and let the arms hang by your sides. If you completely relax them, and let them move forwards and backwards very slightly, they will start to swing in time with the bouncing of the body – backwards with the first bounce, and then forwards with the second bounce. The height that you lift them is entirely up to you; they *can* swing as high as your shoulders when they swing forwards (but no higher). My personal preference is to completely relax them by my sides and hardly move them at all.

Above all, keep the shoulders completely soft and relaxed.

Keep about 70 per cent of your weight on your heels, and relax the back of your neck.

THE YANG TAIJI 24-STEP SHORT FORM

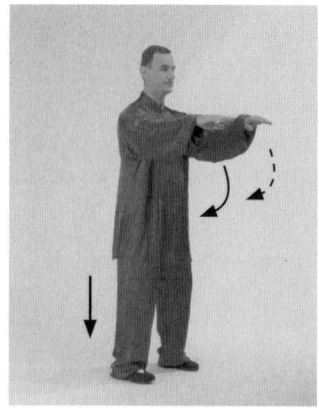
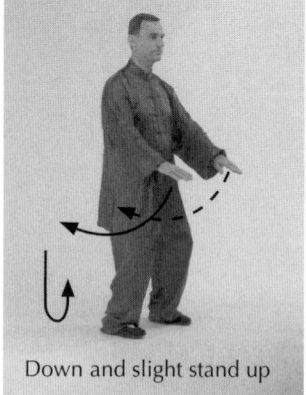
Down and slight stand up
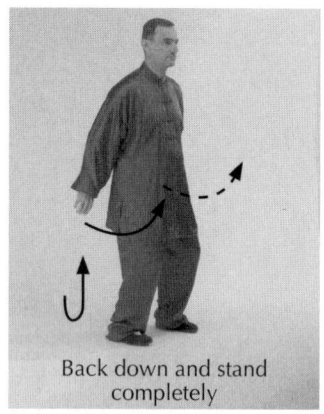
Back down and stand completely

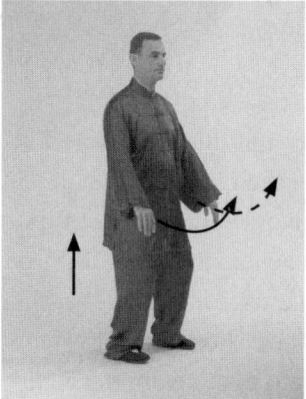
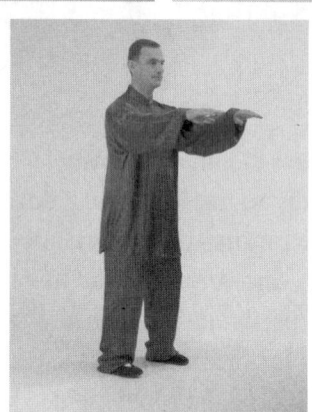

The next level

In this exercise you can feel the centre (dāntián) being moved; all movement of the arms should be governed by this centre-movement. Relax your centre as you bounce, ignoring the arms completely – they don't even have to swing at this stage. Just feel the centre of your body being 'shaken' as you bounce. You can then allow the arms to move, but you might find that it is no longer necessary to raise them so high.

Advanced level

As you sit down for the first bounce, gently pull your lower abdominal muscles in as though you are trying to squeeze into a pair of trousers that is too small. As you do this, let go of the pelvis/hips and allow it/them to tuck under, the small of the back relaxing. Another way to look at it is to feel as though tip of your tailbone (the coccyx) is a long tail. Try to flick your tail right through between your legs to the front, as though to hit yourself on your chest with the tip of the tail. This is doing a *pelvic tilt*.

Keep the abdominal muscles pulled in for the second bounce also, although you can start to ease off the pressure.

Doing the movement this way, you rotate the dāntián in a small vertical circle ahead of you.

This also opens up the small of the back, and gently lengthens the spine when you release the neck. In other words, the coccyx is lengthening downwards and under between the legs, and the neck should respond in the opposite direction – but with great caution. It is very important that this is done without any effort or force; the tailbone gently tucks under, or flexes under, and the neck just releases. Every time that you stand up, the lower spine reverts to its original position.

Do 50 to 100 times.

2. TURNING TO LEFT AND RIGHT

Basic

Place your feet a shoulder's width apart.

Put your hands on your hips/waist.

Without moving your head (keep the eyes fixed on something ahead of you) rotate your hips to the left and then to the right, keeping the body absolutely vertical.

Always keep your head looking straight in front of you, and keep the shoulders completely relaxed. As in the previous exercise, it is tempting to move the weight from the left foot to the right foot; however, it should stay in the middle so that the body is rotating on an entirely vertical axis.

Keep about 70 per cent of your weight on your heels.

The next level

Leave your hands by your sides.

Turn your body to your left and allow your right arm to swing forwards slightly – straight ahead of you to where you are looking. Your left arm will move naturally behind you.

Your head stays looking straight in front of you. As you turn your body to the right, allow your arms to drop to your sides again and straightaway rise up slightly ahead of and behind you again – this time with the left arm ahead of you, and the right arm behind you.

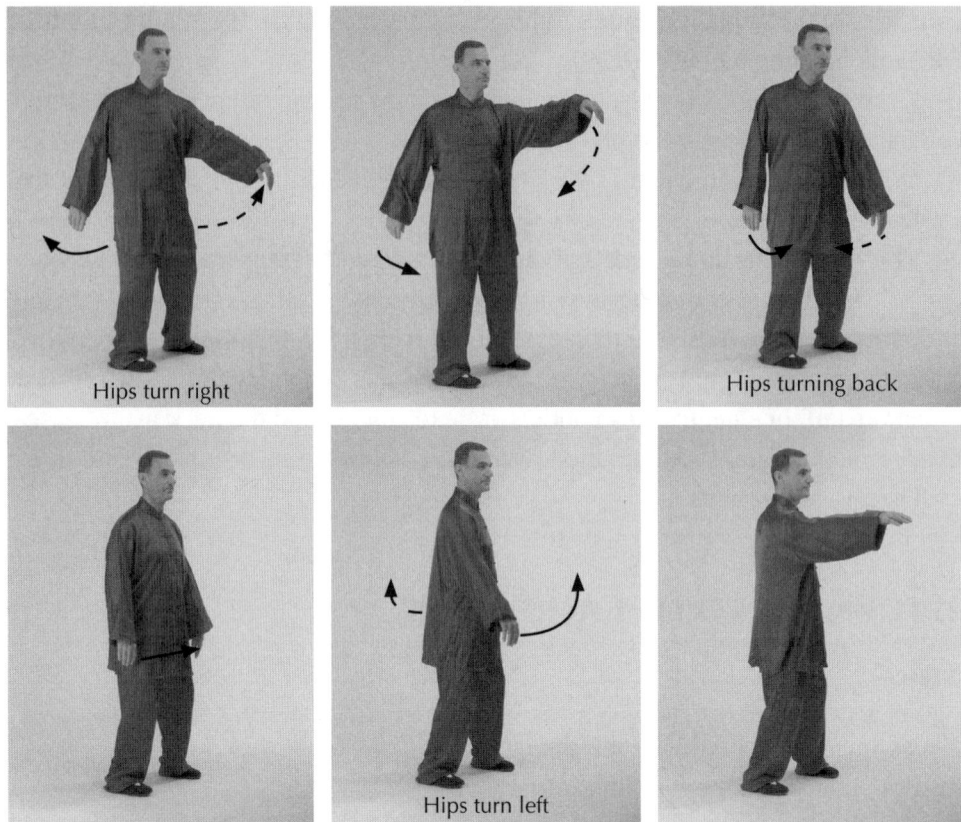

Beginners find this remarkably difficult; they usually want to swing the arms *around* the body, rather than let them swing *forwards* and backwards. It sometimes helps to think of moving the arms as though marching.

Once again, this is an exercise in turning the centre, and all arm movement should be felt as originating from the dāntián. This exercise creates a horizontal circle of the dāntián.

3. ARMS DROP AND SWING

Basic

Place your feet a shoulder and a half width apart.

Raise your arms up on either side of you slightly – perhaps to 45°, or not even that far.

Bend the knees and turn your waist to (for example) the left. As you do so, drop your arms towards the floor. The turn of your waist will carry your right arm in front of your body, and your left arm behind your body.

Turn your body back to the front again and stand up, lifting your arms on either side of you.

Do not turn the *hips*, only turn from the waist so that the hip/legs structure remains constant.

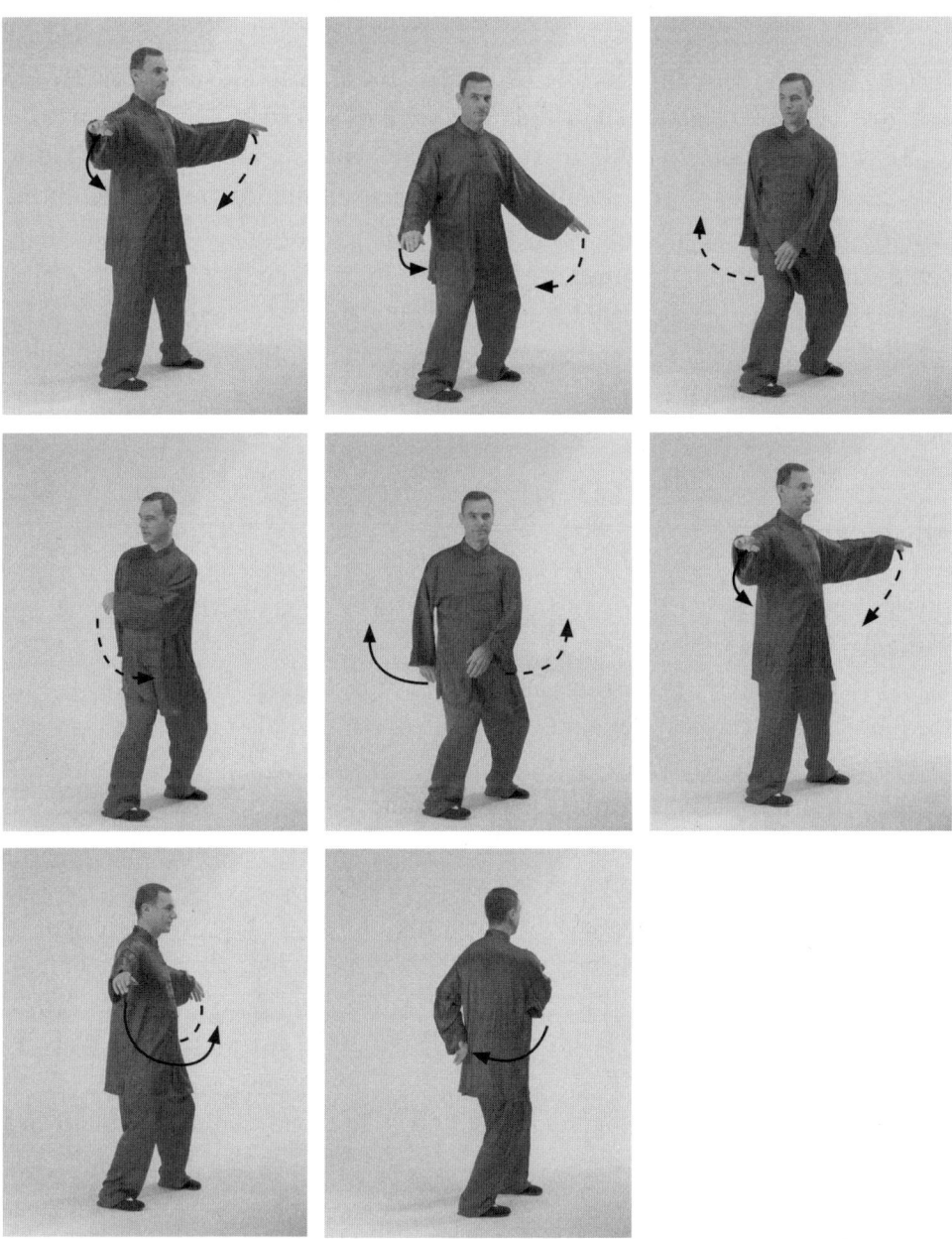

Keep the body upright throughout, and keep 50 per cent of the weight on each foot.

The shoulders should be completely relaxed; it can be tempting to allow them to rise as the arms lift.

The arms *can* lift as high as the shoulders if you like, but it isn't really necessary.

The next level

It is the drop and turn of the centre that causes the arms to move, so you need to feel your centre turning to left or right as your knees bend.

If you find it unavoidable to stop the hips from turning, it is possible to damage your knees if you aren't careful. When turning to (for example) the left, the right knee will have a tendency to collapse inwards, which potentially could cause damage to the inside of the knee joint. Therefore, when dropping and turning left, allow the right knee to open outwards; this exercises the Kuà 胯 (or anatomically, the inguinal groove) by opening it up on the right, whilst simultaneously closing it on the left – very good for the lymphatic system of the body.

Advanced level

It is also possible to use this warm-up to exercise different parts of the spine – in particular to free up the waist.

By not moving the pelvis/hips at all, and by just turning from the waist, only the thoracic and cervical vertebrae are rotated, but there is more to it than just this.

As you sit down, keep the hips facing the front. Some people find this difficult; the hips seem to want to turn. To avoid this, as you turn to (for example) your left, think of turning your left hip towards the front.

However, the most important thing is that as you do this, you also pull in your lower abdominal muscles and again tuck the tailbone/coccyx under, so once again you do a pelvic tilt.

The lower you sit down (within reason!) the easier it is to turn the waist to left or right.

This exercise is a combination of the first and second exercises, and creates a figure eight with the dāntián.

Do 50 to 100 times.

3

Posture

The basic posture is an upright one. The main reason for this is that the amount of energy expended in an upright posture is less than the amount expended in a leaning posture. As humans we move in and out of the upright posture continually, but we usually revert to the upright posture as the body can relax more easily.

In a leaning posture, the body is fighting gravity, and therefore certain muscle-groups will be working harder to ensure that you don't fall over. For example, if your body is leaning forwards at 45°, a large number of the major muscles in your back will be tensed in order to stop the body from falling any further. If you imagine stacking a large pile of plates on a table, the more precisely you stack them, the more you will be able to stack; if the exact centre of each plate is precisely on top of the exact centre of the plate below it, in theory you should be able to stack an endless number.

THE BALANCE POINTS ON THE FEET

The line of gravity passing through the body is over a point just ahead of the heel, where the heel rises up to the arch/instep of the foot. Throughout all movements you should aim to keep gravity passing through this point.

There are a surprising number of benefits from this:

- Your balance is improved.

- The number of muscles being used at any given time is significantly reduced.

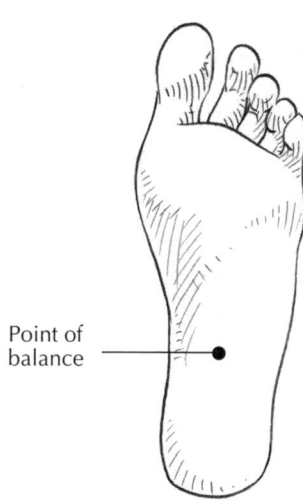

Sole of foot (balance points)

- Because you are no longer using more muscles than are necessary to maintain your balance, tension is released in the legs.

- Because you are using fewer muscles, this has the effect of allowing the legs and feet to relax, the circulation to improve, and the feet and legs to grow warm.

- Because there is less tension, the legs are freed and can stretch more easily – you are no longer holding unnecessary muscles under tension in order to do the job of keeping your balance; therefore those muscles can start to function correctly.

- Because the majority of muscles are relaxed, you can move from a state of non-action to action more easily.

- You feel much more grounded.

- If you follow the rule in a posture such as Bow Stance, i.e. moving the weight over the balance point on the *front* leg, you will find that it is impossible to take the front knee beyond the toes.

- In a posture such as Stork Spreads its Wings, or Play the Pipa, with the weight on the rear balance point, the pelvis tucks under automatically, the neck is automatically released, and the spine *needs* to stay vertical.

- I have found that there are knock-on effects throughout the entire body, for example, the shoulders and back are easier to relax, and the chest does not tighten.

- You are less likely to get knee joint problems.

BODY ALIGNMENT

Although the previous points make this fairly clear, it should be mentioned that, when standing in (for example) a shoulder-width stance, the crown of your head, the perineum and the point midway between the two feet should be aligned on a vertical axis. If your body is directly in line with the force of gravity, your body will be aligned with the absolute centre of the planet. The left shoulder should be directly above the left hip, and the right shoulder directly above the right hip; there should therefore be no vertical twist in the body.

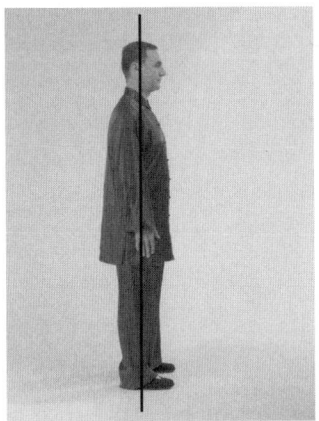
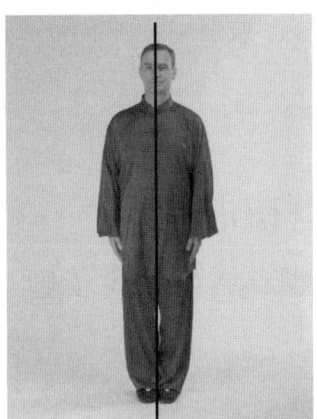

TÀIJÍ AND POSTURE

In Yang Tàijí solo practice, the body is mostly kept upright, although there are certain circumstances when it *is* angled for a specific purpose. When working with a partner on two-person exercises, you are more likely to angle the body slightly.

4

Grounding

The majority of people who have a desk job use their bodies very little, and most of their energy is held in the upper part of their bodies. Everyone is familiar with the symptoms of staying too long on the computer – the blood seems to slow down, and the extremities start to go cold; the body goes into 'sleep' mode, whilst the mind produces all the effort.

The object of this particular exercise is to redress the energy balance, as well as to give you a feeling of stability, solidity and attachment to the earth.

PREPARATION

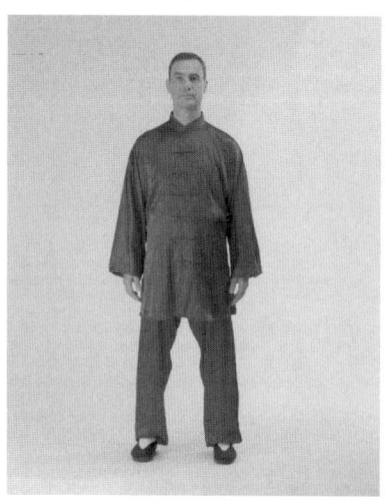

Wearing either completely flat shoes or no shoes at all, stand with your feet a shoulder's width apart. Your eyes can be opened or closed, whichever is the most restful, and whichever makes it easiest to concentrate.

THE FEET

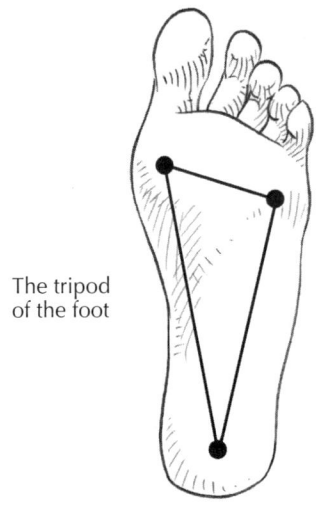

The tripod of the foot

Sole of foot (tripod)

Align your body with the balance points. Feel the weight of your body pressing down into your feet. Feel the 'tripods' of each foot – the heel, the ball in front of the big toe on the sole of the foot, and the ball in front of the little toe (also on the sole of the foot) pressing firmly into the ground, with the weight equally on each point of the tripod.

Relax your toes so that you can feel all of them resting lightly on the floor. Relax the arch of the foot allowing the muscles in the instep or arch of the foot to relax. Bearing in mind that a relaxing muscle will lengthen, allow the toes to lengthen away from you, as though your feet are growing longer and away ahead of you.

Soften and free your ankles.

Keep breathing.

THE KNEES

To find the correct position for the knees, first of all find the 'straight' position where they are neither bent forwards nor locked backwards.

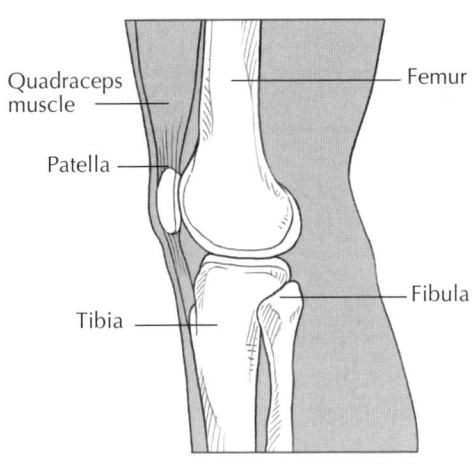

Knee joint (left leg) lateral view

To find this position, bend them slightly forwards, then tense them backwards (so that they can't go any further) and then find the middle position which is on the cusp of flexing.

Having found that point, bend them forwards *very* slightly, so slightly that anyone observing you from the side would be unable to tell that you'd bent them. This allows the small of the back to release more easily.

Keep breathing.

THE HIPS, THE PELVIS AND THE WAIST

Soften the abdomen, the pelvis and, in particular, soften the small of the back. Check that you're not holding any tension in the buttocks (the gluteus muscles) as this can affect the small of the back, and also cause the pelvis to lift upwards behind you. Release any tension in the organs within the pelvis.

Most people find it very difficult to release this area of the body; when releasing, the pelvis will actually make a very slight rotation – the lower edges of the bone moving forwards towards the front of the body rotating on the axis of the iliofemoral joints. Tension at the back of the waist or in the gluteus muscles can cause the pelvis to be rotated backwards and upwards excessively.

Keep breathing.

THE SHOULDERS

Soften the shoulder blades allowing them to fall; have a sensation of their melting and falling first into your pelvis, and then into your feet, and then into the earth. Relaxing the shoulder blades usually helps to relax the shoulder girdle itself.

Try breathing out and relaxing the front of your chest, and you'll find that it releases the shoulders.

Tension in the shoulders is quite often caused by tension of the trapezius muscles. These are triangular shaped muscles on either side of the body which cover much of the upper part of the back. They connect from the upper half of the spine to the 'corners' of your shoulders, and up the back of the neck to the base of the skull. If these are tight they pull the shoulders inwards and upwards, and pull the neck/back of skull downwards.

It quite often helps to think of releasing the *neck* as this has a very definite effect on the shoulders (see 'Freeing the Neck' on p.31).

Keep breathing.

THE HANDS AND ARMS

This also affects the release of tension in the shoulders. Begin by feeling the weight of the hands. Let them hang on either side of you without trying to hold them up; relax them to the extent that you are in effect almost trying to get them to 'fall off'. When they are hanging, try to gauge the weight of each hand. In order to feel this, you have to let go of them as much as possible. Each hand weighs something between 1–2 lbs (0.5–1 kg), i.e. both together would weigh something like a large bag of sugar. Try to *feel* or *gauge* that weight.

The act of feeling the weight of the hands should help you to let go of the wrists, elbows and shoulder joints. It is, after all, very difficult to gauge the weight of the hands if you are tensing up the other joints of the arms.

Keep breathing.

FREEING THE NECK

Freeing the neck allows the crown of the head to rise, and energy to rise up the neck.

There seems to be a number of very definite benefits when this happens:

- The head moves into the correct relationship with the neck, and feels lighter as though it's 'floating' on the neck.
- The breathing can improve.
- The shoulders are better able to relax.
- There is a sensation of warmth rising up the back of the neck, into and over the cranium.
- The entire spine feels as though it is opening and lengthening (which results in a feeling of being more able to breathe) and is generally more relaxed.
- The sensation of energy moving over the head, down, and into the face can result in the sinuses clearing and a feeling of the energy channels in the face clearly opening and functioning from the location below the middles of the lower eyelids and down into the face, as though small streams are running; the nose begins to tingle, and the cheeks feel as though they are glowing.

The method

Freeing and releasing the neck can probably be achieved by many methods, but the following works for me.

The most important point to bear in mind is that when a muscle relaxes, it lengthens.

Continue to relax the shoulders, whilst allowing the arms to hang on either side of you. This will inevitably have an effect on the whole shoulder girdle, which should be allowed to soften. Continue to relax the shoulder blades themselves, letting them drop to their natural position.

Then relax the base of the neck, in particular around the C7 vertebra (this is the vertebra at the base of the neck that protrudes more than the others when you bend your neck forwards). Once again, work on softening every muscle in this area, allowing every fibre to 'melt'.

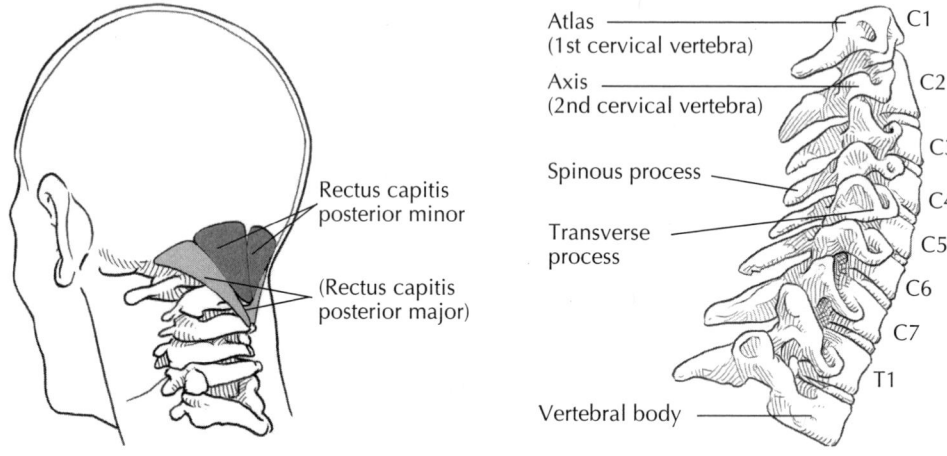

Rectus capitis posterior minor muscles   C7 vertebra and atlas

Whilst still bearing in mind the relaxation of the base of the neck and shoulders, turn your attention to the rectus capitis posterior minor muscles at the base of the skull, where the skull meets the neck. These are deep within the neck and are the muscles that partly control the vertical stability of the head. They connect the skull to the atlas (vertebra). If you have ever dropped off to sleep whilst sitting upright, and have had the sensation of the head dropping forwards when you don't necessarily want it to, this is the result of the rectus capitis posterior minor muscles relaxing. These are also the muscles that, when tensed, push your chin forwards and upwards, stop the neck from being free, and don't allow the crown to rise and the head to 'float'. The important thing is to relax them, not alone, but *in conjunction with* the relaxation of both the base of the neck and the jaw (see the following page).

Finally relax and soften the muscles surrounding the windpipe for the full length of the throat, and also soften the root of the tongue letting the tongue rest on the floor of the mouth.

Keep breathing.

KEEPING THE NECK FREE IN TÀIJÍ

Whilst doing tàijí, there are a number of actions that can cause the neck to become tense. The most notable of these are a) when lifting the hands either to the front or sides, b) when pulling the elbows behind you, c) when your weight is not balanced in the middle of the foot on which you are standing, in particular when the weight is on the toes, d) when over-stepping, i.e. when trying to step too wide or too long, and e) when the small of the back is tense.

THE JAW

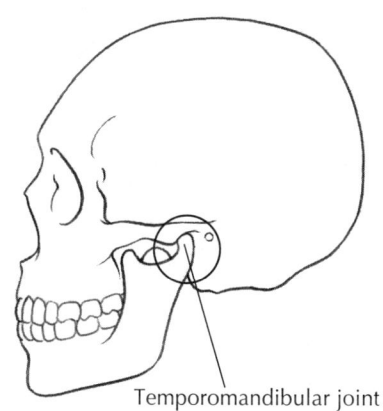

Temporomandibular joint

The jaw exerts control over the entire posture. When tensed and pulled upwards and inwards at the temporomandibular joint (TMJ) it draws the neck forwards, which affects everything below it.

The jaw doesn't release by simply being 'dropped'. Its pivotal hinge joint obviously *can* and *does* open downwards but, in order to release, its natural action is to move *away* and downwards. So when you release the jaw, think of it doing just that – keep your lips closed, and letting the upper and lower teeth part, just think of the jaw both moving away from you and also hanging.

Notice the effect that it has on your neck. When you do it with enough focus, you will probably find that the neck appears to actually move *backwards* a fraction, and seems to *lengthen*. This lets the shoulders sink and connect to the hips, which connect to the knees, which connect to the feet, which connect…etc. And we're back to the feet again…

Keep breathing.

THE CROWN

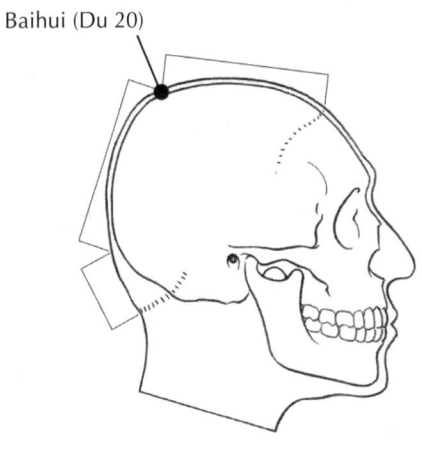

Baihui (Du 20)

Baihui point

This has really been covered in the last paragraph, but should be mentioned anyway as it is something that many tàijí teachers talk about a great deal.

The releasing of the neck (pp.31–2) and allowing the head to 'float' on top of the spine is the meaning of allowing the crown to rise.

Many tàijí teachers teach that you should tuck in the chin to raise the crown, however this merely creates more tension in the neck. By freeing the neck, you will find that the chin automatically tucks in slightly, and that, instead of tension forming in the neck, there is a huge *release* of tension. To get some kind of idea of the right head movement, be aware of your chin and the Bǎihuì 百會 point, and, as though they are two points on a circle, rotate them in the same direction. If you rotate them *lifting* the chin, you will be tilting the head upwards correctly off the atlas; if you rotate them the other way, you will be doing the correct head movement that is referred to in tàijí as 'tucking in the chin', or 'raising the crown', and in the Alexander Technique as 'head forwards and upwards'.

STANDING UP OUT OF THE FEET

As you finish working from the feet to the top of the head in the above components of the exercise, complete the exercise by allowing the body to 'stand up out of the feet'. This is nothing to do with forcing yourself to be taller; instead it is taking an 'overview' of the body.

The body can be thought of as being covered by a thin membranous tissue, just under the skin. This is known as the fascia, and is something like an over-body stocking – if you have ever removed the skin from a piece of fresh chicken, you will have found a thin white tissue between the skin and the flesh; it is similar in texture to this.

As you stand there, feel the entire body being allowed to release and grow, not just in an upwards direction, but downwards also. There is the idea in this part of the exercise in 'connecting Heaven and Earth' – allowing yourself to be an open conduit between the Universe and the planet Earth.

QÌ 气 (氣 TRADITIONAL)

The word 'qì' appears so many times in this book that a brief explanation of both its meaning and its concept might be helpful.

Literally qì translates as any of the following: 'gas / air / steam / vapour / smell / weather / vital breath / to anger / to get angry / to be enraged'. The words that are relevant to the tàijí practitioner are 'air' and 'vital breath'; usually in the West the word is used to mean 'energy' or 'vital energy'.

qì is the vital force without which we would be unable to exist. In the West we would say that someone with a strong constitution has strong qì; it is the power that fuels our bodies and minds, and keeps us healthy.

The Traditional Chinese Medical (TCM) view

Our initial qì is inherited from our parents; this is known as our 'source' Yuán 原 qì or 'congenital' qì. Our own health is dependent upon our ancestors' qì, our own parents' qì, and the health of our mother whilst we are carried in utero. This qì, which is stored in your kidneys, determines your basic constitution, strength and vitality, and is essential to growth and development.

The Chinese believe that although your Yuán qì is your basic building block, you can drain it through misuse, for example by indulging in drugs, alcohol, excessive sexual activity, excessive eating, etc…in fact, anything that makes the body overwork over a prolonged period.

After birth, our functional qì is then provided by the planet in the form of air, water and food; this is usually referred to as 'acquired' qì, and *can* be stored and replenished. In Chinese Medical Theory, the qì from air (Kōng 空 qì), and the qì from food (Gǔ 谷 qì) combine to form Gathering qì (Zǒng 总 qì). These then mix with the Yuán qì to form Zhēn 真 qì (True qì), which is a composite of Nutritive qì (Yíng 营 qì – to 'feed' the body from an energetic and cellular perspective) and Defensive qì (Wèi 卫 qì – to maintain the body's defences against the external pathological factors of wind, summer heat, dampness, dryness, cold and fire).

From a practical point of view therefore, the better the air we breathe, the better the food and water that we take into our bodies, the better the chance we have of being healthy. In addition to this, our breathing can play an important role in the development, circulation and management of our qì.

In TCM theory we can do a small amount to improve our stock of Yuán qì mainly through qìgōng 气功 exercises, but it is only a *small* amount (and some people say that it cannot be replenished at all) and it is therefore important not to deplete the Yuán qì that one has.

However, what we *can* do in both tàijí and qìgōng is to ensure that the 'acquired' qì that we collect works to maximum efficiency, which is where the correct alignment of the body comes in (see earlier in this chapter), and in particular where relaxation and release play an important role (see Chapter 5).

It should also be mentioned that there are a number of tàijí practitioners who perform qì projection 'feats', usually from fingers or palms. I don't have any strong feelings about these 'performers' but I know that many of my contemporaries do, and consider them to be charlatans. I've been on the receiving end of these demonstrations on several occasions, and have also experimented amongst friends, and I have no doubt that it is possible to feel something from the person 'projecting' the qì (or whatever is being projected). However, I have also noticed that not everyone is able to sense it, nor does there appear to be a pattern as to who can or who cannot (that I have been able to observe).

Furthermore, I used to wonder whether it was important to build up an 'energy relationship' between practitioner and 'receptor' for this sensitivity to work, but there have been so many occasions that I have seen an inexperienced or first time receptor sense something, that I don't think this can be a factor. What *is* noticeable though is that it is a skill that can be learned (at least, most people seem to be able to feel something). So I remain open-minded about it. Whether what one is sensing is the practitioner's qì, or perhaps an intensity of the practitioner's focus (in the same way that you might pick up on a bad atmosphere in a room, or when someone stares at you) I can't say…

5

Relaxation and Release

'Relaxation' suggests both relaxation of the mind (i.e. de-stressing) and relaxation of the body (softening of tissue). There is also perhaps the implication of being able to focus or concentrate calmly.

THE MIND

A stressed businessman may be able to focus very effectively, but probably at the expense of his blood-pressure. He is drawing the energy for the concentration or focus from other parts of his body, which is more than likely to be tensed. Calm focus is another matter, and is something that tàijí aims to foster.

One of the reasons that tàijí and many other martial arts are so beneficial for the health is that they bring the mind and body together. You can arrive at a class feeling very stressed-out, but after 15 minutes of working with the body, the mind starts to calm, the breathing alters and your energy starts to sink.

THE BODY

The majority of people think of relaxation as sitting down in an armchair and watching the television – a time when you metaphorically 'switch off'. However, from a body-health point of view, this isn't relaxation; it is collapsing or sagging.

Lengthening of muscles

When a muscle is tense, it has shortened (i.e. contracted); when a muscle relaxes, it naturally lengthens. If you 'sag' into your armchair, your muscles *will* lengthen but without any direction. The result will therefore be a 'sagging' muscle; it's as though the ends of the muscle aren't given the opportunity to move away from each other and, so, as the middle of the muscle relaxes, it has nowhere to go and therefore 'droops'. This is a loss of muscle tone. Therefore a muscle should always relax *with direction*.

This is easy to feel: if you extend your arm in front of you, relax your shoulder, elbow and wrist and, without stretching at all, try to feel the muscles lengthening away from you, allowing the joints of the shoulder, elbow, wrist and each finger joint to expand away from you, you will more than likely have a sensation of the arm 'growing' and 'undoing' as the muscles relax *with direction*.

You may find that the arm starts to feel heavier, and that there is a tingling sensation in the fingers, or the palm, or both. All of this is fine; it is the natural result of letting go in a constructive and creative manner.

Having done this, if you then compare it to the other arm, you may well find that it feels different.

One of the aims of tàijí is that you are able to do this 'controlled' relaxation, not just with one arm, but with the entire body. One of the results of so doing is that the body feels as though it is glowing internally and externally (you 'glow' with health). When this happens there is a sensation of warmth moving around the body, which one can then enhance by softening the body even further with direction.

It is relatively easy to feel this opening out or lengthening in a limb, but is harder when you are trying to relax/release your lower back for example. Suddenly the muscles are not so easy to relate to, they are behind you to start with, and you can't see them.

But it is just a case of practice and, above all, awareness – you can't start to release a muscle until you've noticed that it is tense, and you can't notice that it's tense until you can *feel* it, and you can't feel it because it's become almost numb with tension or habit, and you still need to be aware of it…

So you are in a catch-22 situation, which is where a teacher comes in.

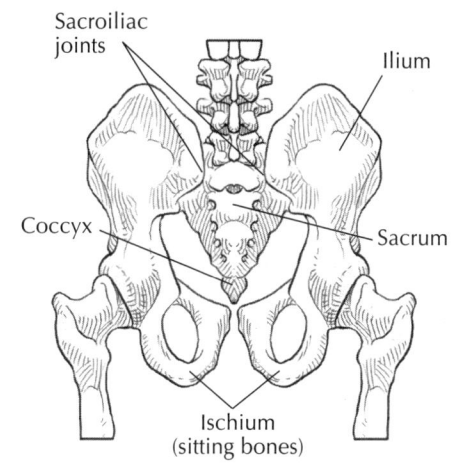

Sinking qì, relaxation and tàijí

This brings us back to the 'Grounding' exercise in Chapter 4. This was a static upright exercise related to posture; when used with movement (i.e. as in tàijí) it is a little harder but the principles are still the same.

'Hollowing' or 'sinking' the chest produces a downwards 'draining' of energy – you can feel this by simply standing or sitting still and closing up the breastbone slightly (i.e. allow the breastbone/sternum to move backwards very slightly towards your spine). As you do it, very gently breathe out and just *feel*. There is a sinking feeling, and a feeling of calmness or tranquillity.

The same principle needs to be applied to the small of the back – the part of the body that most people find *very* difficult to release. You can't hollow the small of the back in the same way, but you *can* soften and release/relax the area around the sacrum. This is like 'hanging' the sacrum from the upper part of the spine; relax the gluteus muscles and try to feel the weight of the pelvis, particularly the central area between the two halves of the ilium.

As a child you might have lain on the ground and 'played dead'; your friends would then try to pick you up. The more dead you managed to be, the heavier you became. If you want to get the feeling of 'sinking your qì', then 'play dead'!

Pelvis and sacrum – rear view

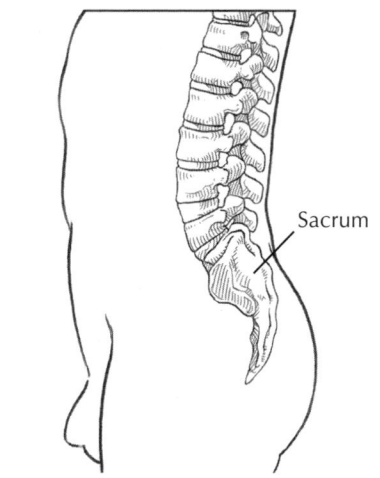

Sacrum and spine – left side view

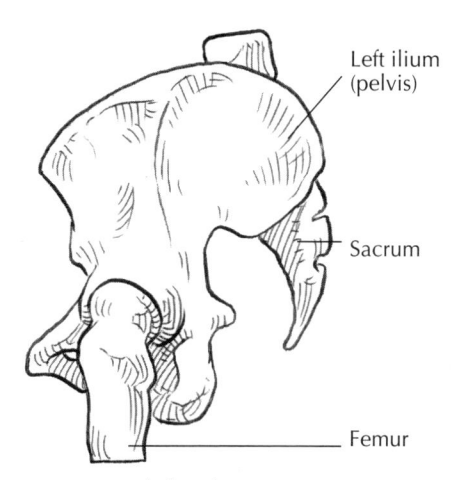

Hip joints – left side view

TÀIJÍ FOR HEALTH

The efficiency of the human body is controlled by the condition of the circulation of blood, the nervous system, the skeletal structure, the muscle-tone and, in TCM thought, by the 'energy system' – the circulation of energy through the channels (meridians) and collaterals.

These channels can be thought of as a series of hosepipes that pump water (energy) continuously around the body, connecting every organ, in many ways not dissimilar to the arterial and venous system of the body. When the hosepipes are open, the water (energy) flows freely and easily, feeding and connecting the viscera of the body.

With a hosepipe, if you twist or bend it, the flow of water becomes impeded and can no longer flow as freely as before. Water may still come out of the hosepipe, but its efficiency is restricted and therefore reduced and certain parts of the pipe may be put under more pressure than usual. In the body, this twisting or bending of the 'hosepipe' is tension – a build up of pressure within the body; tension squeezes the hosepipe; the movement of both blood and energy is restricted, and the nervous system is likely to be cramped and impaired. Everyone is familiar with anxiety or fear causing either 'butterflies in the stomach', or a racing heartbeat, as the heart has to work harder to get the blood through tensed arterial and venous systems, and everyone is familiar with having tensed shoulders and getting a headache as a result.

Tàijí is a method of understanding relaxation and of learning how to control it so that the body can open out/release and undo, enabling the systems of the body (respiratory, digestive, cardiovascular, etc.) to function unimpaired.

TÀIJÍ FOR SELF-DEFENCE

Tàijíquán (or t'ai chi ch'uan) can be translated as 'the Supreme Ultimate Fist'; the art is therefore also a sophisticated method of self-defence. Within the soft and gentle movements are many 'applications' consisting of deflections, punches, kicks, throws, wrist locks and arm lock techniques.

The guiding principle of tàijí self-defence is that you always follow the flow of an opponent's energy, redirecting his energy circularly, and using his own energy against him. An example of this might be during a game of cricket or baseball, where the batsman redirects the ball to the left side or right side, rather than hitting it straight back in the bowler's direction.

All the movements of the Yang Tàijí 24-Step Short Form have applications that usually incorporate an attack and defence, sometimes almost simultaneously.

- There are foot applications such as kicks, trips or blocks.
- There are deflections of strikes.
- There are hand/arm applications such as strikes with the hand, fist, wrist, elbow or shoulder.
- There are arm and wrist locks.
- There are throws.

Many of the connections between the postures can also be used as they are, or adapted to work as applications.

6

The Hands and the Hand Positions

Generally the hands should be held in a relaxed way, with the palms slightly concave, as though holding a beach ball. The fingers are separated slightly, but without any tension either in the palms or fingers. In the Yang Tàijí 24-Step Short Form there are three hand positions.

THE OPEN PALM

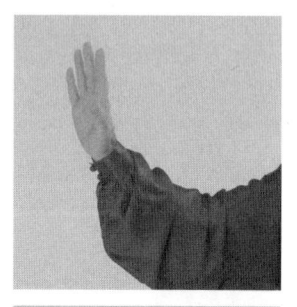

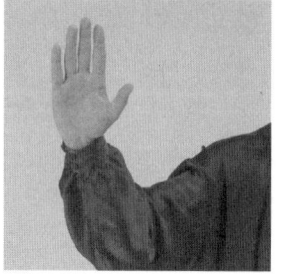

The open palm is the most commonly used hand shape in the Yang Tàijí 24-Step Short Form. It is held at various angles, depending upon its use. For example, in Parting the Wild Horse's Mane, it is held with the palm angled upwards at approximately 45°; in Play the Pipa, it is held with the thumb edge up and the little finger edge down; in Repulse Monkey the hand nearest the body is held with the palm upwards, the other palm is pushing away from you; in certain positions the palm will face the floor, etc.

In all cases, the hand should be relaxed, with the fingers naturally extended and separated, and a slight hollow in the palm as though holding a large beach ball.

THE FIST

The fist is used in two movements in the 24-Step Short Form – Form 14 (Strike (Opponent's) Ears with Both Fists) and Form 21 (Turn, Deflect Downwards, Parry and Punch). The fingers are wrapped into the centre of the palm, and the side of the bent thumb rests on the second or middle bone (phalanx) of the index finger. A tàijí fist is a loosely held fist (no white knuckles!) and there should be a small space in the hollow of the palm.

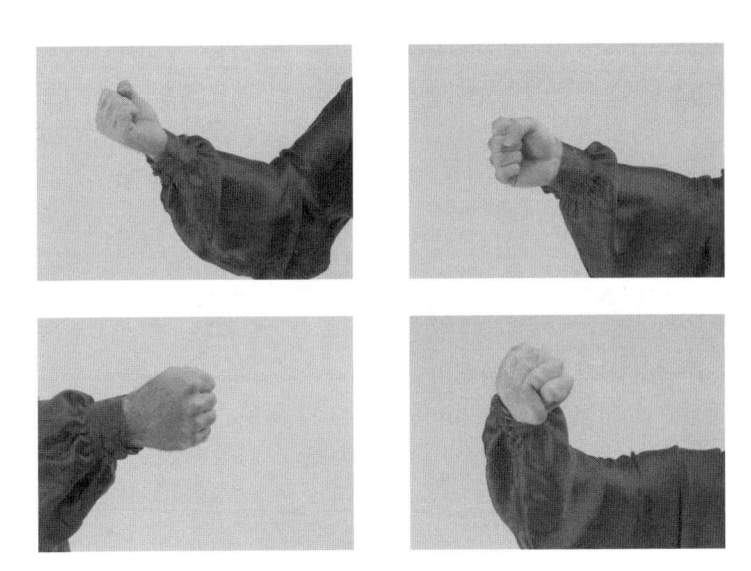

THE CRANE'S BEAK

The crane's beak appears twice in the 24-Step Short Form – Form 9 (Single Whip) and 11 (Single Whip). To make the hand position, bunch the fingers and thumb together of the right palm so that the tips of all five digits are together and forming a five-pointed circle. Then flex the wrist so that the bunched fingers form a 'hook' and pull the tip of the hook back towards the inside of the wrist. In the Yang Tàijí 24-Step Short Form the hook points downwards.

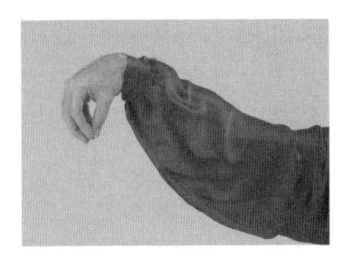

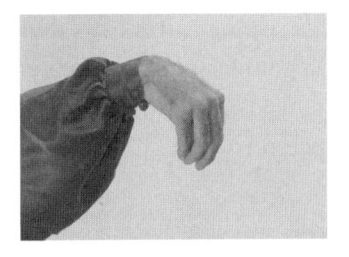

7

The Arms and Shoulders

MOVING THE ARMS

It is particularly important to move the arms in as relaxed a way as possible, with awareness of the shoulder joints and the way in which they function.

1. Over-extension of the arm

Over-extension of the arm should be avoided (i.e. locking or hyper-extending the elbow joint). When pushing the arm either ahead, or down to the floor by the side of the leg (for example as in Parting the Wild Horse's Mane or Brush Knee and Twist Step), straighten the elbow so that there is still a very slight bend in it, but so that it is definitely not hyper-extended. On the other hand, the arm shouldn't be excessively bent either. (See 'Bow of the Arms' on p.347.)

2. Extending the hand/palm ahead of you

Avoid pushing the shoulder joint forwards and also upwards.
   When this happens, it means that the shoulder hasn't relaxed and sunk to the hip, and the shoulder is being treated as part of the arm. This creates tension in the shoulder – the entire shoulder joint is lifted, which lifts and pulls the scapula/shoulder blade forwards.

3. Softening the shoulder joint

- Try relaxing your chest.
- Try relaxing/releasing your neck.
- Think of doing so from inside the armpit. Feel the soft tissue in this very sensitive area, and relax every fibre within the armpit.
- Think of sinking the elbow.

4. Lifting your arm

While lifting your arm avoid lifting the shoulder as well.

When lifting the arms in any direction, allow the shoulders to feel as though they are dropping a corresponding amount. Lifting the shoulder with the arm is a common error with beginners and comes from 'recruiting' muscles. Recruiting muscles is the use of other muscle-groups that are unnecessary to do a job. So, for example, the most common muscle to recruit when lifting the arm is the trapezius, which runs along the top of the shoulder and up into the neck.

5. Opening out the arms

When opening out the arms on either side of you (for example parallel to the ground) retain a 'natural' arm position. A 'natural' open-arm position is such as you might make when standing in front of a large group of people and welcoming them – arms open on either side to perhaps 100–110° wide, with palms up (in the case of welcoming). This would be a 'natural' opening; any more than that and the muscles on the back start to tense, the shoulder blades drawing together, and the muscles on the chest begin to be stretched. Examples of this in the Yang 24-Step Form would be Curve Back Arms on Both Sides, and the positioning of the arms during the kicks.

8

The Knees

LOOKING AFTER THE KNEES

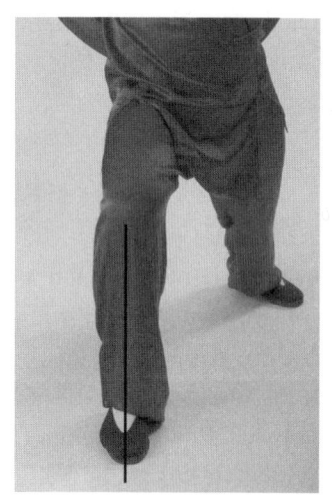

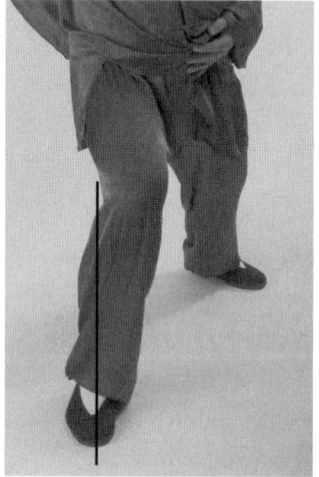

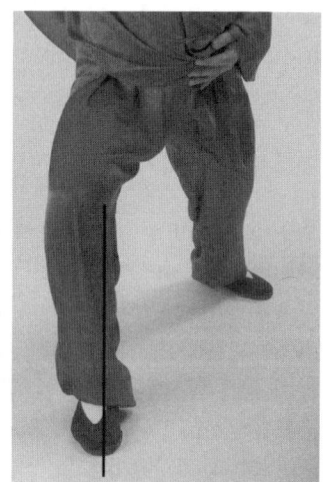

To avoid knee problems, the rule is that the centreline of the top of each thigh should line up with the second toe of the foot. In other words, if you were in a left Bow Stance (p.49) (therefore with the left knee ahead), if it were possible to roll a ball-bearing down the centre of your left thigh, on reaching your knee (which is bent) it would fall over the edge and gravity would take it directly on to the centreline of your foot below (either the second toe, or between the second and third toes). This way, the pressure of the body weight passes directly through the centre of, or weight-bearing part of, the knee joint.

Therefore the stances on the previous page would be potentially damaging to the knee. In the second photograph the weight puts a strain on the medial aspect of the knee joint, and in the third on the lateral aspect.

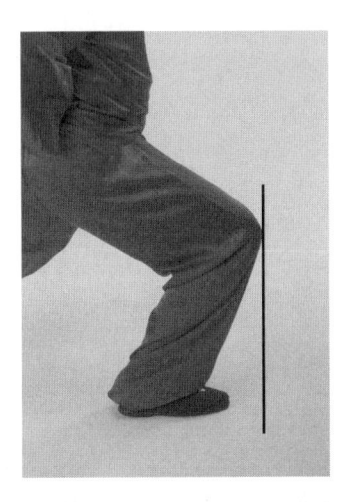

The other rule is that the bent knee should not go beyond the toe; therefore, when viewed from the side, the kneecap should not extend beyond the toes. If it does, once again the knee is not supported.

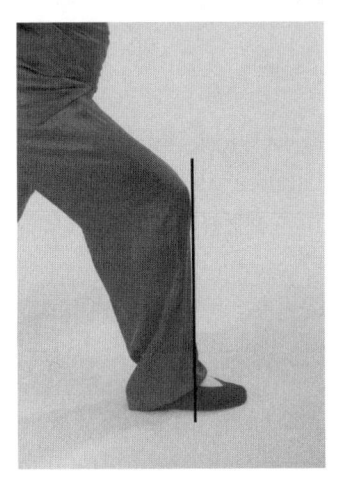

(There is a further school of thought that would argue that the front leg should not even go *this* far, and should go no further than the calf being vertical above the heel.)

9

Stances (步形 Bùxíng)

1. OPEN STANCE (STANDING WITH FEET APART)
开立步 kàilìbù

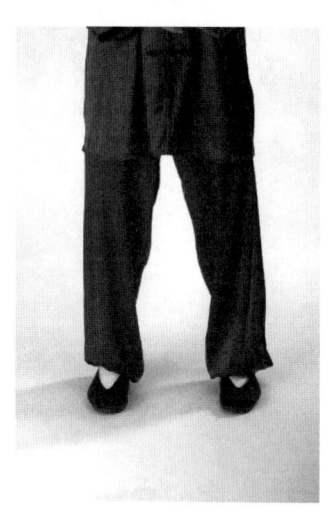

This is the basic 'shoulder-width stance'. The 'perfect' shoulder-width stance is measured as outlined below, and will be very slightly different for every person.

Stand with feet together and, temporarily moving your weight on to your heels, turn both feet outwards to exactly 45°.

Next, move your weight back on to your toes and, lifting your heels, square them up to parallel again. By doing this, the outside edges of your feet are directly below the outside edges of your shoulders, and the inside edges of your feet are directly below the axillary creases – the lines of the armpits.

2. HORSE STANCE

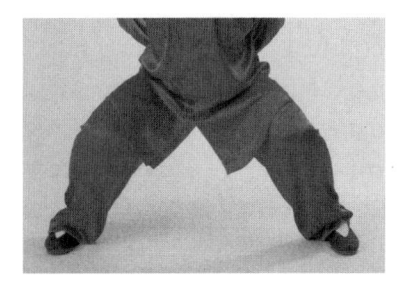

马步 mǎbù

This is also known as a Riding Horse Stance, and is formed from the stance above. From the shoulder-width stance (or it can also be wider, but not in the Yang Tàijí 24-Step Short Form) bend the knees and sit down with the spine upright and with the weight 50/50.

The neck releases and lengthens, the chest relaxes, the shoulders sink to the hips, the buttocks tuck under and the small of the back relaxes and opens, and the knees open over the toes. The photograph shows a wide range

The photograph shows a wide Mǎbù Stance, but it doesn't have to be this wide (e.g. see p.81).

3. BOW STANCE

弓步 gōngbù

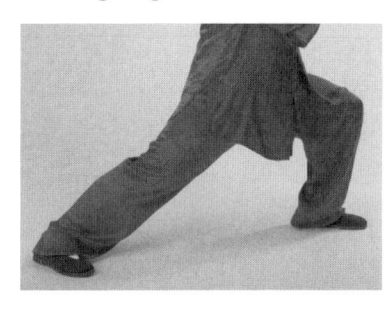

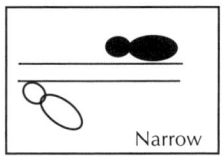

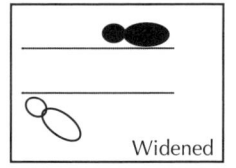

Narrow

Widened

Also known as a Bow and Arrow Stance, this is the most common stance in tàijí.

The shape of the posture is: one foot ahead of the other, with approximately 70 per cent weight on the front foot; the front knee bent, the back leg naturally straightened.

In order to get into a Bow Stance, stand with your feet a shoulder's width apart and with both feet pointing straight ahead. Turn your right foot outwards to 45°, and then, with your weight on your right foot, and bending your right knee, move your left foot *directly* ahead (as though sliding it parallel to the side walls of a room). Don't allow the left foot to move to the right as you move it forwards, and it is *very* important to keep the toes pointing straight ahead. Next, move 70 per cent of your weight on to the left foot, keeping both feet flat on the ground.

This is a very narrow left Bow Stance. As mentioned, the toes of the left foot *must* point straight ahead; the toes of the right foot pointing outwards at 45°. The left knee is bent forwards like a bow so that it is vertically above the toes; the right leg is extended straight and naturally.

The width between your heels *laterally* is determined by the posture, but is usually anything from 4–12 inches (10–30 cm). For example, if you are in a right Bow Stance (with the right foot forwards) and you are thrusting with the sword (i.e. with your right hand) this will tend to be a narrower stance because the arm and leg on the same side of the body are forwards. A left Bow Stance with the same right-handed thrust will tend to have a wider stance.

The weight distribution is usually 70/30, but can also be found as 60/40.

(Note on the 'straightening' of the back leg: the rear leg *is* bent, but the bend is achieved by the relaxation/release of the pelvis, rather than by bending the actual knee. To get the feel of it, go into the posture described above and then lock the rear leg. Next, try relaxing the pelvis particularly around the area of the sacrum, and the rear leg will bend slightly, but in the same way that an archer's bow will bend.)

The body might be completely square to the front (for example Brush Knee and Twist Step) or it might be turned to the side depending upon the posture. For example, in Péng (in Grasp the Bird's Tail) the turn is only about 15°, in Parting the Wild Horse's Mane it is about 30°, and in Single Whip the angle might be as much as 45°.

As you move into Bow Stance and 'complete' the posture, there is a sensation of allowing the energy to the four limbs and also to the top of the head and tip of spine. Generally, the Bow Stances are performed with an exhalation, and it helps to feel as though you are exhaling into the limbs and to both ends of the spine. This should be done with great softness, and a feeling of flexibility.

4. EMPTY STANCE

虚步 xūbù

In an Empty Stance, all the weight is on one leg, which is bent; the other leg is extended ahead of you and is 'empty' of weight. The toes of the foot can touch the floor (1) (as in Stork Spreads its Wings), or the heel can touch the floor (2) (as in Play the Pipa), or the front foot can be virtually flat (3) (as in Repulse Monkey).

Stand with both feet together. Turn the toes of your (for example) right foot outwards by 30–45°, and move your weight on to your right foot. Bending your right knee, move your left foot as far ahead of you as possible, putting the foot flat on the floor with no weight on it. Alter the toes/heel as required.

STANCES (步形 BÙXÍNG)

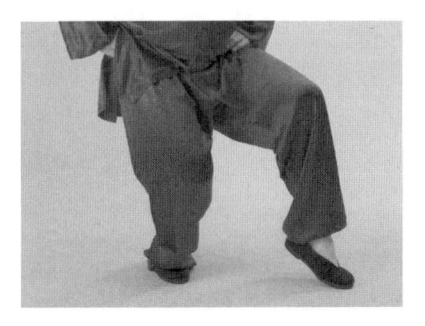

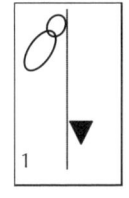

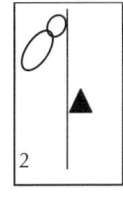

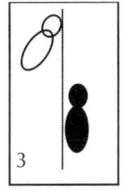

Foot completely flat

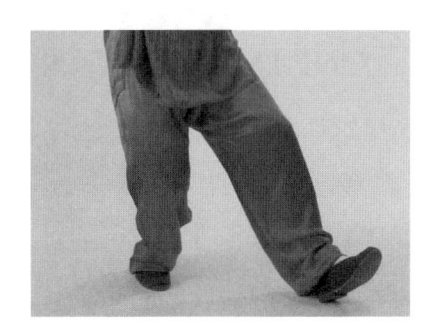

5. T-STANCE

丁步 dīngbù

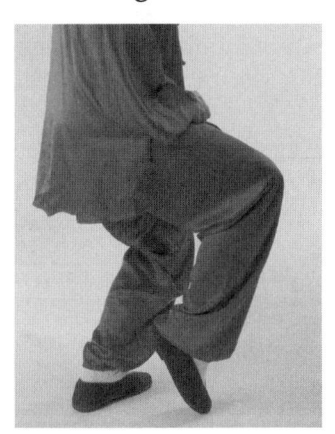

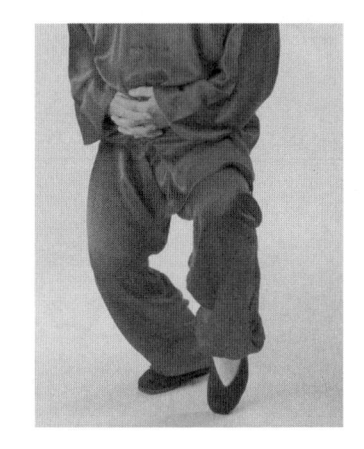

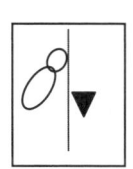

To form a T-Stance, place all of your weight on one foot and then place the toes of the other foot by the side of it, with little or no weight on it. This is a type of Empty Stance. The T-Stance is also a fast way of changing the weight distribution from one foot to the other.

Stand with both feet together. Turn the toes of your (for example) right foot outwards by 30–45°, and move your weight on to your right foot. Bending your right knee, lift the left heel; there should be little or no weight on the left toes.

(Dīng in Chinese is a 'nail'. Not only does the character for the word closely resemble a nail, but the way in which the foot is held in this stance also copies the shape of a nail – with the toe touching the ground.)

51

6. ONE-LEGGED STANCE
独立步 dúlìbù

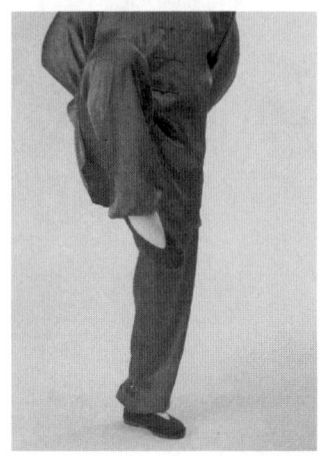

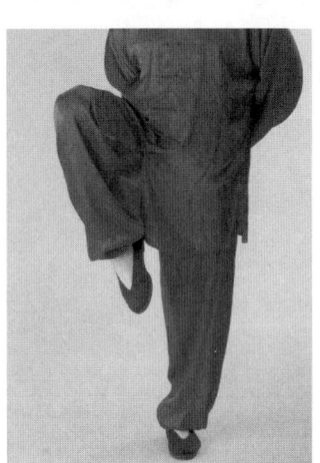

This posture appears twice in the Tàijí Yang 24-Step Short Form.

With feet together, turn one foot outwards by 30–45° and move your weight on to it. Lift the other leg up as high as possible with a relaxed calf (i.e. just lift up the knee) and leave the toes hanging downwards. The supporting leg should be straight, but not locked.

The leg on which you are standing, is straight; the knee should neither be locked backwards, nor bent forwards.

The raised leg and toes should be slightly curved inwards, creating the feel of a circle in front of you – 'Péng' of the leg. Ideally the knee should be a minimum of parallel to the ground, and preferably higher.

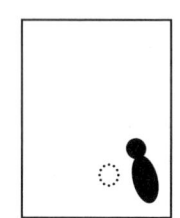

7. CROUCH STANCE (LIKE A SERVANT)
仆步 púbù

To form a Crouch Stance, stand with both feet together (with your back to a wall in order to get the angle of the feet correct in the posture) and about one foot's length away from the wall; your toes point to (for example) 12.00.

STANCES (步形 BÙXÍNG)

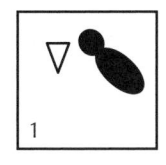

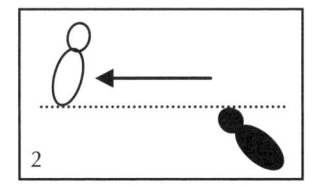

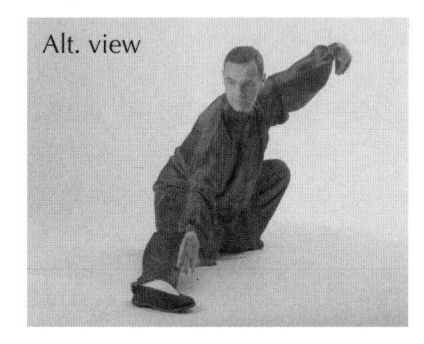

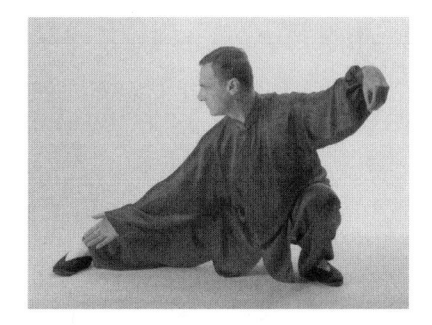

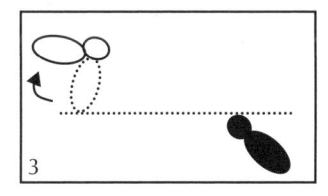

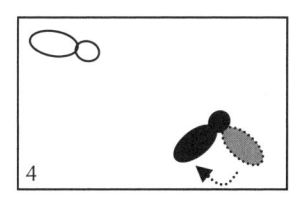

1. Turn the toes of your (for example) left foot outwards by 30–45° (to point to 10.30/11.00) and move your weight on to your left foot.

2. Lift up your right foot, and touch the toes against the back of the heel of your left foot (this is in order to get the line of the right foot in the next movement). Then, keeping your weight completely on your left foot, slide your right foot sideways along an imaginary line to 9.00, that starts at your left heel, and which is parallel to the wall (in other words, your right heel would lightly brush along the wall, if it were touching it).

   As you do this, sink down into your left heel, bending your left knee as much as possible. Keep the left knee over the left toes, and keep the soles of both feet flat on the ground. The tip of your spine – your coccyx – should be as directly above your left heel as possible.

   As the foot slides out to 9.00, the body turns to 45° into the space between the thighs. The body can lean slightly forwards, but preferably not as much as 45°.

   As the knee of the fixed foot should remain over the toes of the same foot (in order to avoid knee problems), a good 'turn-out' (as in ballet) is very helpful.

3. To move out of a Crouch Stance, as your weight moves forwards on to your right foot, turn your right *toes* outwards so that they point to 3.00 or 3.30, then…

4. turn the toes of your left foot to point to 1.30, pivoting on the *heel*.

10

Footwork Techniques (步法 **Bùfǎ**)

Examples of the footwork techniques are:

FORWARDS STEP

上步 shàngbù

The rear leg is moved forwards one step, or the front leg is moved half a step forwards.

BACKWARDS STEP

退步 tuìbù

The front leg is moved back one step. (For example Form 6: Curve Back Arms on Both Sides.)

WITHDRAWING STEP

撤步 chèbù

The front leg or the rear leg is moved back half a step. Some practitioners use this in Stork Spreads its Wings, Play the Pipa, and High Pat on Horse.

SWING STEP

摆步 **bǎibù**

As the foot comes down on the ground after a forwards step, the heel is placed first and then the toes are turned outwards and placed on the ground so that the feet form an outwards Chinese figure eight shape \ /. (For example moving into Bān in Form 21: Bānlánchuí.)

GRINDING STEP

碾步 **niǎnbù**

With the heel as an axis, the toes are turned outwards or inwards; or, with the ball of the foot as an axis, the heel is turned out. (For example the right foot at the end of Form 1 as you complete the first Bow Stance.)

TURNING-IN STEP

扣步 **kòubù**

As the foot comes down on the ground after a forwards step, the heel is placed first and then the toes are turned inwards and placed on the ground so that the feet form a Chinese figure eight shape / \. (For example the connection between Forms 16 and 17.)

11

The Process of Stepping

1. HOW TO STEP

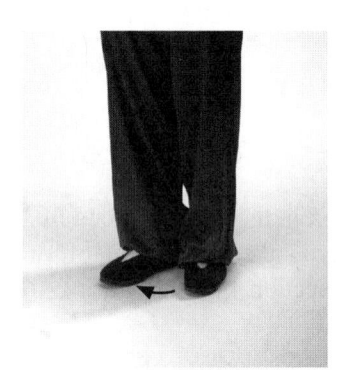

When stepping forwards from a feet together position, turn (for example) your right foot out to 45°.

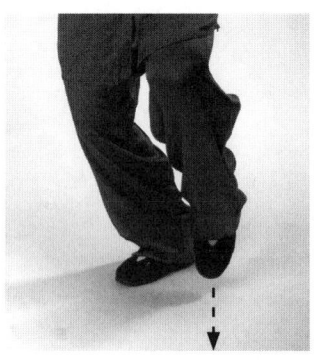

Bending both knees, move all your weight on to the right foot; lift your left foot up slightly and completely relax the right hip/buttock with a feeling of its sinking into your right ankle. The left ankle should be relaxed and the leg completely 'empty'; if there is any tension in the lifted leg, the hip will tend to lock.

When you're ready to step, move the left foot forwards, touching the heel lightly on the floor ahead of you and, transferring the weight on to the left foot, place the sole flat. In the majority of cases, avoid lifting the rear heel.

THE PROCESS OF STEPPING

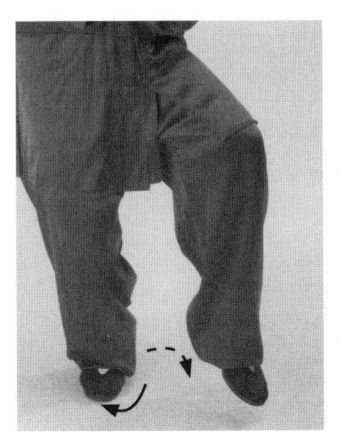

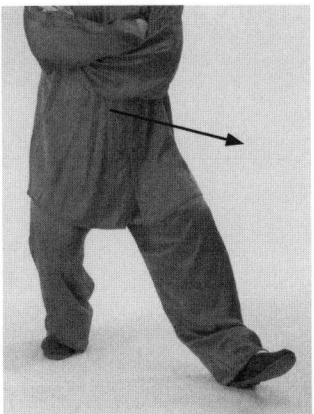

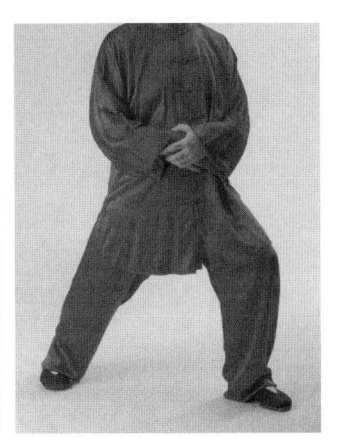

The expression for stepping sideways with toes still pointing ahead is 'Diǎnqǐ, diǎnluò 点起点落'. This is the *method* of stepping and translates as 'point, rise, point, fall'. The *feeling* of stepping is 'Qīngqǐ, qīngluò 轻起轻落', which translates as 'gently rise, gently fall'.

This means that if your feet are together and you are about to step sideways (for example when either beginning the Tàijí Form, or in Cloud Hands):

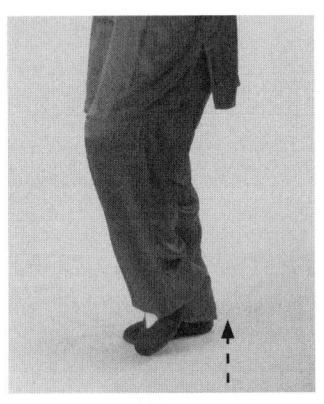

1. Lift the heel thereby pointing the toes.

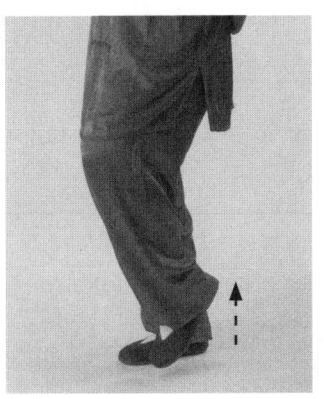

2. Lift your foot off the ground.

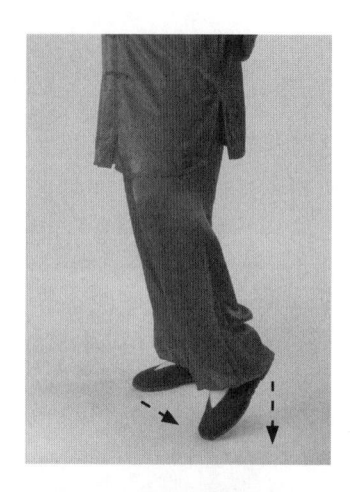

3. When you place your foot, point the toes.

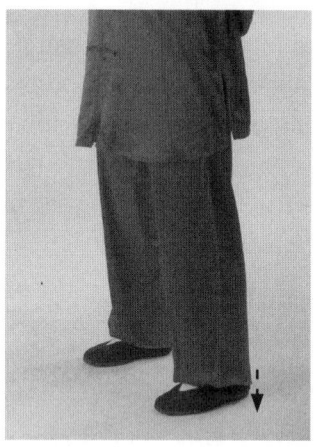

4. Then place the foot joint by joint, sinking the foot into the ground.

The *feeling* is of always stepping 'gently' with an awareness of where the weight is on the foot, and without falling or dropping into the step. The transfer of weight is therefore always under control.

2. PROBLEMS IN STEPPING

Beginners have a tendency to over-step and *fall* into the front foot. This can be for a number of reasons:

1. Because they are trying to step too far.

2. Because, as they move one leg forwards to step, the other leg is not strong enough to support their full weight.

3. Because they try to stand up *as* they step.

3. FINDING THE RIGHT STEPPING DISTANCE

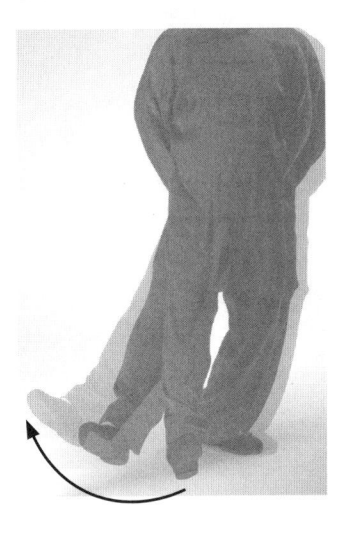

Visualize your legs as being like a pair of geometric compasses for drawing an arc.

The stepping 'rule' is that if you bend one leg (this is the 'point' of the compass on the paper) and then move the leg with which you are stepping forwards (this is the compass opening) you can then place your stepping heel anywhere within the radius of that compass arc – forwards, backwards, sideways, diagonally, etc., *whilst still maintaining your balance on the standing leg.*

The idea is that, wherever you step, you keep the point (or pin) of the compass (i.e. your leg that you are balancing on) upright. To get the feel of it, just swing your leg around in a large compass arc without putting it on the floor, *then* place the heel somewhere on the line of the arc. Avoid standing up to do so; keep the knee that you are standing on bent, and keep the body low and upright.

This avoids over-stepping.

Over-stepping occurs either when you stand up just as you are stepping, or when you fall forwards on the standing leg.

To actually step, bend the leg on which you are standing just at the moment that you are going to place the stepping heel, but without moving the weight on to it. The second that it has landed, you can transfer the weight.

4. STEPPING TO PUSH

If you want (for example) to step into and push a partner who is very solidly rooted, there is a way of stepping that grounds you better than if you were to simply lift up your leg and step into him. With the foot *almost* on the floor (but not quite), step by *sliding* your foot forwards as though floating the foot over the surface of the floor, and without lifting the toes.

This has the effect of 1) keeping your pelvis free so that it doesn't lock up, and 2) keeping your energy sunk – stepping by lifting the foot off the ground tends also to lift your energy unless you are careful.

12

Breathing in the Form

The advice that I was given as a beginner is 'Don't worry about breathing; breathing will happen automatically.'

I've found that this is true, and I have also found that when trying to make breathing patterns fit the Form you actually end up tensing the body far more than you would do if you just let it happen.

But, for those who want to know how it works, there are Yang moves in the Form – the moves that have a feeling of expansiveness and which usually give the movement its name, and there are Yin moves that lead into the Yang moves.

As an overall rule, you exhale as you move into a posture, and when you have finished exhaling, you start to inhale…and that's it! Once you get to know the moves, it becomes a completely automatic and natural way of breathing – in fact you will find it difficult to breathe in any other way.

It's quite difficult to do it incorrectly; try pushing against a partner's body as you breathe *in*!

There are many different ways to breathe, and the easiest to use is abdominal breathing; qìgōng and yoga will offer many other alternatives, but they are beyond the scope of this book. Abdominal breathing really needs to become second nature; you shouldn't need to think about it whilst practising tàijí. So when you are learning, it is best just to breathe naturally, and not worry about it.

ABDOMINAL BREATHING EXERCISE

- Sit in a chair.

- Inhale and exhale gently. Inhale as though you are smelling a flower; exhale as though you are trying not to disturb the air in front of your nostrils.

- Aim to slow your breathing down, particularly the out-breath.

- Observe the breath leaving the body, in particular the tail-end of the breath.

- Watch how the breath gradually ceases until you appear to be breathing neither in nor out.

- The softer you are with the breath, and the closer you observe the tail-end of it, the better you will feel what is taking place. You may notice that the abdomen appears to be *rising* at this stage.

- Repeat this several times, and just breathe in when you need to. Never *force* the out-breath.

- The next time that you are about to breathe in, just before doing so, release the abdomen and abdominal muscles *first* before you breathe in, allowing the abdomen to have a sensation of dropping or sinking. Concentrate on the sinking abdomen, and allow the breath to just follow.

The more that you are able to relax and let the abdomen drop rather than *push* it down, the better the results will be.

If you are doing it correctly, you will feel several things:

- It will start to feel as though the body is 'breathing itself'.

- It will feel as though your abdomen is rising and falling, acting like a pump.

- Your breath will be deeper.

- It might make you feel dizzy; this is nothing to worry about, it probably means that your usual way of breathing is much shallower. You are now putting more oxygen into your system, therefore the dizziness. Revert to your normal breathing briefly until it passes and then go back to the abdominal breathing.

13

Definitions

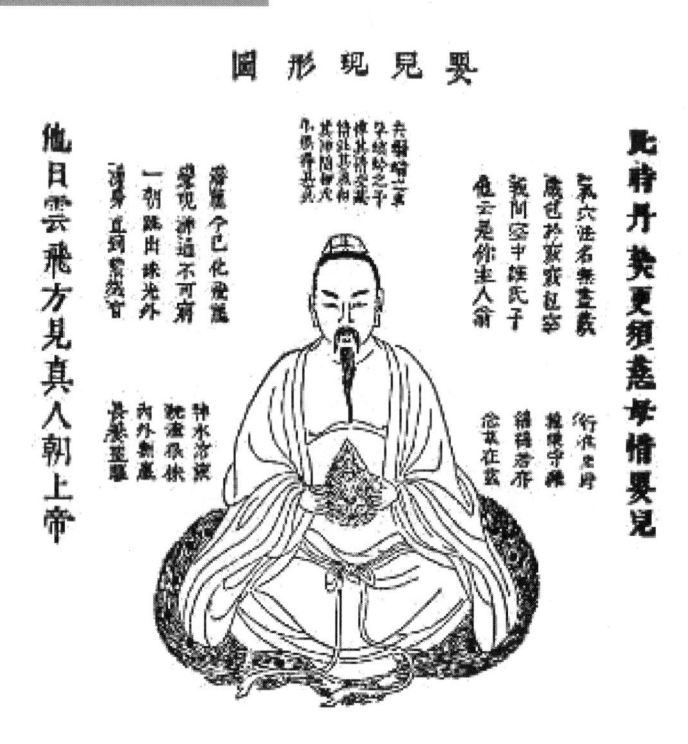

THE CENTRE, CENTRE-TURN AND THE CENTRELINE OF THE BODY

The *centre* refers to the dāntián, 1–2 inches (2.5–5 cm) below the navel, and approximately one third inwards towards the centre of the body. (See also 'Location' on p.335.)

Centre-turn, or the expression 'turning your centre', refers to the way in which you turn this core of the body.

The *centreline* of the body simply refers to a line that equates with the Ren channel (Conception Vessel) running down the front of the body. It is used to describe which way the body is facing. (See also the additional information in Chapter 17, 'Beyond the Basics', on p.316.)

SITTING BACK

Moving the weight backwards on to the rear leg is a weight shift that occurs often in tàijí. (See also 'Full (solid) and Empty Stance; transferring the weight' on p.324.)

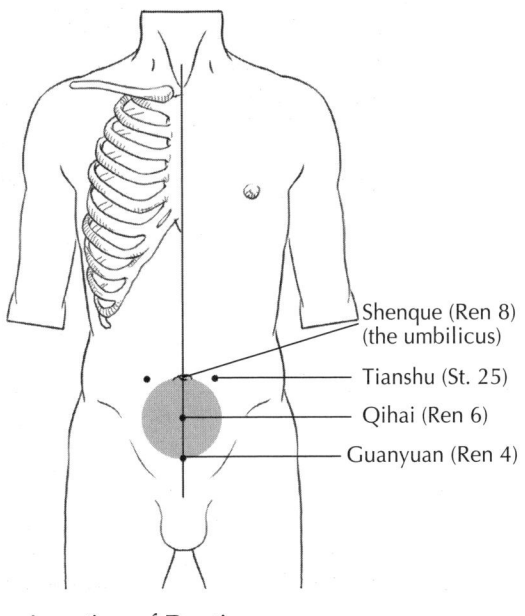

Shenque (Ren 8) (the umbilicus)
Tianshu (St. 25)
Qihai (Ren 6)
Guanyuan (Ren 4)

Location of Dantian

HOLDING THE BALL

This is an overused phrase that regularly crops up in tàijí but which is misleading as it implies that 'holding the ball' is an actual posture.

There *are* certain places throughout the Tàijí Form where the arms do *appear* to be holding a ball, and when teaching beginners the expression can be quite useful as the concept approximately gives the correct shape to the arms…but there is no 'ball' as such.

In the Yang Tàijí 24-Step Short Form there is only one place where you do actually 'hold the ball' – Form 18, Jade Lady Weaves Shuttles. In every other instance, the ball symbolizes the moment between the arms 'opening' and 'closing', but is not a feature in itself.

'Holding the ball' in places other than Form 18 stagnates the energy of those movements, breaking the smooth transition between 'opening' and 'closing', Yin and Yang. (See also Chapter 18, 'Open and Close'.)

TUCKING UNDER/COCCYX/TAILBONE/PELVIC TILT/ PULL IN LOWER ABDOMINAL MUSCLES

This refers to Chapter 18, 'Open and Close'.

SLIPPING THE (REAR) HEEL

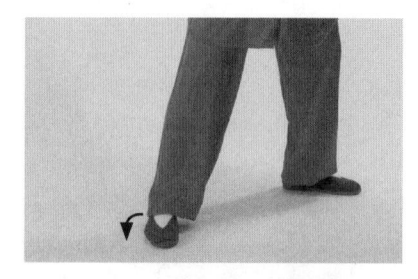

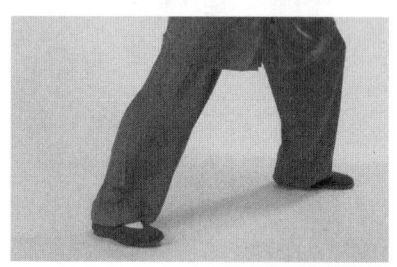

When moving into certain postures, it is necessary to adjust the rear foot, so that the two feet do not form an angle of 90°.

In tàijí, there are two ways of doing this, either by lifting the toes of the rear foot and turning them inwards by 45° (this is what might be called the 'traditional' way), or by leaving the toes in place and pushing the heel backwards by 45° (the 'modern' way).

Both have their merits, but in the Yang Tàijí 24-Step Short Form the latter method is used more often than the former.

SCREWDRIVER TURN OF THE HAND

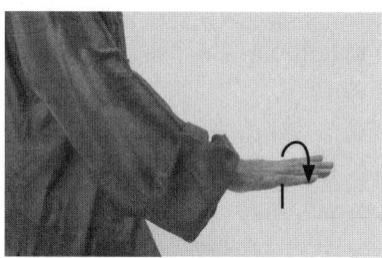

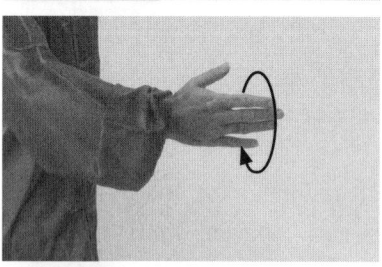

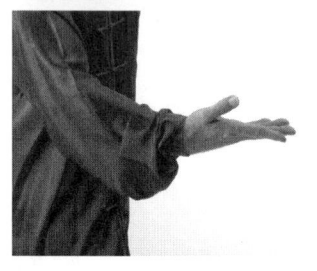

This means that when turning the palm upwards (for example), the arm and hand act together like a screwdriver, the forearm (handle of the screwdriver) rotating, and the hand/palm (blade) turning over. In other words, there is no independent flexion of the wrist.

THE CLOCK SYSTEM OF DEFINING DIRECTIONS

The usual method of defining directions in tàijí is the compass points, and normally this assumes a starting direction of South. This works moderately well, but runs into problems when you need to describe a 30° turn from one of the cardinal points.

I have therefore used the clock system as opposed to the compass points, as I think it is easier to understand. The clock system always refers to the hour hand, and assumes that you start with the body facing 12 o'clock (12.00). A 90° turn to your right will therefore take you to 3 o'clock (3.00) and a further 45° turn will take you to 4.30, etc.

The clock system has the added advantage of easily defining 30° turns, as every hour is at 30°.

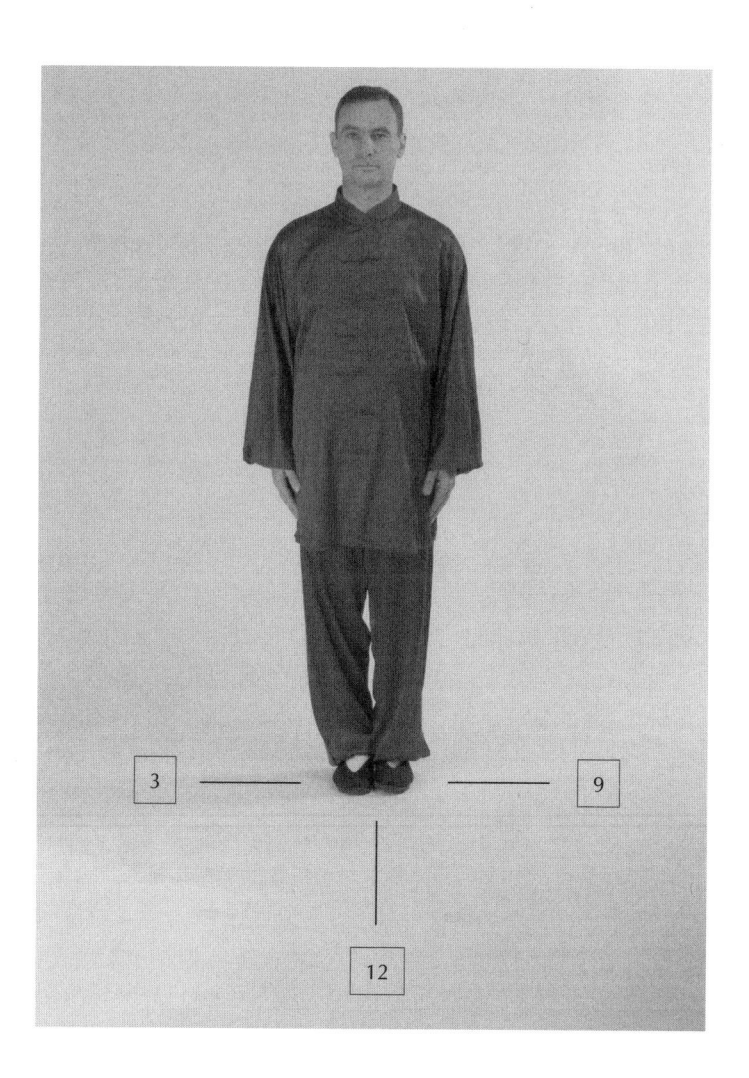

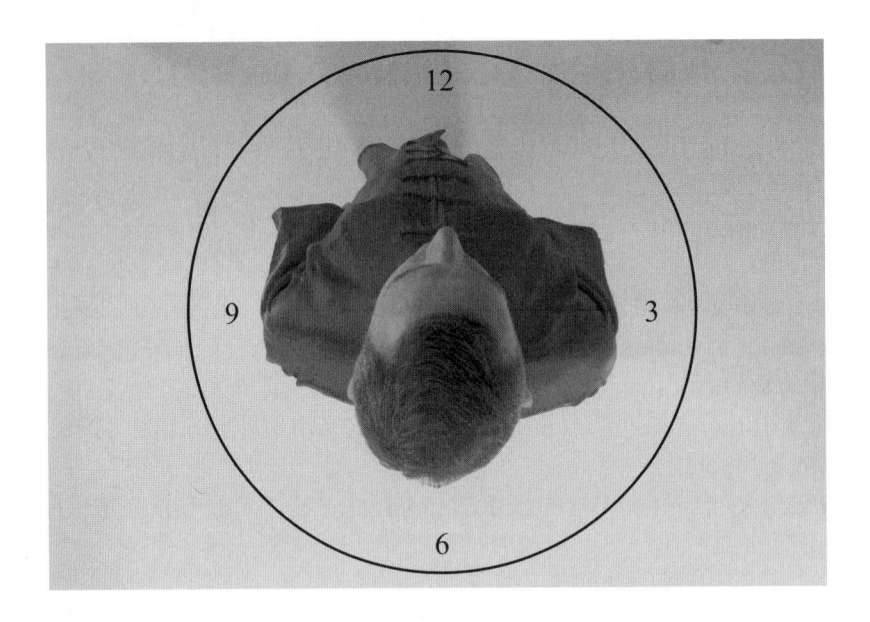

THE YANG TAÌJÍ 24-STEP SHORT FORM

THE KUÀ 胯

This translates as 'thigh/crotch' and refers to the area between the pelvis and the upper thigh – the diagonal 'crease' leading from the outer pelvis to the crotch, or the join where the leg meets the body/pelvis. Anatomically this is the 'inguinal groove'.

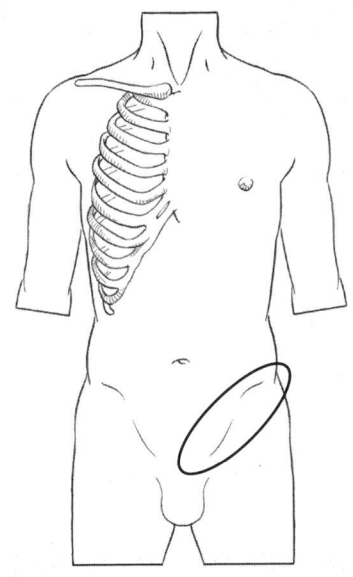

The Kuà (anterior view)

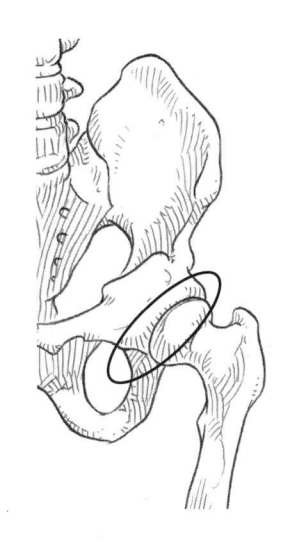

The Kuà (anterior view)

In dance, or in ballet, the ability to open the thigh outwards to the side whilst keeping the pelvis facing the front would be called 'turn out'. It is very easy to forget to relax this part of the body, which locks the thighs and makes the movements of the lower body rather rigid.

THE HYPOTHENAR EMINENCE

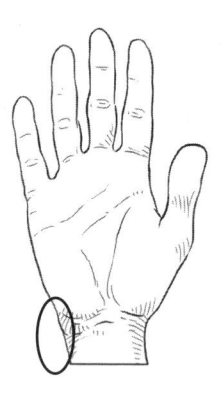

There are several references in the text to the hypothenar eminence, as this part of the hand often completes the push.

KEY TO FOOT PATTERNS

Left foot = ■● **Direction of step:** Black dotted arrow e.g. ┈┈┈▶

Right foot = ○○ **Direction of step:** Black solid arrow e.g. ⟶

The arrow, depending upon its positioning, refers either to the direction of the next step, or to where the foot has come from.

A double arrow ⟹ signifies the rotation of the body.

▲▼ or ▽△ signifies toes *down* or toes *up*, and the colour again refers to left (black) or right (white).

▼⋯ (or e.g. ⋯▽) shows the angle of the foot when on the ball of the foot.

● or ○ signifies the foot raised off the ground – the colour again referring to left (grey) or right (white).

'Slipping the heel' is shown by a small arrow which starts from the heel, dotted for the left foot, and solid for the right foot. The previous foot position is shown in feint: or

'Turning the toes' is shown by a similar method:

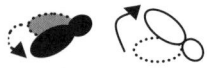

NOTE ON PRONUNCIATION OF CHINESE WORDS

The Chinese language uses four 'tones', or inflections of the voice, and one 'neutral' tone, and these have been rendered in the text as closely as possible.

Tone 1 (a flat tone):	āēīōū
Tone 2 (a rising tone):	áéíóú
Tone 3 (a falling/rising tone):	ǎěǐǒǔ
Tone 4 (a falling tone):	àèìòù
Tone 5 (a neutral tone):	aeiou

Therefore, a word such as 行步 xing2bu4 will be written as xíngbù.

YANG TÀIJÍ 24-STEP FORM WITH MUSIC

Traditionalists are usually horrified at the idea of doing tàijíquán to music, and having trained in the traditional style myself, before the introduction of music to almost every form of Chinese exercise, I understand the sentiment. It certainly seems to grate with the 'quán' aspect of tàijíquán, although perhaps it's more pertinent to the 'tàijí' side!

However in China, performing tàijí to music has become the norm. When you go to the parks in the mornings, every practice area will have music blasting out at full volume for every different form of exercise taking place. This is tàijí for the general public, and there seems to be no shortage of participants.

So whilst I am not particularly keen on it, I have to admit that it does have some very definite benefits, those being that it undoubtedly relaxes people, and it allows them to enjoy the movements without getting too intense about them – and this, for the vast majority, is a very good thing.

Bearing in mind that most people do tàijí for relaxation, or because it's something a little different, or for gentle exercise, or to meet like-minded people, or any number of other reasons, then it's actually a very good idea – and most seem to love it!

So I use music in some classes, but in the higher level classes I avoid it.

There is 'official' music for this set of movements. This is because in the 1990 Asian games (the eleventh), in order that several hundred performers (approximately 1200) could work together simultaneously, it was decided that the only way to do this was to use music to which the performers could time their movements. The story as I have heard it is that this was quite problematic and the initial attempt meant that some of the tàijí movements had to be performed too quickly as some of the individual parts of the music were too short (or in one case too long) for the relevant movement.

If you look at the 'No. of beats' column in Yang 24-Step music on p.362, it's fairly clear which those were. Overall, each movement is given a certain number of beats, usually eight, but in some cases this has had to be extended to ten, or shortened to six. Even then some of the movements are a little too fast.

For those of you who have had a musical education, the music is in 4/4 time, with two bars (usually) designated for each movement, for example Parting the Wild Horse's Mane 1 is two bars of four, and ditto for Parting the Wild Horse's Mane 2, etc.

14

Structure of the Standardized Yang Tàijí 24-Step Short Form

Preparation/Ready position
预备势 (Yùbèishì)

SECTION 1 (3 MOVEMENTS)

1. **Commencing Form**
   起势 (Qǐshì)
2. **Parting the Wild Horse's Mane (Left and Right)**
   左右野马分鬃 (Zuǒyòu Yěmǎ Fēnzōng)
3. **Stork (White Crane) Spreads (Flashes) its Wings**
   白鹤亮翅 (Báihè Liàngchì)

SECTION 2 (3 MOVEMENTS)

4. **Brush Knee and Twist (Side) Step on Both Sides (Brush Aside Over the Knee in Reverse Forwards Stance) (Left and Right)**
   左右搂膝拗步 (Zuǒyòu Lōuxī Àobù)
5. **Play the Pipa (Strum the Lute/Guitar)**
   手挥琵琶 (Shǒuhuī Pípā)

6. **Curve Back Arms on Both Sides (Repulse Monkey on Both Sides) (Step Back and Curl the Arms) (Left and Right)**
   左右倒卷肱 (Zuǒyòu Dàojuǎngōng)

SECTION 3 (2 MOVEMENTS)

7. **Grasp the Bird's (Sparrow's/Peacock's) Tail (Left Style)**
   左揽雀尾 (Zuǒ Lǎnquèwěi)

8. **Grasp the Bird's (Sparrow's/Peacock's) Tail (Right Style)**
   右揽雀尾 (Yòu Lǎnquèwěi)

SECTION 4 (3 MOVEMENTS)

9. **Single Whip (Single Biān)**
   单鞭 (Dānbiān)

10. **Cloud Hands (Wave/Move the Hands Like Clouds)**
    云手 (Yúnshǒu)

11. **Single Whip (Single Biān)**
    单鞭 (Dānbiān)

SECTION 5 (4 MOVEMENTS)

Two are about footwork, one about the palm, and one about the fist.

12. **High Pat on Horse (Pat Horse from on High) (Gauge the Height of the Horse) (Strike the Face with the Palm)**
    高探马 (Gāotànmǎ)

13. **Kick with Right Heel (Separate Right Foot)**
    右蹬脚 (Yòu Dēngjiǎo)

14. **Strike (Opponent's) Ears with Both Fists**
    双峰贯耳 (Shuāngfēng Guàn'ěr)

15. **Turn and Kick with Left Heel (Separate Left Foot)**
    转身左蹬脚 (Zhuǎnshēn Zuǒ Dēngjiǎo)

THE YANG TAÌJÍ 24-STEP SHORT FORM

SECTION 6 (2 MOVEMENTS)

These movements have different directions of performance.

16. **Push Down and Stand on One Leg (Left Style) (Snake Creeps Down) (Golden Cockerel/Rooster on One Leg)**
    左下势独立 (Zuǒ Xiàshì Dúlì)

17. **Push Down and Stand on One Leg (Right Style) (Snake Creeps Down) (Golden Cockerel/Rooster on One Leg)**
    右下势独立 (Yòu Xiàshì Dúlì)

SECTION 7 (3 MOVEMENTS)

18. **Jade Lady Weaves Shuttles (Fair Lady Weaves her Shuttle Left and Right) (Shuttle Back and Forth) (Move the Shuttle Left and Right) (Work at Shuttles on Both Sides)**
    左右穿梭 (Zuǒyòu Chuānsuō)

19. **Needle at Sea Bottom**
    海底针 (Hǎidǐzhēn)

20. **Flash Arms (Fan Through Back) (Send a Flash Through the Arms)**
    闪通臂 (Shǎntōngbì)

SECTION 8 (4 MOVEMENTS)

21. **Turn, Deflect Downwards, Parry and Punch (Turn the Body, Deflect, Block and Punch)**
    转身搬拦捶 (Zhuǎnshēn Bānlánchuí)

22. **Apparent Close-Up (Appearing to Seal and Close) (Pull Back then Push, as if to Close)**
    如封似闭 (Rúfēng Sìbì)

23. **Cross Hands**
    十字手 (Shízìshǒu)

24. **Closing Form**
    收势 (Shōushì)

15

Description of the Yang Tàijí 24-Step Short Form

I have divided the description of the Form into three sections:

1. BRIEF
   Thumbnail notes of the Form, mainly for beginners who are unable to remember what comes next.

2. DETAILS
   More detail such as hand rotations, directions of turn, etc.

3. NOTES
   For the more advanced practitioners, in particular for those who want to understand the feeling and the energetic flow of the movements, the more subtle turns of the hands, the 'opening' and 'closing' of the movements, etc. In this section there are also a number of 'Variations' for some of the movements, because not all practitioners do the movements with exactly the same feeling. None of the 'Variations' are *right* or *wrong*, there are only preferences; occasionally I state which is my personal preference. However, it's important to understand that more often than not a 'Variation' merely implies a different martial application, and little else.

Yang Tàijí doesn't require the more extreme postures and compressions of Chen and Sun style tàijí, and yet the same ideas are inherent in Yang style.

I have described the 'open' and 'close' movements and the method of *thinking* them (usually the connections between the shoulders and hips, elbows and knees, and wrists and ankles), but in actual performance you should hardly show these ideas in Yang style; it would be the equivalent of playing a piece of Mozart in the style of Beethoven – too dramatic!

Therefore, when practising Yang Tàijí, you *feel* it, but you don't *show* it.

I have done the best that I can with the descriptions, but the more detail that I try to describe, and the more that I try to explain the 'feeling' that lies behind the movements, the more I realize that language (or my grasp of it) is often totally inadequate.

PREPARATION/READY POSITION

预备势 (Yùbèishì)

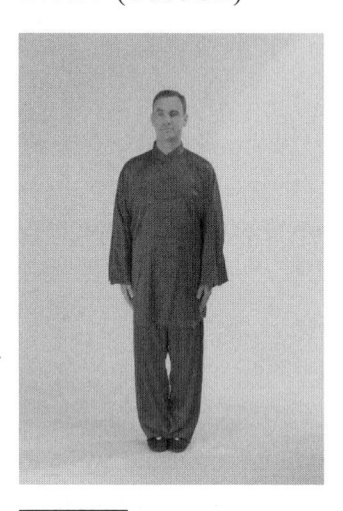

BRIEF
Feet together; the body faces 12.00.

DETAILS
Sometimes referred to as 'raising the spirit': body upright, allowing the crown to rise.

NOTES
Preparation prior to stepping:

- **The weight:** Even before you step, your weight should be about 70 per cent on the heels.

- **The body** should be completely relaxed, with the hands on either side of the body fingers pointing downwards.

- **The back of the neck** should release as though being gently drawn upwards. This will cause the chin to tuck under slightly, but without any tension.

- **The knee joints** are 'soft', with the knees not tensed or locked backwards. However, as in the 'Grounding' exercise on p.28, the knees are *very* slightly bent forwards, as this has the effect of relaxing the hips/pelvis.

- **The tip of the tongue** is placed in the roof of the mouth. If you place the tip of your tongue just in front of the upper teeth and then brush it backwards over the upper palate (towards the throat), you reach a point where the tip appears to go up a steep incline. There is also a point where it 'tickles' slightly more than other places. *This* is where you place the tongue; it is the connection point between two acupuncture channels: the Du channel (Governing vessel) and the Ren channel (Conception vessel).

Once the tongue is in place, relax the root of it completely.

- **The eyes** look straight ahead.
- **Breathe** naturally.

SECTION 1

(3 MOVEMENTS)

1. **Commencing Form**
   起势 (Qǐshì)

2. **Parting the Wild Horse's Mane (Left and Right)**
   左右野马分鬃 (Zuǒyòu Yěmǎ Fēnzōng)

3. **Stork (White Crane) Spreads (Flashes) its Wings**
   白鹤亮翅 (Báihè Liàngchì)

FORM 1: COMMENCING FORM

起势 (Qǐshì)

BRIEF 1
Step left.

DETAILS
Move the weight on to the right foot, raise the left heel (relaxing the ankle so the toes point downwards), lift the left knee (the foot rises) and place the left toes a shoulder's width to the left (relaxing the ankle so the toes point downwards), place the left heel and move the weight between the feet (sink the foot).

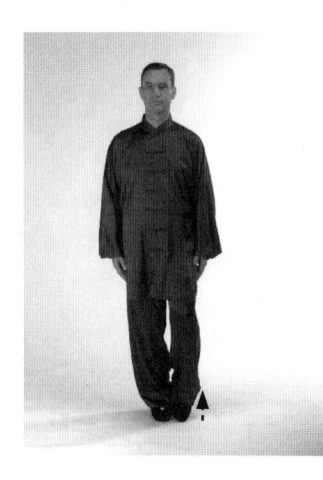

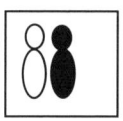

NOTES

- **To initiate the sideways step:**
    - Hollow or soften the chest slightly, and use the firming of the abdominal muscles to bend the left knee prior to stepping, i.e. use

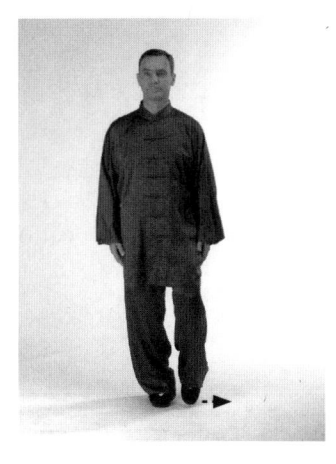

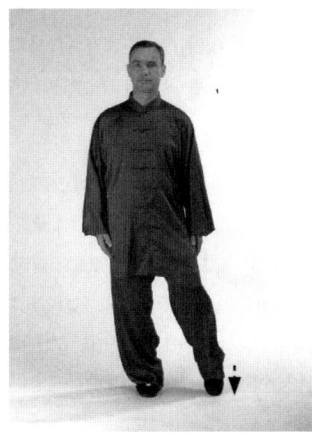

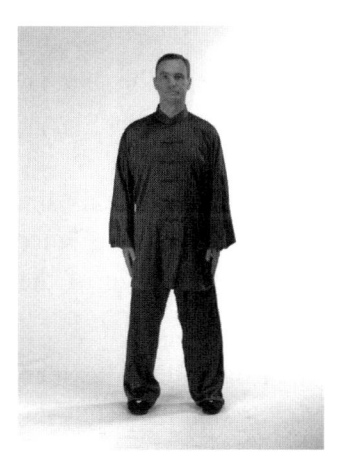

the centre to lift the leg. (If you place your palms on your lower abdominal muscles and try to lift your knee *without* involving your abdominal muscles, you'll find that it is almost impossible – they automatically come into play. Just make it a conscious process.)

- Feel a slight pushing down with the tips of the fingers.

- **Stepping:**

    - The expression for stepping sideways is 'Diǎnqǐ, diǎnluò 点起点落'. This is the method of stepping and translates as 'point, rise, point, fall'.

      'Fall' is perhaps an unfortunate translation; 'sink' the foot would probably be better. The toes should be placed, and then, joint by joint, the weight should be transferred.

    - The feeling of stepping is 'Qīngqǐ, qīngluò 轻起轻落', which translates as 'gently rise, gently fall'; the key word is 'gently'.

    - As you place the right heel, the weight moving 50/50, soften the hips and the upper body.

    - As you place the weight on to the left foot, sink the qi: feel the shoulders sink into and connect with the hips.

- **Allow the spine to lengthen:** Release the neck and raise the crown (Bǎihuì 百會).

- **Coordination:** Complete control of balance and weight distribution is important.

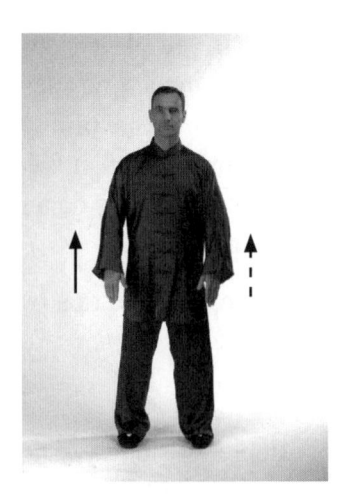

Brief 2
Raise the hands.

Details
Relax the shoulders as you raise the wrists to no higher than shoulder-height.

Notes

- In many respects, this is one of the most complicated movements in the Form. The problem that beginners find is how to lift the arms whilst involving the entire body and, in particular, the centre.

  - **Sinking the qi:** As the left heel presses into the ground (50/50 in the 'Preparation' on p.74), feel the sinking of the weight into the heels (70%) and combine it with further relaxation of the chest that you began when stepping out in the previous movement. This creates the Bow of the Arms before you start to lift them.

  - **Release the pelvis:** Soften the knees, slightly pulling up your pelvic floor (your perineum) and also gently pulling in the lower abdominal muscles. If you relax the small of the back at the same time, this latter action should cause the lower edge of the pelvis to roll/tilt forwards.

  - **The arms:** Simultaneously lengthen/extend the fingertips downwards before lifting the wrists ahead of you. (The palms, which initially face the sides of your thighs, will turn downwards after lifting approximately 3–4 inches (8–10 cm) ahead of you). (See 'The slight "pushing down" of the wrists/fingertips' note on the following page.)

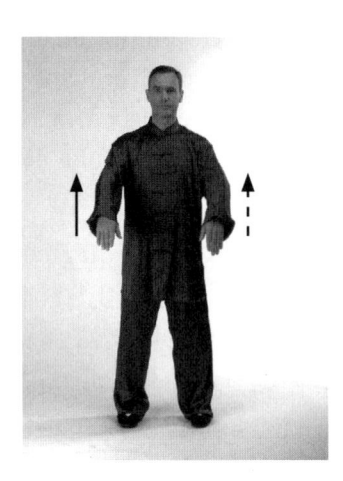

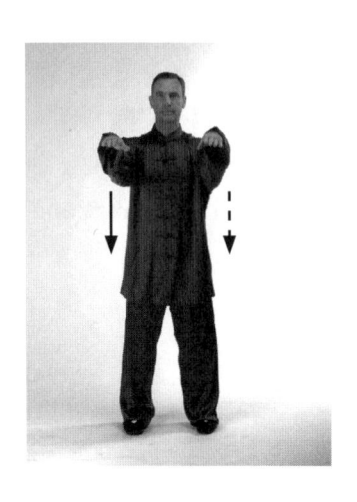

- **The knees and elbows:** As you start to lift the arms, the knees and elbows rotate outwards slightly. This should not be obvious, in that anyone watching you would be unaware of what you were doing. The feeling should be of almost rotating the flesh around the bone of the limbs, rather than rotating the bones themselves.

- **The neck** should gently lengthen upwards, and the tip of the spine (because you are slightly pulling in the perineum) should lengthen downwards.

- **The slight 'pushing down' of the wrists/fingertips** at the start of the movement creates a small vertical circle moving away from you – downwards, away and upwards.

  The effectiveness of this can be felt if a partner pushes against your wrists prior to your moving them:
  - Just push your wrists straight ahead of you against his push, and then…
  - do the fractional push downwards first forming a circle that curls ahead of you – against his push.

  You might also feel this slight extension downwards causing the chest to hollow.

- **The wrists** are relaxed as you raise them and move them away from the body towards 12.00.

- **The elbows:** The arms and therefore the elbows will rotate outwards as they are lifted; this is a natural rotation on the arms, and it is important not to bend the elbows so that they stick out sideways.

- **The weight:** Keep the feeling of the weight on the heels; you will otherwise tend to rock forwards on to the toes because of the weight of the arms rising ahead of you.

- **'Centre back':** Your centre will actually move backwards as you lift the arms.

- **'Opening':** This is an 'opening' movement.

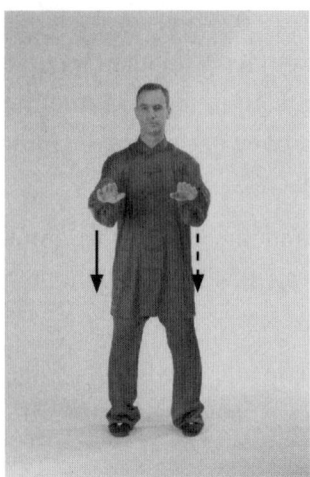

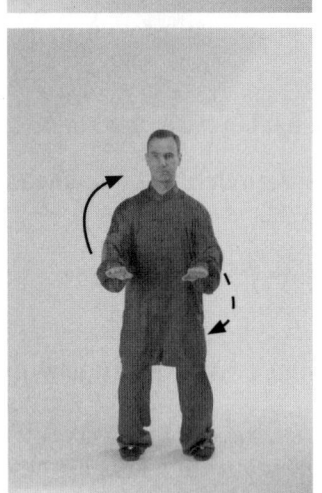

Brief 3
Bend knees; lower the hands.

Details
Bend the knees and sit down, gently flexing the wrists.

The elbows draw halfway back towards the body and the forearms lower until they are approximately parallel to the ground (but also see 'Variation' note on the following page).

The eyes look straight ahead.

Centre forwards.

Notes

- **Using the centre:** The downwards movement of the body comes entirely from the centre.

    Continue the movements that you began in Brief 1 on p.76: pulling in the perineum and the lower abdominal muscles, releasing the neck. By engaging the entire structure the apparent downwards push down of the arms is therefore achieved by integrating the entire body (also see note below).

- **Coordination** of the movement is important; the lowering of the arms needs to take place at the same time as sitting down.

    When lowering the hands, connect:

    - **shoulders to hips**, then
    - **elbows to knees**, and then think
    - **wrists to ankles**.

    The tucking under of the hips and 'closing' of the centre initiates the entire process.

- **The elbows** rotate downwards as you sit down (part of the 'closing').

- **The hands** will be 'in' at the wrists, so the palms will face the floor. Avoid the wrists becoming limp.

- **The neck:** Release the back of your neck.
- **The posture** is Horse Stance (马步 Mǎbù) (see p.49).
- **The spine** should be vertical as you sit, allowing the small of the back to open as the coccyx tucks under.
- **The weight** should be about 70 per cent on the heels.
- **'Closing':** This is a 'closing' movement.
- **Variation:** Some practitioners do not stop with the hands at waist height; they take them almost down to the thighs. This is the same as in the Traditional Long Form (see p.17).

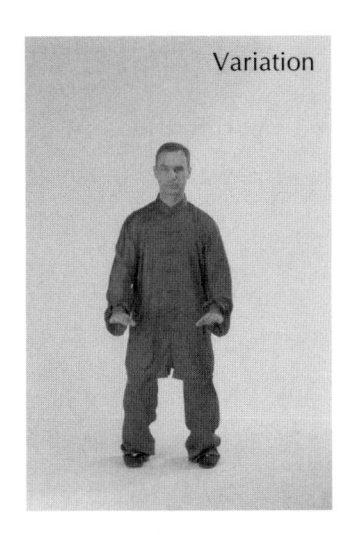

Variation

FORM 2: PARTING THE WILD HORSE'S MANE (LEFT AND RIGHT)

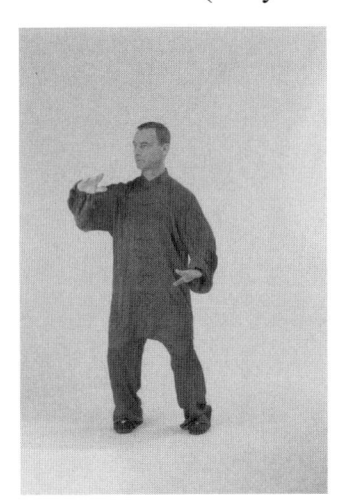

左右野马分鬃 (Zuǒyòu Yěmǎ Fēnzōng)

Brief 1
Slight turn to 12.30/1.00, 'splitting' or separating the hands; right hand lifts up and left hand pushes down; weight begins to move on to the right foot.

Details
Start to take the weight on to the right foot and, as you turn the body no further than 1.00, raise the right wrist to shoulder-height (palm down) and push the left hand downwards.

Keep both feet flat on the ground. The eyes look slightly right beyond the right hand.

Centre right.

NOTES

- **Coordination:** When shifting the weight on to the right foot, and turning slightly to the right, beginners tend to push their arms to the right also. In fact the left hand (low) almost stays in exactly the same position in space that it was on the previous move, so that, in the move that follows, you rotate the body back towards it.

- **The left hand:**
  - Although the left hand is quite close to the body, avoid the left armpit closing up; keep a small relaxed space there.
  - The left hand, which is sinking, begins very slightly to turn palm upwards at this point, although it doesn't complete its turn until the end of the next move below.
  - The left hand is at pelvis/waist height, and the right hand is at throat height.

- **Opening the arms:** The lowering of the arms at the end of Form 1 was a 'closing' movement. This move is therefore a small 'opening' one; allow the chest and arms to relax and open.

- **Posture:** Keep the body upright.

- **Variation:** Some practitioners do not make a turn to the right here at all but turn left to immediately hold the ball (see pp.87–88).

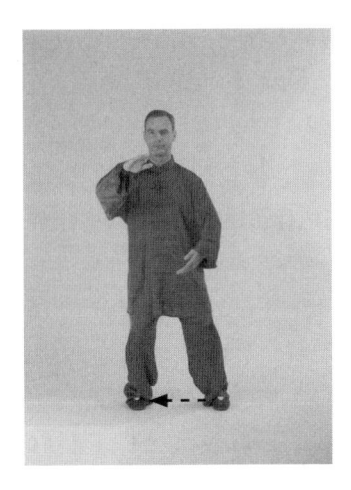

BRIEF 2
Turn; palms face each other; left foot in.

DETAILS
Three things happen simultaneously:

- Turn your body back towards 12.00.
- Complete turning the bottom hand palm upwards.
- Draw the left foot into the right foot.

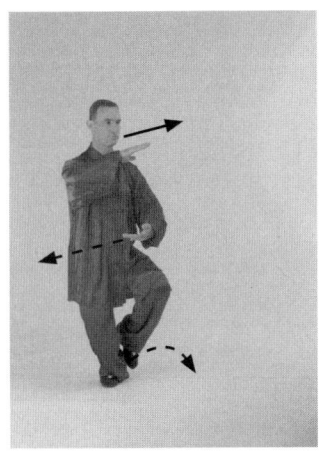

The eyes continue to look over the right hand. Centre left.

NOTES
Please note: In reality this move and the one above are a single move and the above description is aimed at beginners.

- **The left palm**, which is sinking, begins to rotate palm upwards (screwdriver turn) at this point.
- **The left hand:** Although the hand is quite close to the body, avoid the left armpit closing up; keep a small relaxed space there.

- **The arms/hands** are in the shape that is often referred to as 'holding the ball' with the upper wrist at shoulder-height, and the lower wrist just below waist height. Note, however, that this is not a static posture but one which the body is moving through. (See 'Holding the ball,' p.63.)
- **The arms** are about 8–12 inches (20–30 cm) from the body.
- **The weight** should now be completely on the right foot; the body rotates to 10.30 on a vertical axis (crown and right foot).
- **The right leg:** Avoid straightening the leg at this point – beginners tend to want to stand up here.
- **Posture:** Continue to keep the body upright, rotating it on a *vertical axis* (crown and right foot).

THE YANG TAIJI 24-STEP SHORT FORM

- **Variation:** Some teachers say that it is not necessary to bring the left foot in before stepping to 9.00 in the following movement. (See 'To test it' on p.89.)

Brief 3

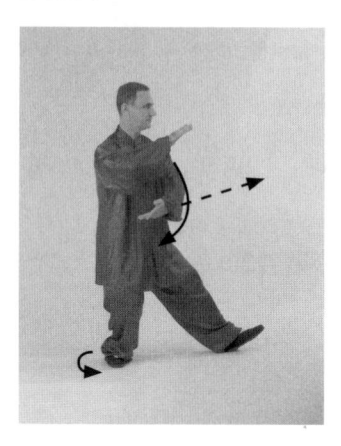

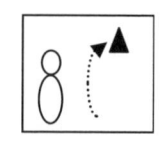

Step to 9.00 (the left side) with the left heel.

Details

Step to 9.00 with the left heel making sure that it is a shoulder's-width step. (See Chapter 11, 'The Process of Stepping'; also see 'Width of step' on p.86.)
  Start to extend the left arm towards 11.00/12.00
  Sink the right elbow.
  The body stays facing 11.30/12.00.

Notes

- **Sink** further into the right foot.

- **The neck** should remain relaxed.

- **The right knee:** Watch the tendency to allow the right knee to 'collapse' inwards; apart from the fact that it is not good for the knee, it also weakens the balance.

- **Width of step:** See 'Width of step' note on p.86.

- **'Closing':**

  - **Tuck the tailbone:** As you place the left foot, 'close' the body by starting both to tuck the coccyx under, and to pull in the lower abdominal muscles.

  - **The elbows** begin to compress slightly inwards towards each other, thereby 'closing' the chest. This will cause the hands to move in opposite directions; sink your right elbow and start to lift the inside elbow crease of your left arm. In effect you will be lifting the left upper arm towards approximately 12.00.

  - **The arms:** Bear in mind that you are in the process of creating an anti-clockwise horizontal circle with the left hand, and a downwards push with the right hand. This should govern the direction of the closing.

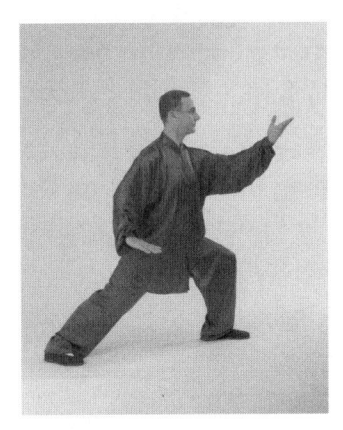

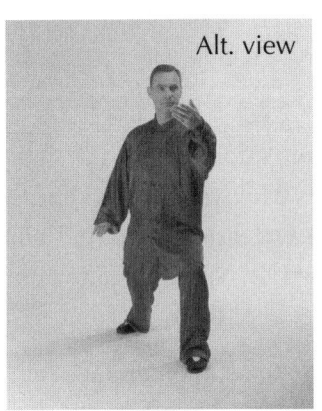

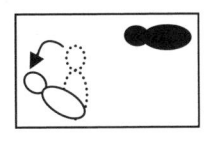

BRIEF 4

Left foot flat; weight forwards; left palm out to 9.00; push down right palm, slip rear heel.

DETAILS

As you transfer the weight on to the left foot, turn the body and sweep the left hand out (with palm still facing up), moving it diagonally upwards from your right side to 9.00.

Push the right hand downwards so that the arm is almost straight.

As the weight moves on to the left foot, use the turn of the hips to slip the right heel. (For 'Slipping the rear heel' see p.64.)

The eyes look beyond the left hand to 9.00.

Alt. view

NOTES

- **The final posture:**
  - Your left foot is facing straight ahead to 9.00.
  - Your right foot is turned outwards at 45°, i.e. pointing to approximately 10.30.
  - Your hips and torso are turned approximately 30° to the right – can be fractionally more.
  - Your left hand is at chin height and on the line between your head and 9.00. (The line of your left thumb is between you and 9.00, pointing to 9.00.)
  - The palm of your left hand is turned upwards at 45° or more.
  - The fingers of your right hand should be approximately between the two thighs when the posture is looked at from the side (as in the photograph).
  - There should be a relaxed space under the right armpit, and the hand should be approximately 6 inches (15 cm) away from the side of your body.

- **Width of step:** This should be 8–12 inches wide (20–30 cm), but will depend upon the frame of the practitioner. If it is too narrow, the turn of the body to the left at the start of Parting the Wild Horse's Mane 2 (p.89) will be almost impossible.
  - **Testing the width of the step:** A test for finding this is based on the strength of the legs. Ask a partner to place his knee outside and against your left knee; he should then try to push your knee inwards.
- **Sink the right hip** so that the bow of the rear leg is formed.
- **Spiralling in the posture:**
  - **The legs** spiral outwards, in other words the knees should feel as though they are both opening outwards.
  - **The left palm** twists anti-clockwise.
  - **The right hand:** In the final posture the predominant feeling of the right hand is of pushing downwards, but it also pushes backwards. In addition, the hand twists inwards (not visibly to anyone watching), but the right elbow doesn't twist outwards; therefore the wrist will flex outwards slightly (the hypothenar eminence or the ulnar side of the wrist).
- **Directions of arms/hands:** Both hands should feel as though they are extending away from each other – the left hand away to the left (9.00) and the heel of the right hand downwards and backwards.
- **The left hand movement** is 'liě' (pinyin) 挒 (or 'lieh' in the Wade-Giles (WG) system of Romanizing Chinese) – a horizontal-sideways, sweeping or 'splitting' movement of the arm.

  This is not, as performed by some beginners, a lifting-ahead-of-you movement.

  The right hand movement is 'Cǎi' 采, or 'Tsai' (WG) – usually translated as 'plucking' – as in plucking an apple from a tree.
- **The energy of the movement** should be in the outside of the left forearm.
- **Turning the body:** When performing this movement, there is initially a feeling in this posture of barging with the shoulder (Kào) towards 7.30/8.00, the lifting of the left upper arm serving to enhance the power of the movement.

  (It should be noted, however, that a great number of tàijí movements can be used as Kào, and that this is not the predominant energy of Parting the Wild Horse's Mane.)

The turn of the body 'liě' 挒 comes towards the end of the movement – in other words don't make the turn of the body too early, move the weight at least halfway forwards before turning the body.

Variation to Briefs 1 and 2

The following two movements are alternatives to Parting the Wild Horse's Mane 1, Briefs 1 and 2 (pp.81–84). The differences between the two are very small, but alter the feeling of the movement and are preferred by some practitioners. Neither is 'right' or 'wrong', but the martial application alters depending upon which one is performed.

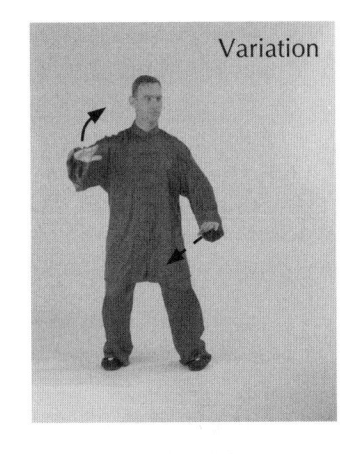

BRIEF 1
Slight turn to 11.30 'splitting' or separating the hands; right hand lifts up and left hand pushes down.

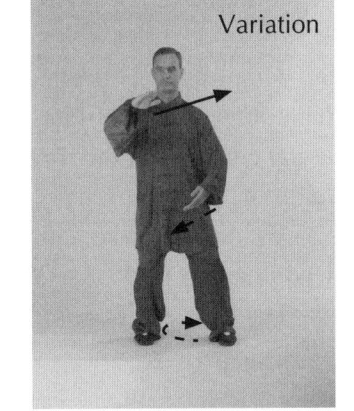

DETAILS
Turn the body slightly left and separate the hands. The back of the right hand will rise ahead of you, and the left hand (palm down) will move sideways with the turn of the body.

Turn the centreline back to 12.00 simultaneously lifting the back of your right hand (to shoulder-height) and pushing your left hand downwards (see also Notes for Brief 2 on p.88). Keep your weight between the feet still.

Keep both feet flat on the ground.
The eyes look slightly right towards the right hand.
Centre left.

NOTES

- **Opening the arms:** The lowering of the arms at the end of Form 1 was a 'closing' movement. This move is therefore a small 'opening' one; allow the chest and arms to relax and open.

THE YANG TAIJI 24-STEP SHORT FORM

- **Shifting the weight on to the right foot:** Some practitioners shift the weight on to the right foot at this point. It is fine to do so, but from a martial arts point of view can weaken your movement (see 'To test it' note on p.89).

BRIEF 2

Turn back; left palm upwards; begin to move weight on to the right foot.

DETAILS

Three things happen simultaneously:

- Turn your body back to 12.00.

- Complete turning the bottom hand so that both palms face each other.

- Shift the weight on to the right foot (see 'Weight-shift' note on p.89).

As you turn the centreline back to 12.00, your right hand arrives at shoulder-height and begins to fold at the elbow with the forearm approximately parallel to the ground.
Your left hand rotates palm up and the fingertips lead towards 12.00 (see also Notes below).
The eyes continue to look over the right hand.
Centre right.

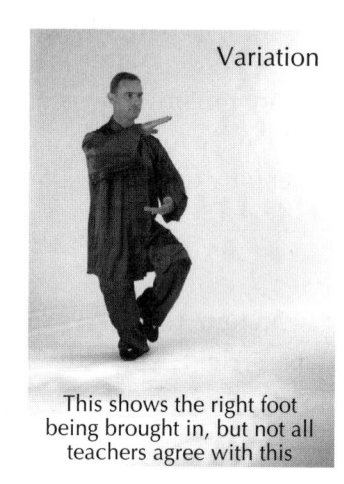

Variation

This shows the right foot being brought in, but not all teachers agree with this

NOTES

- **The left palm** rotates palm upwards (screwdriver turn) and starts to thread towards 12.00 under the right arm.

- **The left hand** (palm up) completes this movement at pelvis/waist height, and **the right hand** (palm down) at throat height.

- **The arms** are about 8–12 inches (20–30 cm) from the body.

- **Bringing in the left foot:** Not all teachers bring the left foot into the right foot before stepping to 9.00 in the third movement. There are arguments on both sides, but see note on the following page about testing the martial aspect of the movement.

- **Weight-shift:** Some teachers argue that there is little point in shifting any weight on to the right foot until the moment of actually stepping with the left foot (Brief 3).

  - The amount of weight that you shift on to the right foot can be minimal.
  - Therefore, having completed Form 1, start to rotate the body to the left with the weight still equally between the feet (Brief 2), then just before stepping with the left foot, shift the weight on to the right foot (blending Briefs 2 and 3).

    This is my personal preference. From a martial point of view the movement is weakened if the weight is placed on the right foot too early as any force applied to your body from the left side will unbalance you.

  - **To test it**, begin from the end of Form 1 (arms lowered) and ask a partner to push your left shoulder towards 3.00 as you try to complete the movements that follow. If your balance is easily upset, something is wrong.

Moving into Parting the Wild Horse's Mane 2

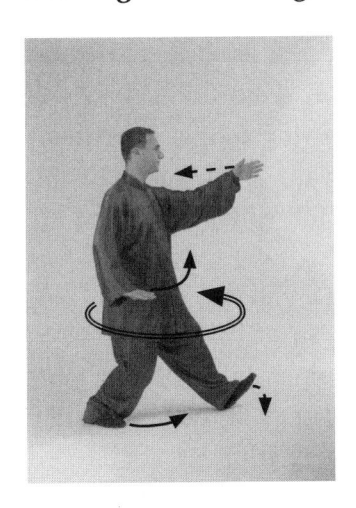

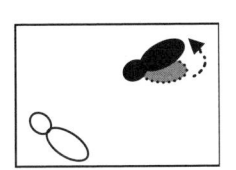

BRIEF 1
Sit back turning to the corner; turn the left hand.

DETAILS
Sit back on to your right foot lifting the left toes; turn both the hips and the left toes to the left diagonal, i.e. towards 7.30.

Rotate the left palm to face downwards, and let the arm move with the turn of the body.

Allow the right hand to release, relaxing the wrist and, without independently moving it, let it move with the body.

The eyes follow the left hand.

NOTES

- **The left hand:** When rotating the left hand, avoid bending the wrist; it should turn as though the hand were the blade of a screwdriver, with the tips of the fingers turning the screw.

- **The right hand:** As you sit back, there is a very small anti-clockwise circle drawn by the right palm facing the floor. Feel it yourself, but don't make it obvious.

- **Sitting back:** It is not necessary to sit back completely – just sit back enough to turn the toes of the foot.

- **The pelvis:** Sit back by gently pulling up the pelvic floor, pulling in the lower abdominals, and sinking the buttocks. Release the neck as you do so.

- **Advanced:** See additional note at end of Brief 2 (pp.91–2) for more advanced method of performing both this and the next movement.

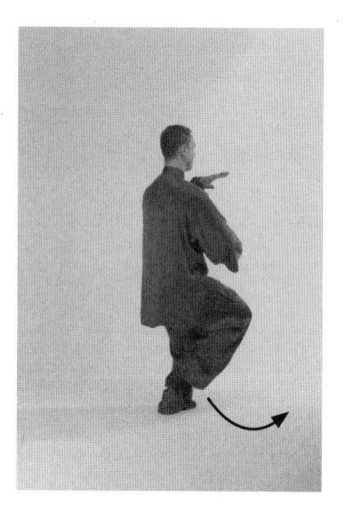

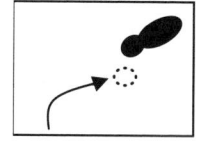

BRIEF 2
Weight forwards; bend left arm; right foot in.

DETAILS
Move the weight forwards (left foot is placed and turned on the diagonal towards 7.30) and draw the right foot in alongside the left with the toes just off the ground.

The left hand turns palm down and the arm folds in front of the chest.

As you transfer the weight on to the left foot, release the right wrist and start to rotate the palm upwards leading with the fingertips.

The eyes are still looking towards the left hand.

NOTES

- **The left foot:** Turning the left foot to 7.30 is the minimum amount; it can be turned even further.

- **Turning the body** to the left (and eventually bringing in the right foot) is easier if you think of either bringing your right shoulder towards your left hip, or of turning the centre towards the left knee.
- **The left leg:** Beginners often straighten the left leg at this point. Keep it bent, it helps to maintain the balance.
- **The arms:**
  - **The upper wrist** is at shoulder-height.
  - **The left elbow** has folded so that the thumb edge of the hand is just below the throat.
  - **Both arms** are very relaxed and approximately 6 inches (15 cm) from the body.
  - **The right arm:** Try to avoid 'doing' too much with the right arm; it is virtually in position before you begin this part of the movement, so you almost need to do nothing more than turn the palm upwards and push the arm (fingertips leading) below the left arm (but see below for a more advanced method).
- **More advanced method for Briefs 1 and 2:**
  - **Brief 1:**
    'Opening': As you sit back, turn the body to the *right* – a very small turn. This is an 'opening' of the body. There should be a feeling of the left fingertips opening/pushing towards 9.00. Don't turn the body to the left yet.

    The right hand moves slightly backwards with the turn of the body (the start of a small anti-clockwise circle).
  - **Brief 2:**
    The left hand: As you turn to the left and move the weight on to the left foot, the left hand screwdriver-turns over, the left elbow bending, the thumb edge starting to move towards you, and the wrist flexing outwards slightly (the little finger – lateral – edge of the wrist stretching slightly). The left hand (now palm down) has folded in front of your chest (see 'Testing' on the following page).

    The right hand: As you move forwards turning the body left, the right hand/palm completes its small anti-clockwise circle, and then screwdriver-turns palm up so that the fingertips are leading the hand to the left (except that it is the shifting of the weight on to the left foot that makes it appear as though the hand is moving).

Testing the feeling of the left hand in this movement: As you move the weight on to the left foot, have a partner gently pull your left fingertips. Relax the left wrist and left shoulder, and pull your partner forwards. In order to make the movement work, you will be compelled to use the connection of the centre to the left shoulder.

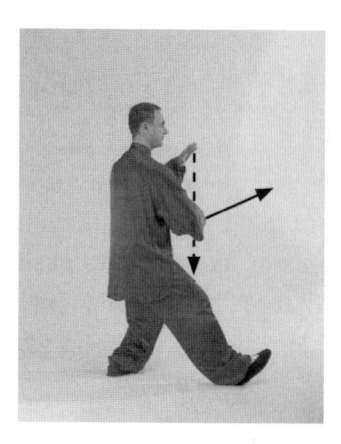

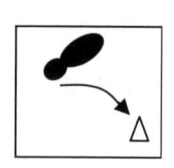

BRIEF 3

Step to 9.00 (the right side) with the right heel.

DETAILS

Step to 9.00 with the right heel making sure that it is a shoulder's-width step. (See Chapter 11, 'The Process of Stepping'.) The body stays facing 7.30.

Extend the left arm towards 6.00/7.00.

Sink the right elbow.

NOTES

- **Sink** further into the left foot.

- **The neck** should remain relaxed.

- **The left knee:** Watch the tendency to allow the left knee to 'collapse' inwards; apart from the fact that it is not good for the knee, it also weakens the balance.

- **Width of step:** See note on p.94.

- **'Closing':**

  - **Tuck the tailbone:** As you place the right foot, 'close' the body by starting both to tuck the coccyx under, and to pull in the lower abdominal muscles.

  - **The elbows** begin to compress slightly inwards towards each other, thereby 'closing' the chest. This will cause the hands to move in opposite directions; sink your left elbow and start to lift the inside elbow crease of

DESCRIPTION OF THE YANG TÀIJÍ 24-STEP SHORT FORM

your right arm. In effect you will be lifting the right upper arm towards approximately 6.00.

- **The arms:** Bear in mind that you are in the process of creating a clockwise horizontal circle with the right hand, and a downwards push with the left hand. This should govern the direction of the closing.

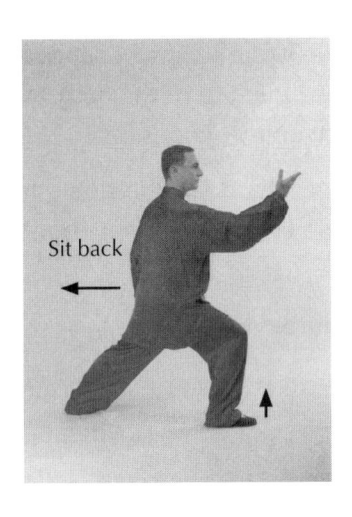

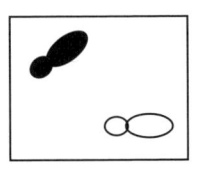

Sit back

BRIEF 4
Right foot flat; weight forwards; right palm out to 9.00; push down left palm, slip rear heel.

DETAILS
As you transfer the weight on to the right foot, turn the body and sweep the right hand out (with palm still facing up), moving it diagonally upwards from your left side to 9.00.

Push the left hand downwards so that the arm is almost straight.

As the weight moves on to the right foot, use the turn of the hips to slip the left heel. (For 'Slipping the rear heel' see p.64.)

The eyes look beyond the right hand to 9.00.

NOTES

- **The final posture:**

  - **Your right foot** is facing straight ahead to 9.00.

  - **Your left foot** is turned outwards at 45°, i.e. pointing to approximately 7.30.

  - **Your hips and torso** are turned approximately 30° to the left – can be fractionally more.

  - **Your right hand** is at chin height and on the line between your head and 9.00. (The line of your right thumb is between you and 9.00, pointing to 9.00.)

- - The palm of your right hand is turned upwards at 45° or more.
  - The fingers of your left hand should be approximately between the two thighs when the posture is looked at from the side (as in the final posture of Parting the Wild Horse's Mane 1 on p.85).
  - There should be a relaxed space under the left armpit, and the hand should be approximately 6 inches (15 cm) away from the side of your body.
- **Width of step:** This should be 8–12 inches wide (20–30 cm), but will depend upon the frame of the practitioner. If it is too narrow, the turn of the body to the right in Parting the Wild Horse's Mane 3 will be almost impossible.

  Testing the width of the step: A test for finding this is based on the strength of the legs. Ask a partner to place his knee outside and against your right knee; he should then try to push your knee inwards.
- **Sink the left hip** so that the bow of the rear leg is formed.
- **Spiralling in the posture:**
  - **The legs** spiral outwards, in other words the knees should feel as though they are both opening outwards.
  - **The right palm** twists clockwise.
  - **The left hand:** In the final posture the predominant feeling of the left hand is of pushing downwards, but it also pushes backwards. In addition, the hand twists inwards (not visibly to anyone watching), but the left elbow doesn't twist outwards; therefore the wrist will flex outwards slightly (the hypothenar eminence or the ulnar side of the wrist).
- **Directions of arms/hands:** Both hands should feel as though they are extending away from each other – the left hand away to the left (9.00) and the heel of the left hand downwards and backwards.
- **The right hand movement** is 'liě' (pinyin) 挒 (or 'lieh' in the Wade-Giles (WG) system of Romanizing Chinese) – a horizontal-sideways, sweeping, or 'splitting' movement of the arm.

  This is not, as performed by some beginners, a lifting-ahead-of-you movement.

  The left hand movement is 'Căi' 采, or 'Tsai' (WG) – usually translated as 'plucking' – as in plucking an apple from a tree.
- **The energy of the movement** should be in the outside of the right forearm.

- **Turning the body:** When performing this movement, there is initially a feeling in this posture of barging with the shoulder (Kào) towards 10.00/10.30, the lifting of the right upper arm serving to enhance the power of the movement.

  (It should be noted, however, that a great number of tàijí movements can be used as Kào, and that this is not the predominant energy of Parting the Wild Horse's Mane.)

  The turn of the body 'liě' 挒 comes towards the end of the movement – in other words don't make the turn of the body too early, move the weight at least halfway forwards before turning the body.

Moving into Parting the Wild Horse's Mane 3

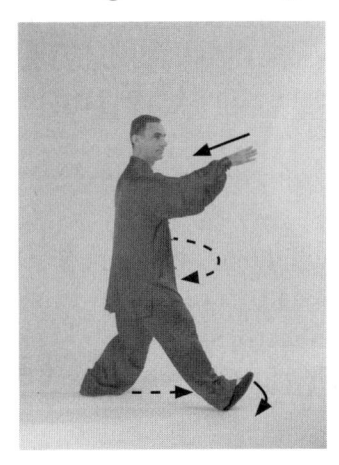

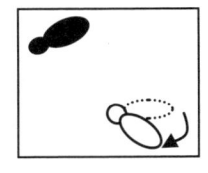

BRIEF 1
Sit back, turning to the corner; turn the right hand.

DETAILS
Sit back on to your left foot lifting the right toes; turn both the hips and the right toes to the right diagonal, i.e. towards 10.30.

Rotate the right palm to face downwards, and let the arm move with the turn of the body.

Allow the left hand to release, relaxing the wrist and, without independently moving it, let it move with the body.

The eyes follow the right hand.

NOTES

- **The right hand:** When rotating the right hand, avoid bending the wrist; it should turn as though the hand were the blade of a screwdriver, with the tips of the fingers turning the screw.

- **The left hand:** As you sit back, there is a small clockwise circle drawn by the left palm facing the floor. Feel it yourself, but don't make it obvious.

- **Sitting back:** It is not necessary to sit back completely – just sit back enough to turn the toes of the foot.

The pelvis: Sit back by gently pulling up the pelvic floor, pulling in the lower abdominals, and sinking the buttocks. Release the neck as you do so.

- **Advanced:** See additional note at end of Brief 2 (p.97) for a more advanced method of performing both this and the next movement.

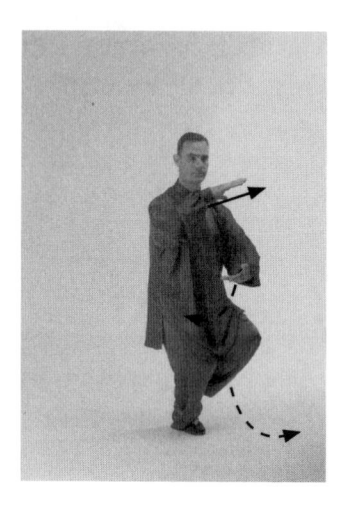

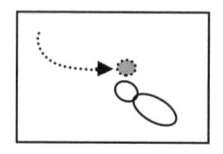

BRIEF 2

Weight forwards; bend right arm; left foot in.

DETAILS

Move the weight forwards (right foot is placed and turned on the diagonal towards 10.30) and draw the left foot in alongside the right with the toes just off the ground.

The right hand turns palm down and the arm folds in front of the chest.

As you transfer the weight on to the right foot, release the left wrist and start to rotate the palm upwards leading with the fingertips.

The eyes are still looking towards the right hand.

NOTES

- **The right foot:** Turning the right toes to 10.30 is the minimum amount; it can be turned even further.

- **Turning the body** to the right (and eventually bringing in the left foot) is easier if you think of either bringing your left shoulder towards your right hip, or of turning the centre towards the right knee.

- **The right leg:** Beginners often straighten the right leg at this point. Keep it bent, it helps to maintain the balance.

- **The arms:**

  - **The upper wrist** is at shoulder-height.

  - **The right elbow** has folded so that the thumb edge of the hand is just below the throat.

- **Both arms** are very relaxed and approximately 6 inches (15 cm) from the body.

- **The left arm:** Try to avoid 'doing' too much with the left arm; it is virtually in position before you begin this part of the movement, so you almost need to do nothing more than turn the palm upwards and push the arm (fingertips leading) below the right arm (but see below for a more advanced method).

- **More advanced method for Briefs 1 and 2:**

  - **Brief 1:**

    'Opening': As you sit back, turn the body to the *left* – a very small turn. This is an 'opening' of the body. There should be a feeling of the right fingertips opening/pushing towards 9.00. Don't turn the body to the right yet.

    The left hand moves slightly backwards with the turn of the body (the start of a small clockwise circle).

  - **Brief 2:**

    The right hand: As you turn to the right and move the weight on to the right foot, the right hand screwdriver-turns over, the right elbow bending, the thumb edge starting to move towards you, and the wrist flexing outwards slightly (the little finger – lateral – edge of the wrist stretching slightly). The right hand (now palm down) has folded in front of your chest (see 'Testing' below).

    The left hand: As you move forwards turning the body right, the left hand/palm completes its small clockwise circle, and then screwdriver-turns palm up to that the fingertips are leading the hand to the right (except that it is the shifting of the weight on to the right foot that makes it appear as though the hand is moving).

    Testing the feeling of the right hand in this movement: As you move the weight on to the right foot, have a partner gently pull your right fingertips. Relax the right wrist and right shoulder, and pull your partner forwards. In order to make the movement work, you will be compelled to use the connection of the centre to the right shoulder.

THE YANG TAIJI 24-STEP SHORT FORM

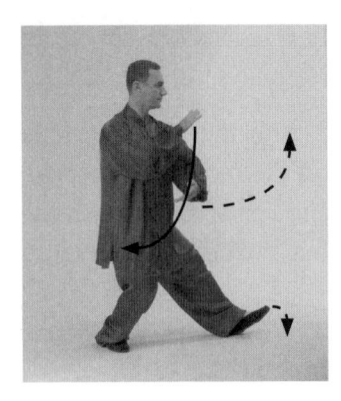

Brief 3
Step to 9.00 (the right side) with the left heel.

Details
Step to 9.00 with the left heel making sure that it is a shoulder's-width step. (See Chapter 11, 'The Process of Stepping'.) The body stays facing 10.30.
Extend the right arm towards 11.00/12.00.
Sink the left elbow.

Notes

- As in Parting the Wild Horse's Mane 1 (p.84).

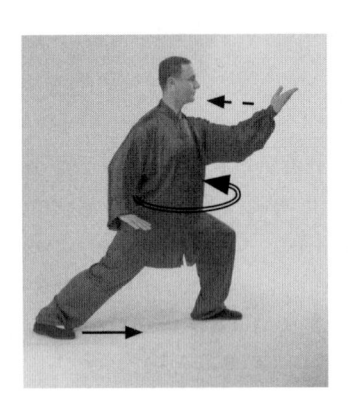

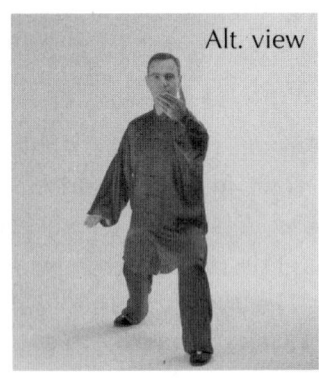

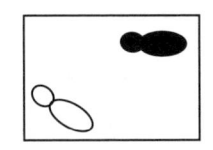

Brief 4
Left foot flat; weight forwards; left palm out to 9.00; push down right palm, slip rear heel.

Details
As you transfer the weight on to the left foot, turn the body and sweep the left hand out (with palm still facing up), moving it diagonally upwards from your right side to 9.00.

Push the right hand downwards so that the arm is almost straight.

As the weight moves on to the left foot, use the turn of the hips to slip the right heel. (For 'Slipping the rear heel' see p.64.)

The eyes look beyond the left hand to 9.00.

Notes

- As in Parting the Wild Horse's Mane 1 (p.85).

FORM 3: STORK (WHITE CRANE) SPREADS (FLASHES) ITS WINGS

白鶴亮翅 (Baíhè Liàngchì)

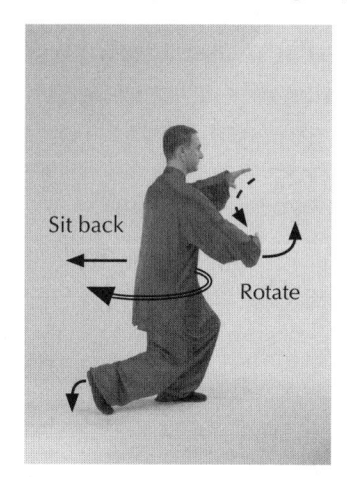

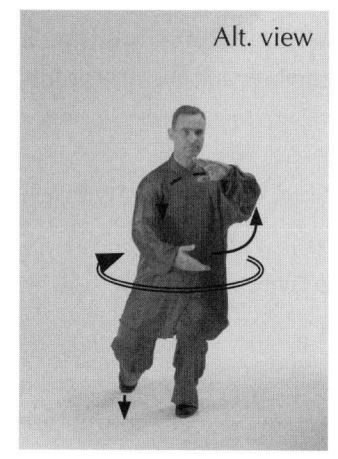

BRIEF 1
Weight forwards; turn left; back foot a half pace in; hold the ball.

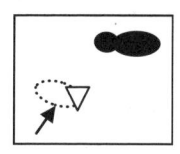

DETAILS

Start to turn the centre towards the left knee (i.e. towards 7.30); as the body turns, lift the right heel so that only the ball is touching the floor.

Simultaneously, start to bend your left elbow and turn your left palm down.

Your right palm starts to turn palm up (screwdriver turn of the hand).

Move the weight fully over the left foot and lift your right foot half a pace forwards towards 9.00. As the right foot arrives in its new position, both hands have completed turning over and the body has turned slightly to the 7.30 direction. The left hand will be in front of your upper chest, and the right hand will be approximately ahead of your right thigh.

The eyes look beyond the left hand.

Centre left.

NOTES

- **The turn of the body:** In the previous posture (Parting the Wild Horse's Mane 3) the pelvis is turned to the right at approximately 30°. When bringing in the rear foot, the right hip will move forwards so that the pelvis squares to 9.00. There is then a turn to the left from the waist upwards.

- **The right knee:** Avoid the right knee collapsing inwards towards the left knee when turning the body to the left and bringing the right foot forwards.
  (For those familiar with the Sun style of tàijí, this is not dissimilar to a Sun style following-step.)

- **The left hand:** As you move forwards, the left palm rotates (screwdriver turn) and the elbow bends so that the arm folds in front of your upper chest.

- **The right hand:**
  - Use the momentum of the turn of the body to move the right hand.
  - The hand moves below the left elbow, leading with the fingertips, but there should be an awareness of the upward direction that the fingertips are about to take.
  - Some practitioners keep the right fingertips leading up to outside the elbow or even to outside the upper arm during this movement.

- **'Closing':** This is a 'closing' move; feel the right shoulder closing towards the left hip.

- **The feeling of the movement:** The turn of the body is as though the back of your right shoulder were being pushed (from behind). You are turning the body and moving with the push – almost like shrugging your shoulder, but without lifting it.

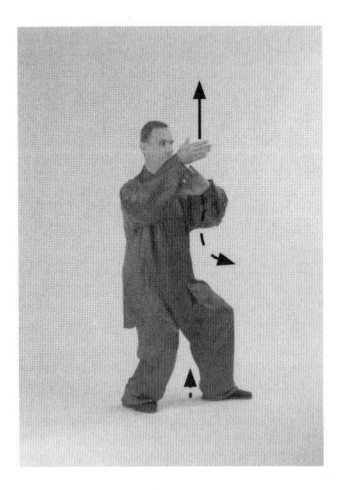

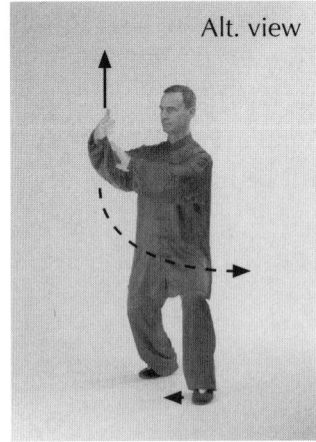

BRIEF 2
Sit back; turn right; fingertips towards the wrist crease.

DETAILS
Turn the centre/hips to the right diagonal (10.30) and sit back on to the right foot, pivoting the right foot on the ball of the foot so that it also turns to point at 10.30.

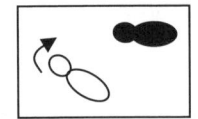

Simultaneously, start to raise the right fingers (see 'The right hand' below) and move the left palm downwards towards and then past the right wrist crease/forearm (see 'The hands' below). The two hands will pass each other approximately in front of the centreline of your body, which is facing the right diagonal.

The eyes look to the right.

Centre right.

Notes

- **The right foot:** Rather than turn the right toes to 10.30, beginners tend to turn them further to 12.00. This causes problems in Brief 3 where the hips need to be squared to 9.00.

- **The hands:** The simplest way for beginners to do this is to place the left fingertips on the right wrist, with the hands at chest/heart height, as you turn to face the right diagonal.

  In fact, from a timing point of view, by the time that the body has turned to the right, the arms will have bypassed each other.

  It is also unimportant whether the left fingertips have passed the wrist, forearm or elbow of the right arm.

  - **The right hand:** Use the momentum of the turn of the body to the right to move the right hand. If they haven't already begun to do so, the right fingertips lead up to outside the sinking left elbow or even to outside the upper arm during this movement. There should be an awareness of the upwards direction of the fingertips.

  - **The left hand:** Use the momentum of the turn of the body to the right to move the left hand. The left elbow is sinking, with a feeling of sinking towards the right hip.

- **The timing** in this transitional move can be difficult. There is a weight shift, a body rotation on the vertical axis, pelvic rotation (tucking under), and opposing directions of hand movement all simultaneously.

- **The 'feel' of this movement** needs to be combined with the previous brief (1) to understand it:

  - **Brief 1**: Partner pushes your shoulder from 12.00 (as discussed previously); roll with it, but then…

  - push off your left foot and 'roll' your shoulder back the other way against him.

The 'feel' is not one from the forearms therefore, but one from the body and back of right shoulder and upper right arm; you should feel as though the back of the right shoulder and upper right arm is exerting a backwards push and rotation.

- **Application:** Having said the above, there is an excellent application that uses the forearms and wrists, but the movement comes entirely from the centre!

- **The hips/centre:** As you sit on to the right foot, start to pull in the perineum and lower abdominals, releasing the small of the back, and tucking the pelvis under.

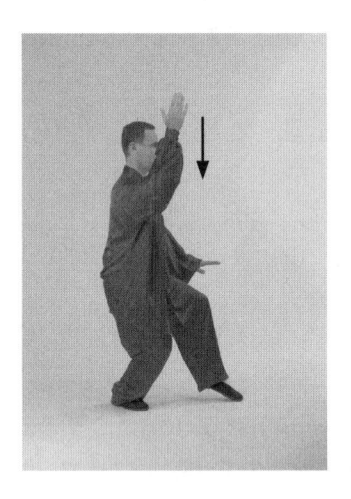

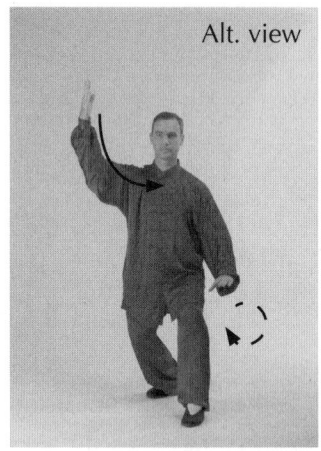

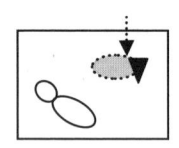

BRIEF 3
Square to 9.00; separate hands up and down; left toes into the centreline.

DETAILS
Turn the body to face 9.00. Direct the right fingertips upwards on your right side and the heel of the left palm downwards to your left side.

The palm of the right hand faces left towards 6.00 (see 'The right hand' on p.103), with the hand above your head. The arm should be angled upwards at approximately 45–50°.

The heel of the palm of the left hand pushes down on your left side at waist height; the fingers should be pointing towards 9.00.

As the arms arrive in position, move your left toes into the centreline, with a small amount of weight on them.

The eyes look to 9.00.

Centre back.

NOTES

- **The hips/pelvis:** As you arrive in the final posture, pull in the pelvic floor and the lower abdominals further, tucking the coccyx/tailbone under. Sit down into the right foot.

    The pelvis should be square to 9.00.

- **Posture:** The back should be relaxed and upright; release the neck. Beginners often tend to lean backwards.

- **The right shoulder** should be relaxed and soft.

- **The Bow of the Arms:** There should be a smooth arc from one hand, around the back and shoulders, and up to the other hand – the fingers of the right hand to the tip of the left little finger. Make sure therefore that the elbows don't protrude backwards by keeping the creases of both elbows very slightly ahead of the body. See also pp.347–8.

- **The left hand** should be close to the left thigh. It should feel as though it is pushing downwards, but there should still be a feeling of 'Péng' in the arm so there is a very slight bend in the elbow, and the little finger edge of the wrist crease (the hypothenar eminence – the ulnar side of the wrist crease) expands outwards slightly.

- **Direction of energy in the arms:** This movement has a downwards and upwards feel of the arms (but see 'The right hand' below).

- **The right hand:** When doing this movement, if your partner stands at 12.00 and gently pushes your right elbow as you raise it, he should feel not only an upwards movement, but also a slight bowing outwards movement (i.e. a slight 'Péng' of the upper arm).

    This is a 'diagonally upwards and forwards' movement with the fingertips leading.

- **The 'toes' in the centreline** at the end means that the ball of the left foot should be on the ground, but the heel is slightly raised off the floor – an Empty Stance. You can place about 10–20 per cent of weight on this foot.

- **Completion of the posture:**
    - Having arrived in Brief 3, sit down into it a little further sinking your qì.
    - Simultaneously push the heel of the left palm downwards, whilst pushing the right fingertips upwards.

- Without actually doing so, twist the right palm slightly further clockwise. This sounds like a contradiction but, if you do it, you'll feel the hypothenar edge of the hand extending outwards (as mentioned above).

- Simultaneously twist the left fingertips slightly inwards, without pushing the elbow outwards.

- It is at *this* point that you place a little more weight on to the toes (10–20%).

- **Point of interest re. the hand shapes:** If you look at the movements of the arms starting from the first movement to the last of Stork Spreads its Wings, you can see that the left arm draws a semi-circular clockwise line.

   The line of the right hand is more complex though; it creates a reverse 'S'.

   I have never been told whether this is intentional or not, but the combination of the left and right hands therefore shapes the Yin/Yang symbol, the right hand making the reverse 'S', and the left hand drawing the circle around it (almost!).

SECTION 2

(3 MOVEMENTS)

4. **Brush Knee and Twist (Side) Step on Both Sides (Brush Aside Over the Knee in Reverse Forwards Stance) (Left and Right)**
   左右搂膝拗步 (Zuǒyòu Lōuxī Àobù)

5. **Play the Pipa (Strum the Lute/Guitar)**
   手挥琵琶 (Shǒuhuī Pípā)

6. **Curve Back Arms on Both Sides (Repulse Monkey on Both Sides) (Step Back and Curl the Arms) (Left and Right)**
   左右倒卷肱 (Zuǒyòu Dàojuǎngōng)

FORM 4: BRUSH KNEE AND TWIST (SIDE) STEP ON BOTH SIDES (BRUSH ASIDE OVER THE KNEE IN REVERSE FORWARDS STANCE) (LEFT AND RIGHT)

左右搂膝拗步 (Zuǒyòu Lōuxī Àobùi)

BRIEF 1
Centre left; right palm twist and down centre.

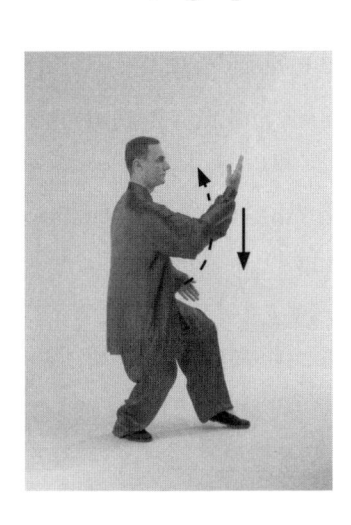

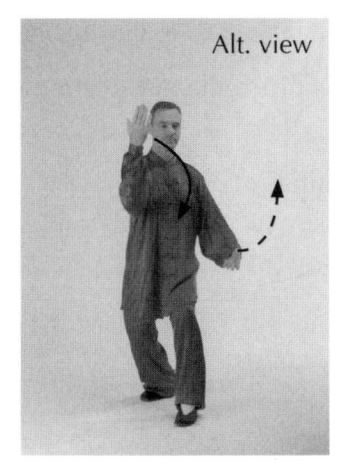

DETAILS
Close your right shoulder towards your left hip, simultaneously turning the right palm to face you. Because of the contraction of the centre, the right hand will move between your body and 9.00; start to lower the back of the right hand.

105

THE YANG TAIJI 24-STEP SHORT FORM

The left hand does a screwdriver turn, and the palm rotates to face upwards. As the right hand starts to lower, the fingers of the left hand extend out to 7.30 and the palm starts to rise.

The eyes continue to look to 9.00.

Centre left.

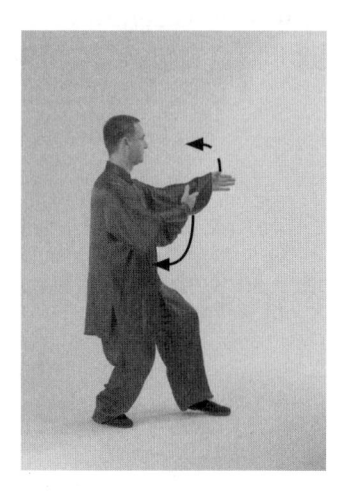

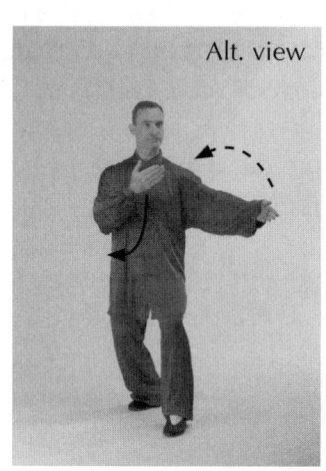

NOTES

- **The palms** turn at the same time because the elbows are rotating together (see next note). Twist the hands simultaneously.

- **'Closing'**: The drawing in of the centre initiates the inwards rotation of the elbows.

- **The right arm:**

  - The inwards movement of the right arm comes from the turn of the waist.

  - Keep the hips square to 9.00; only move the waist and above.

  - To initiate the right arm movement to the left side, sink the right elbow towards the left knee, simultaneously turning the palm further to face you. You can also think of this as closing the right shoulder to the left hip.

  - The feeling here is of the elbows rotating inwards and moving towards each other.

- **The right palm** will initially face you, and the back of the hand will then drop directly downwards between your body and 9.00 (with the palm upwards when down by your waist).

- **The left fingers** lead the movement of the left hand by extending out to the side, the palm simultaneously rising.

- **Yin and Yang of the arms:** When lowering the right arm and raising the left arm, feel the downwards and upwards movements of the arms working together like a seesaw.

- **The head** looks towards 9.00; avoid turning it to the left.

- **The weight:** Keep the majority of the weight on the right foot; beginners often shift the weight forwards on to the left foot at this point.

BRIEF 2
Left palm pushes across at mouth height from left to right; right hand (palm up) swings out to right side.

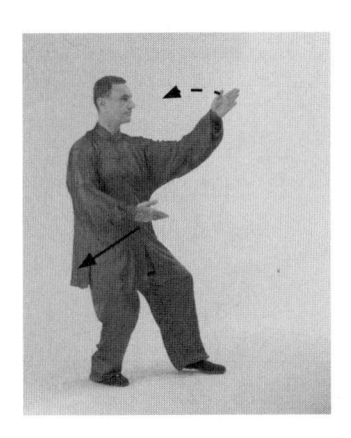

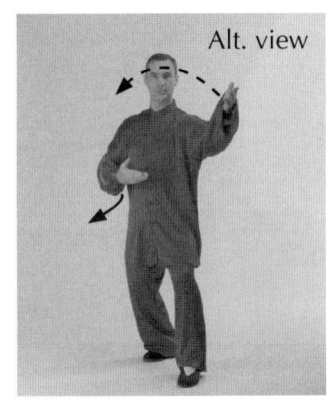

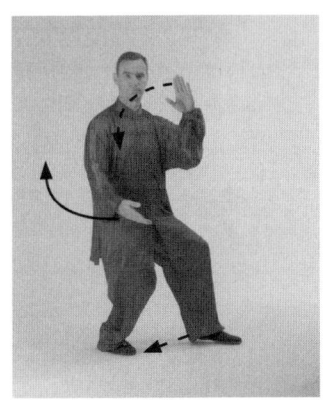

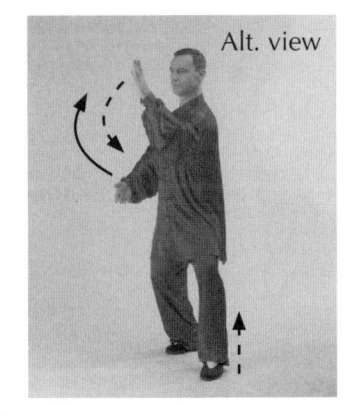

DETAILS
The left palm continues to rise and then pushes across your front (at mouth height between your body and 9.00) in the direction of your right side (with the palm facing to the right and with the left fingers pointing upwards).

The right hand continues to lower and swings out to your right side with the palm up.

The eyes look beyond the left hand (i.e. still to 9.00).

Centre right.

NOTES

- **The hips** begin to turn to the right during this part of the movement; feel the elbows and hips working together.

To get the feeling of the hips and elbows working together, try doing the above movements keeping your elbows as close as you can to your hips. Having felt this, you can lift your arms away from the hips, but continue to maintain the feeling of connection.

- **The turn of the centre** makes the arms move; beginners often circle the arms without involving the trunk.

  If you try the above exercise 'gluing' the elbows to the hips, you'll find that you have to move the body in order to get the arms into the correct position.

BRIEF 3

Right hand out to the side (palm up); left hand (palm down) in front of chest; left foot in.

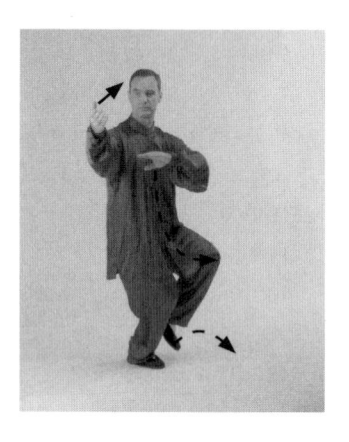

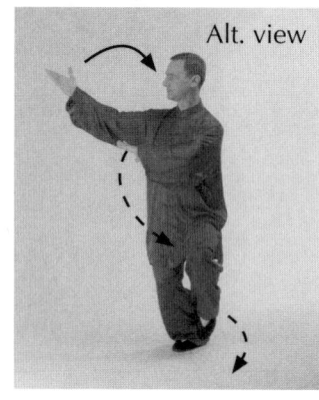

DETAILS

The left hand pushes down in front of your body with the palm turned down.

The right hand rises to your right side with the palm up.

As both hands arrive in position, free the left foot and draw it back towards the right foot.

The eyes look in the direction of the right hand.

Centre right.

NOTES

- **Turn the centreline** towards 10.30 or further, i.e. the line of your right foot.

- **The right hand:**

  - As you push the hand out to the side, be aware of the line of connection between right elbow and right hip.

- The movement of the right hand is led by the *fingertips*; it should feel as though you are extending the arm, not lifting the palm; the arm should extend well out to the side with the palm up.
- The right wrist will be approximately at the height of your right shoulder.

- **The left hand:**
  - As you push the hand down, lead the downwards movement of the arm/hand with the elbow, i.e. sink the elbow.
  - There should be feeling of pushing the hand down towards the right elbow crease.
  - Avoid squashing the arm against the body; there should still be a small space in the left armpit.
- **Yin and Yang of the arms:** When lowering the left arm and raising/extending the right arm, feel the downward and upward movements of the arms working together like a seesaw.

BRIEF 4
Fold right arm; left hand pushes down; keep the left foot relaxed; look to 9.00.

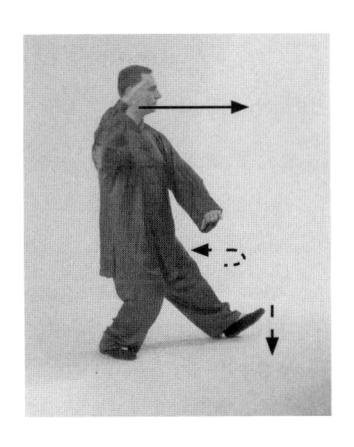

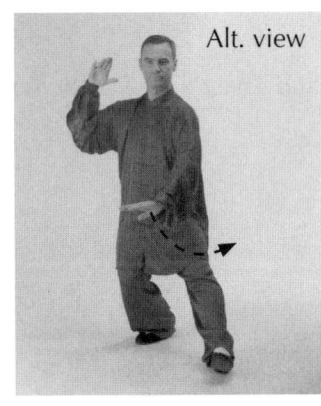

DETAILS
Dropping and bending your right elbow, fold your right arm so that your hand starts to move towards the centreline at approximately throat height; then start to turn your head to look towards 9.00.

The left hand pushes vertically down the body.
Keep your weight on the right foot, completely releasing the left ankle; be prepared to step to 9.00.
The head is starting to turn to look towards 9.00.
Centre is still facing the right side, but is starting to turn left.

NOTES

- **The feeling of 'closing':** Sink into your right foot and start 'closing' by tucking the coccyx under, and by closing the chest. There is a feeling of the elbows closing towards the knees (see also the following notes). There should be a feeling of the central 'spring' having been fully loaded.

- **Hollow the chest**, the shoulders relaxing.

- **The right arm:** When 'folding' the right arm, do so by sinking the elbow towards the right hip; this also helps to relax the shoulder. Be aware of the elbow/hip connection.

    The right wrist should be relaxed with the hand angled as though to push forwards with the fingertips – beginners tend to flex the wrist so that the fingers are vertical.

    The right shoulder should remain relaxed and sunk.

- **The left hand** continues to push downwards towards the right hip, but be aware of the connection between left elbow and left knee.

- **The left ankle** should be relaxed so that it 'hangs'; don't place it yet and keep the right hip relaxed and free.

BRIEF 5

Step to 9.00; Brush Knee and Twist Step 1 with the right hand pushing.

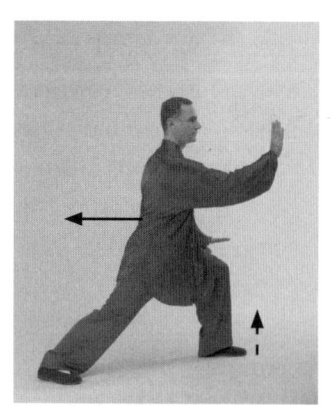

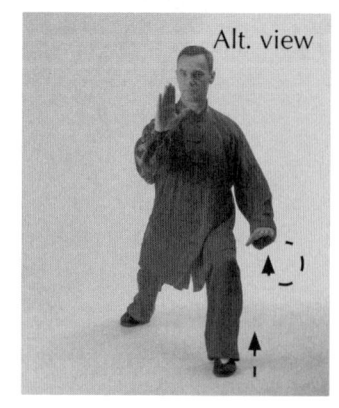

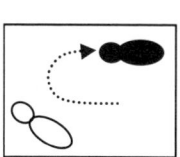

DETAILS

Place the left foot at 9.00 in a wide stance, and transfer the weight from the right foot into a left Bow Stance.

At the same time the left hand, following the turn of the body from right to left, circles from the centreline of the body to the left side of the thigh with palm down, to finish with fingers pointing ahead to 9.00.

Simultaneously, the right hand pushes to 9.00, the fingers initially leading and the heel of the palm pushing forwards as the arm extends.

The eyes look to 9.00.

Centre forwards.

NOTES

- **The stance** should be a wide one, so it is important to step about 12 inches (30 cm) wide – a shoulder-width stance.

- **The push:**
  - It is the *fingertips* of the right hand that lead in the push initially, and only when the arm is getting near to its extension does the heel of the hand actually push (i.e. the fingers lift).
  - Keep the wrist soft throughout until the end.
  - At the end of the movement, it is the little finger side of the heel of the right hand (the hypothenar eminence) that does the push.

- **The right elbow** should sink when pushing; beginners often lift it outwards.

- **The left hand movement:**
  - This is one of pushing *down* and moving around to the left side; use the turn of the body to achieve this.
  - Feel the connection of the left wrist to the stepping left ankle.
  - Feel the connection of the left elbow and left hip working together in the turn.
  - The energy of the 'sweep' around the front of the left knee ('brush knee' without actually doing so) is focused in the side of the left wrist (the hypothenar eminence). There should be a feeling of the skin stretching on the outside edge of the little finger, hand and wrist. The Chinese describe this as a feeling of the stretching of the cloth of an umbrella when it is opened.

- **The fingertips of the left hand** finish level with the front knee, with the palm facing the floor. Some practitioners like to finish with the fingers further forwards than the knee.

- **Final posture:**

  - **The centreline** is either straight to 9.00 or turned towards 8.30 – a very slight twist towards the left knee. It is important not to overdo this.

  - **The right index finger** finishes at the height of, and ahead of, the tip of the nose; this is achieved by the slight turn of the centre to 8.30 (but see 'Variation' immediately below).

    In other words, when the body is square to 9.00, the index finger should be slightly to the right of the centreline of the body, ahead of the side of your right cheek, and it is the turn of the centre that brings it in line with the tip of the nose.

  - **Variation:** Not all practitioners agree with this turn to 8.30; some say that the centreline should be square to 9.00, and therefore the index finger will complete the movement to the right of the centreline of the body. (As with all of these slight differences, it usually depends upon the application of the movement.)

- **'Primary' and 'secondary' hands:** Although it appears that the push is the main objective of the movement, and although both hands actually move together with the turn of the body, in a way the 'primary' hand is the left hand.

  By this I mean that, although both hands move simultaneously with the turn of the body, the left hand will *appear* to be moving first. A good way to get the feel of this is to try moving out of the previous movement (Brief 4) and do nothing with the arms other than to allow the elbows to move with the hips. It becomes clear that the arms actually do very little – you almost have to only 'extend' them slightly throughout movement (Brief 5).

- **The 'feeling' of the final movement in the arms:**

  - Both hands finish by pushing with the heels of the hands, the left hand downwards, and the right hand away from you. There should be a feel of stretch from one hand to the other across the shoulders (see 'Bow of the Arms', pp.347–8).

  - From a different perspective: As the right palm pushes away, feel as though you are gently pushing the upper thoracic vertebrae (i.e. from between the shoulder blades and upwards to the height of the shoulders) backwards. In other words, create 'Péng' in the arm.

    At the same time, let the neck lengthen as you push.

- **Relax the waist and the hips** allowing the buttocks to sink – in particular the right hip.

- **Posture:** The body should be upright at the end of the movement.

Moving into Brush Knee and Twist Step 2

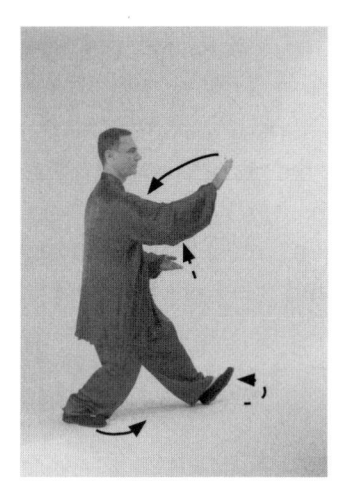

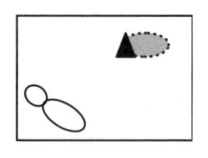

BRIEF 1
Sit back; turn left palm upwards.

DETAILS
Sit back on to your right foot, turning your centreline (but *not* your pelvis) to the left diagonal (7.30).

The left heel doesn't move but lift the left toes without turning them yet.

Simultaneously, release and soften both wrists. Allow the right elbow to soften and 'close' (i.e. sink it towards your left knee), the palm will turn to face left.

Because you've released the left wrist, the left fingers point downwards and you then turn the left palm upwards using a screwdriver turn of the hand. There will be a feeling of the left elbow rotating inwards.

Centre left and back.

NOTES

- **Turning the waist:** The hips do *not* turn, but the waist/torso *does*. Close the centre by bringing the right shoulder towards the left hip (see also next note).

- **'Closing' the chest:** Feel as though the elbows are compressing together.

- **Tuck under as you sit back:** As you sit back on to the right foot, bend the knee, and allow the tailbone to tuck under slightly, allowing the spine to stay straight or even slightly rounded. Beginners often incorrectly stand up slightly at this point.

- **The right hand:** Continue the feeling of pushing with the right hand as you sit back, but start to sink the right elbow and slightly lift the hand. You'll feel the right shoulder softening as you do so.

THE YANG TAIJI 24-STEP SHORT FORM

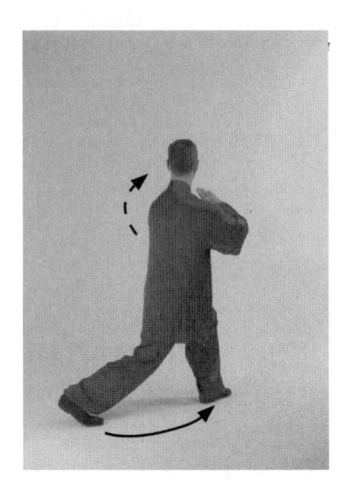

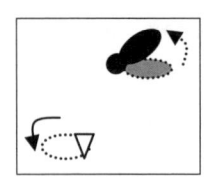

BRIEF 2
Pelvis left; weight forwards.

DETAILS

Push off your right foot and simultaneously turn your hips and your left toes to the left diagonal (7.30). Lift your rear heel.

The elbows follow the turn of the hips.

Because of the turn of the body, your arms also start to move leftwards.

Continue the feeling of the elbows moving together; start to lift the left palm out to the side; keep sinking the right arm/elbow.

The eyes look left with the turn of the body.

Centre left.

NOTES

- **Turning the body left:** Balance can be an issue here. Think of either turning your centreline towards your left knee, or think of bringing your right shoulder towards your left hip as you move forwards.

- **The left foot:** Having turned the left foot out to a minimum of 45°, place it at this angle (or turn it out even further as you move the weight on to it). Beginners often turn it back to point at 9.00 again.

  The angle of the left foot: The minimum amount to turn the foot out by is 45°, but more is quite acceptable, and in fact has the advantage of making you turn the body more.

- **The left elbow** should move with the left hip.

- **The right elbow:** There's a feeling of starting to sink the right elbow towards the left knee.

- **The fingertips of the left hand** lead outwards.

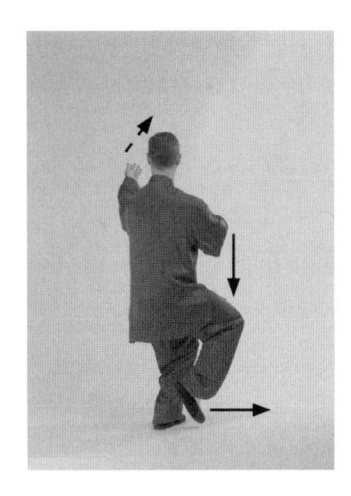

Brief 3

Left arm out; draw the right foot in.

Details

As you start to transfer your weight fully on to your left foot, the left hand (with the fingertips leading) moves out to your left side (approximately 6.00, but it depends upon how much you have turned the left foot) with the palm up.

The right hand pushes towards your left elbow (with the palm facing down).

As both hands arrive in position, draw in your right foot with toes just off the ground.

The eyes look in the direction of the left hand.
Centre left.

Notes

- **Turn the centreline** towards 7.30 or further, i.e. the line of your left foot.

- **The left hand:**

  - **Connections:** As you push the hand out to the side, be aware of the connection of left elbow to left hip.

  - **The movement of the left hand** is led by the *fingertips*; it should feel as though you are extending the arm, not lifting the palm; the arm should extend well out to the side with the palm up.

  - **The left wrist** will be approximately at the height of your left shoulder.

- **The right hand:**

  - As you push the hand down, lead the downwards movement of the arm/hand with the elbow, i.e. sink the elbow.

  - There should be feeling of pushing the hand down towards the left elbow crease.

  - Avoid squashing the arm against the body; there should still be a small space in the right armpit.

THE YANG TAIJI 24-STEP SHORT FORM

- **Yin and Yang of the arms:** When lowering the right arm and raising/extending the left arm, feel the downwards and upwards movements of the arms working together like a seesaw.

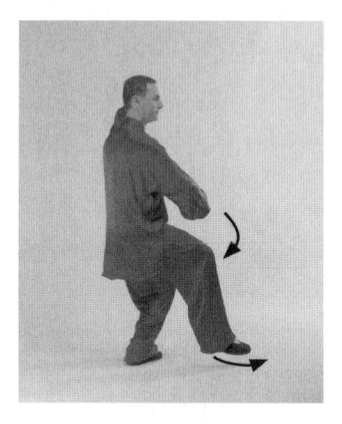

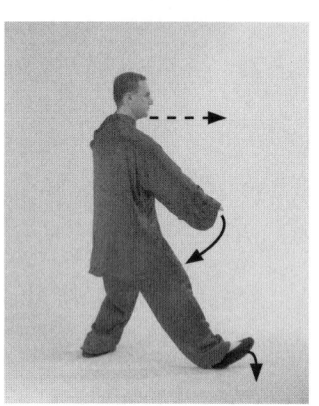

Brief 4

Fold left arm; right hand pushes down; keep the right foot relaxed; look to 9.00.

Details

Dropping and bending your left elbow, fold your left arm so that your hand starts to move towards the centreline at approximately throat height; then start to turn your head to look towards 9.00.

The right hand pushes vertically down the body.

Keep your weight on the left foot completely releasing the right ankle; be prepared to step to 9.00.

The head is starting to turn to look towards 9.00.

Centre is still facing the left side, but is starting to turn right.

Notes

- **The feeling of 'closing':** Sink into your left foot and start 'closing' by tucking the coccyx under, and by closing the chest. There is a feeling of the elbows closing towards the knees (also see 'The left arm' and 'The right hand' notes below). There should be a feeling of the central 'spring' having been fully loaded.

- **Hollow the chest**, the shoulders relaxing.

- **The left arm:** When 'folding' the left arm, do so by sinking the elbow towards the left hip; this also helps to relax the shoulder. Be aware of the elbow/hip connection.

The left wrist should be relaxed with the hand angled as though to push forwards with the fingertips – beginners tend to flex the wrist so that the fingers are vertical.

The left shoulder should remain relaxed and sunk.

- **The right hand** continues to push downwards towards the left hip, but be aware of the connection between right elbow and right knee.

- **The right ankle** should be relaxed so that it 'hangs'; don't place it yet and keep the left hip relaxed and free.

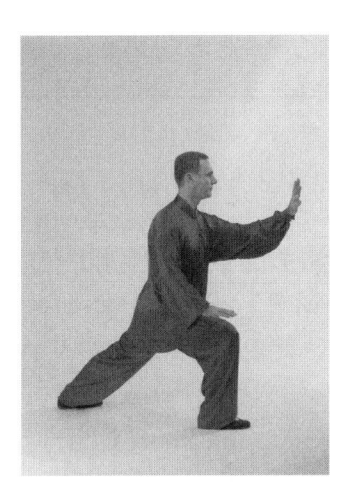

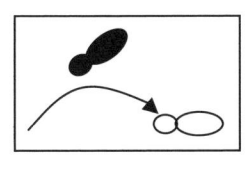

BRIEF 5
Step to 9.00; Brush Knee and Twist Step 2 with the left hand pushing.

DETAILS
Place the right foot at 9.00 in a wide stance, and transfer the weight from the left foot into a right Bow Stance.

At the same time, the right hand, following the turn of the body from left to right, circles from the centreline of the body to the right side of the thigh with palm down, to finish with fingers pointing ahead to 9.00.

Simultaneously, the left hand pushes to 9.00, the fingers initially leading and the heel of the palm pushing forwards as the arm extends.

The eyes look to 9.00.

Centre forwards.

NOTES

- **The stance** should be a wide one, so it is important to step about 12 inches (30 cm) wide – a shoulder-width stance.

- **The push:**
  - It is the *fingertips* of the left hand that lead in the push initially, and only when the arm is getting near to its extension does the heel of the hand actually push (i.e. the fingers lift).
  - Keep the wrist soft throughout until the end.

- At the end of the movement, it is the little finger side of the heel of the left hand (the hypothenar eminence) that does the push.
- **The left elbow** should sink when pushing; beginners often lift it outwards.
- **The right hand movement:**
  - This is one of pushing *down* and moving around to the right side; use the turn of the body to achieve this.
  - Feel the connection of the right wrist to the stepping right ankle.
  - Feel the connection of the right elbow and right hip working together in the turn.
  - The energy of the 'sweep' around the front of the right knee ('brush knee' without actually doing so) is focused in the side of the right wrist (the hypothenar eminence). There should be a feeling of the skin stretching on the outside edge of the little finger, hand and wrist. The Chinese describe this as a feeling of the stretching of the cloth of an umbrella when it is opened.
- **The fingertips of the right hand** finish level with the front knee, with the palm facing the floor. Some practitioners like to finish with the fingers further forwards than the knee.
- **Final posture:**
  - **The centreline** is either straight to 9.00 or turned towards 9.30 – a very slight twist towards the right knee. It is important not to overdo this.
  - **The left index finger** finishes at the height of, and ahead of, the tip of the nose; this is achieved by the slight turn of the centre to 9.30 (but see 'Variation' immediately below).

    In other words, when the body is square to 9.00, the index finger should be slightly to the left of the centreline of the body, ahead of the side of your left cheek, and it is the turn of the centre that brings it in line with the tip of the nose.
  - **Variation:** Not all practitioners agree with this turn to 9.30; some say that the centreline should be square to 9.00, and therefore the index finger will complete the movement to the left of the centreline of the body. (As with all of these slight differences, it usually depends upon the application of the movement.)

- **'Primary' and 'secondary' hands:** Although it appears that the push is the main objective of the movement, and although both hands actually move together with the turn of the body, in a way the 'primary' hand is the right hand.

  By this I mean that, although both hands move simultaneously with the turn of the body, the right hand will *appear* to be moving first. A good way to get the feel of this is to try moving out of the previous movement (Brief 4) and do nothing with the arms other than to allow the elbows to move with the hips. It becomes clear that the arms actually do very little – you almost have to only 'extend' them slightly throughout movement (Brief 5).

- **The 'feeling' of the final movement in the arms:**
  - Both hands finish by pushing with the heels of the hands, the right hand downwards, and the left hand away from you. There should be a feel of stretch from one hand to the other across the shoulders (see 'Bow of the Arms', pp.347–8).
  - From a different perspective: As the left palm pushes away, feel as though you are gently pushing the upper thoracic vertebrae (i.e. from between the shoulder blades and upwards to the height of the shoulders) backwards. In other words, create 'Péng' in the arm.

    At the same time, let the neck lengthen as you push.

- **Relax the waist and the hips** allowing the buttocks to sink – in particular the left hip.

- **Posture:** The body should be upright at the end of the movement.

Moving into Brush Knee and Twist Step 3

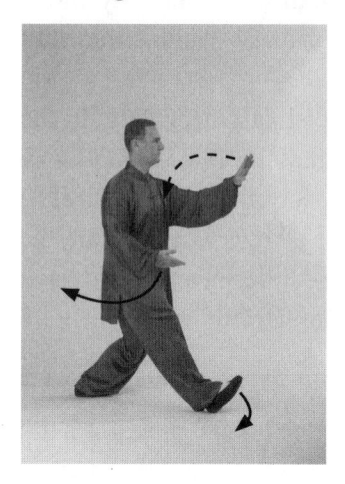

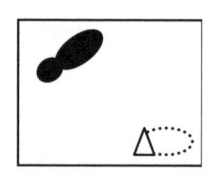

BRIEF 1
Sit back; turn right palm upwards.

DETAILS

Sit back on to your left foot, turning your centreline (but *not* your pelvis) to the right diagonal (7.30).

The right heel doesn't move but lift the right toes without turning them yet.

Simultaneously, release and soften both wrists. Allow the left elbow to soften and 'close' (i.e. sink it towards your right knee), the palm will turn to face right.

Because you've released the right wrist, the right fingers point downwards and you then turn the right palm upwards using a screwdriver turn of the hand. There will be a feeling of the right elbow rotating inwards.

Centre right and back.

NOTES

- **Turning the waist:** The hips do *not* turn, but the waist/torso *does*. Close the centre by bringing the left shoulder towards the right hip (see also next note).

- **'Closing' the chest:** Feel as though the elbows are compressing together.

- **Tuck under as you sit back:** As you sit back on to the left foot, bend the knee, and allow the tailbone to tuck under slightly, allowing the spine to stay straight or even slightly rounded. Beginners often incorrectly stand up slightly at this point.

- **The left hand:** Continue the feeling of pushing with the left hand as you sit back, but start to sink the left elbow and slightly lift the hand. You'll feel the left shoulder softening as you do so.

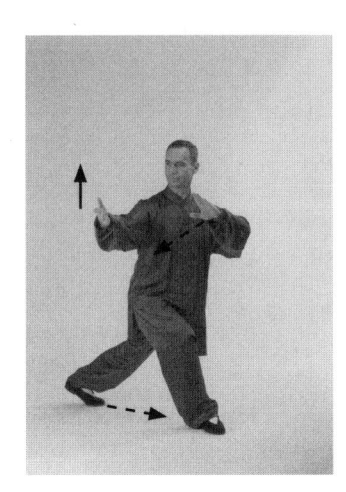

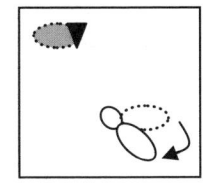

DESCRIPTION OF THE YANG TÀIJÍ 24-STEP SHORT FORM

BRIEF 2
Pelvis right; weight forwards.

DETAILS

Push off your left foot and simultaneously turn your hips and your right toes to the right diagonal (7.30). Lift your rear heel.

The elbows follow the turn of the hips.

Because of the turn of the body, your arms start to move to the right also.

Continue the feeling of the elbows moving together; start to lift the right palm out to the side; keep sinking the left arm/elbow.

The eyes look left with the turn of the body.

Centre right.

NOTES

- **Turning the body right:** Balance can be an issue here. Think of either turning your centreline towards your right knee, or think of bringing your left shoulder towards your right hip as you move forwards.

- **The right foot:** Having turned the right foot out to a minimum of 45°, place it at this angle (or turn it out even further as you move the weight on to it). Beginners often turn it back to point at 9.00 again.

  The angle of the right foot: The minimum amount to turn the foot out by is 45°, but more is quite acceptable, and in fact has the advantage of making you turn the body more.

- **The right elbow** should move with the right hip.

- **The left elbow:** There's a feeling of starting to sink the left elbow towards the right knee.

- **The fingertips of the right hand** lead outwards.

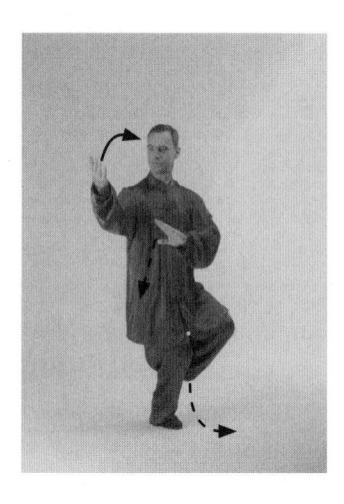

Brief 3
Right arm out; draw the left foot in.

Details
As you start to transfer your weight fully on to your right foot, the right hand (with the fingertips leading) moves out to your right side (approximately 6.00, but it depends upon how much you have turned the right foot) with the palm up.

The left hand pushes towards your right elbow (with the palm facing down).

As both hands arrive in position, draw in your left foot with the toes just off the ground.

The eyes look in the direction of the right hand.

Centre right.

Notes

- **Turn the centreline** towards 10.30 or further, i.e. the line of your right foot.

- **The right hand:**

  - **Connections:** As you push the hand out to the side, be aware of the connection of right elbow to right hip.

  - **The movement of the right hand** is led by the *fingertips*; it should feel as though you are extending the arm, not lifting the palm; the arm should extend well out to the side with the palm up.

  - **The right wrist** will be approximately at the height of your right shoulder.

- **The left hand:**

  - As you push the hand down, lead the downwards movement of the arm/hand with the elbow, i.e. sink the elbow.

  - There should be feeling of pushing the hand down towards the right elbow crease.

  - Avoid squashing the arm against the body; there should still be a small space in the left armpit.

- **Yin and Yang of the arms:** When lowering the left arm and raising/extending the right arm, feel the downwards and upwards movements of the arms working together like a seesaw.

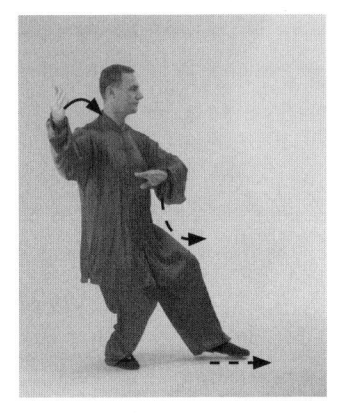

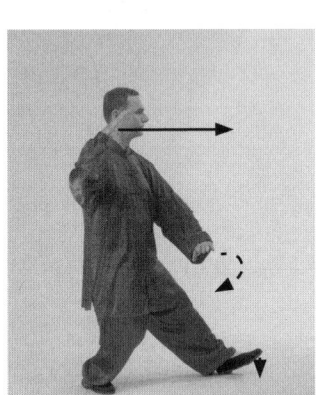

Brief 4

Fold right arm; left hand pushes down; keep the left foot relaxed; look to 9.00.

Details

Dropping and bending your right elbow, fold your right arm so that your hand starts to move towards the centreline at approximately throat height; then start to turn your head to look towards 9.00.

The left hand pushes vertically down the body.

Keep your weight on the right foot completely releasing the left ankle; be prepared to step to 9.00.

The head is starting to turn to look towards 9.00.

Centre is still facing the right side, but is starting to turn left.

Notes

- As in Brush Knee and Twist Step 1 (p.110).

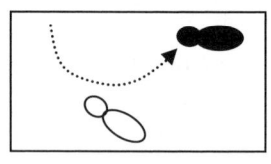

THE YANG TAIJI 24-STEP SHORT FORM

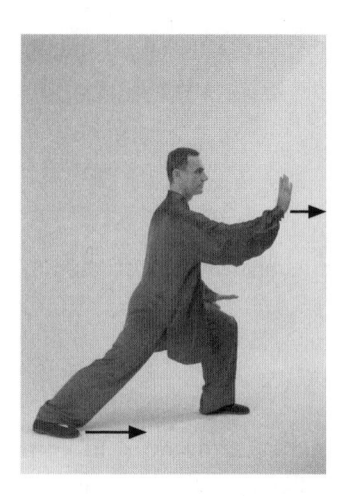

BRIEF 5
Step to 9.00; Brush Knee and Twist Step 3 with the right hand pushing.

DETAILS
Place the left foot at 9.00 in a wide stance, and transfer the weight from the right foot into a left Bow Stance.

At the same time, the left hand, following the turn of the body from right to left, circles from the centreline of the body to the left side with palm down, to finish with fingers pointing ahead to 9.00.

Simultaneously, the right hand pushes to 9.00, the fingers initially leading and the heel of the palm pushing forwards as the arm extends.

The eyes look to 9.00.

Centre forwards.

NOTES

- As in Brush Knee and Twist Step 1 (p.111).

FORM 5: PLAY THE PIPA (STRUM THE LUTE/GUITAR)

手挥琵琶 (Shǒuhuī Pípā)

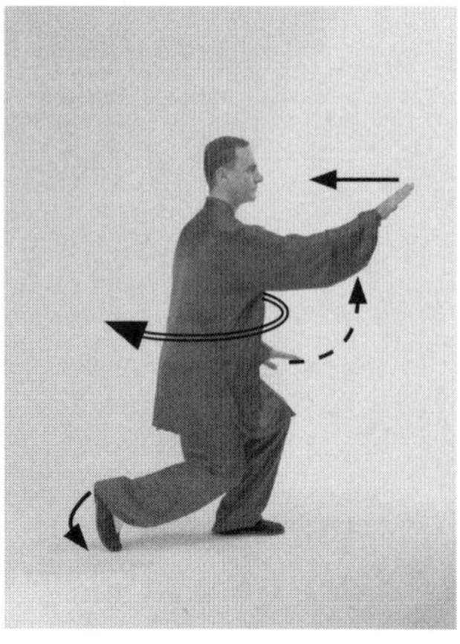

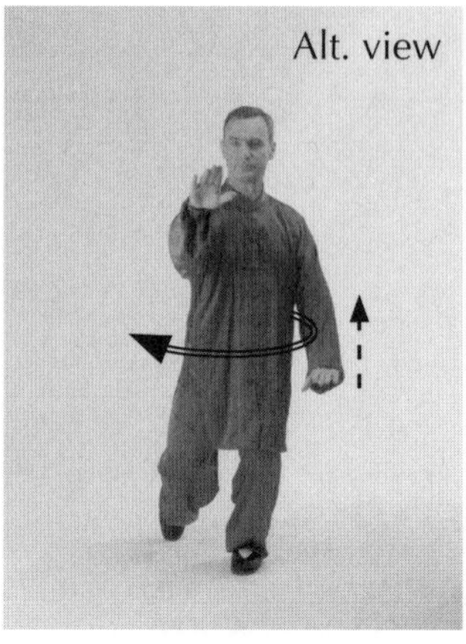

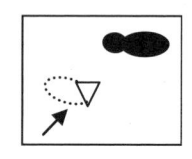

BRIEF 1
Back foot half a pace forwards.

DETAILS

Gently pushing the right palm forwards and relaxing the wrist, move the weight fully on to the front foot, bringing the right foot half a step forwards.

The eyes continue to look to 9.00.

Centre left.

NOTES

- **Method of moving the weight forwards:**

  - **Push with palms and rear foot:** In order to move the weight over the left foot and bring the right foot forwards, push the left palm gently downwards at the same time as pushing with the right hand. This is therefore a three-way push – both palms and also the ball of the rear foot. (See also 'Addendum to the push (the right hand)' below.)

  - **Left foot:** As you move forwards, press the left foot into the ground, feeling the weight sinking into it.

  - **Transfer of weight:** When bringing the rear foot forwards, avoid 'jumping' off the back foot. Be conscious of the weight transferring fully on to the left foot as the rear foot 'unpeels' from the ground; the rear foot should then be free and can be lifted and placed to complete the movement.

- **Addendum to the push (the right hand):** As in all connection moves it is important to be aware of the direction of energy of the previous movement and to make use of it in the movement that follows.

  The previous movement was the actual 'push' of Brush Knee and Twist Step, so all that you are doing at the start of this move is to continue the forwards energy of the right hand.

  At the end of the continued push, as the forwards momentum 'runs out', relax the right wrist so that the palm faces the floor.

- **The step:** There is a feel here of a Sun style forwards step. The right foot moves forwards to about one foot-length's distance behind and to the right of the left foot.

- **Yin and Yang:** Notice the working of opposites – the right hand pushing forwards, and the right foot pushing backwards into the ground.

- **'Closing':** This is a 'closing' movement.

THE YANG TAIJÍ 24-STEP SHORT FORM

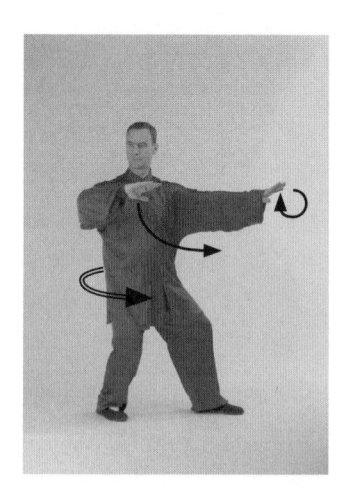

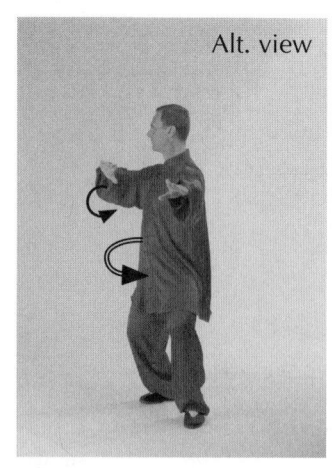

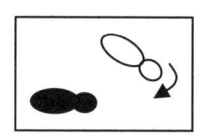

BRIEF 2
Sit back; change hands (left arm up; right arm back).

DETAILS
Sit back on to the right foot turning your centreline to the right diagonal (10.30). As you do so, pivot the right foot on the ball of the foot, placing it so that the toes point to 10.30.

As you turn your body to the right, bend the right arm at the elbow, releasing the right wrist so that the palm faces downwards; by the time that you have put your weight on to the right foot, the right hand will be approximately opposite your sternum.

The left hand lifts with palm down and arm pointing towards 9.00.
The eyes can look either to 9.00 or towards 10.30.
Centre right.

NOTES

- **The right arm** is often a problem for beginners. It *looks* as though the arm pulls backwards, but in fact, relative to the body, the wrist stays in exactly the same place, i.e. opposite the sternum (breastbone). The appearance of movement is caused by turning the body to the right and just bending the right elbow.

  The right hand shouldn't be held too close to the body, there should be slightly more than 90° at the elbow joint.

- **Variations:** Minor variations for the right hand are:
  1. Palm facing the floor.
  2. Rotation of the right palm to face outwards, i.e. thumb downwards and palm facing away from the body slightly.

- **Coordination of the joints in the turn:**
  - Coordinate the turning of the *hips* with the movements of both *elbows*.
  - Coordinate the left elbow with the left knee, and the right elbow with the right knee.
- **The left leg:** Avoid the left leg 'collapsing' inwards as you turn to the right; this is an 'opening' move for the legs.

  The left foot can either remain flat or the heel can begin to lift.
- **The left arm** can circle out slightly to the left as it lifts.

  The left wrist and arm, when arriving with the arm parallel to the ground, are completely relaxed.
- **Posture:** Keep the body upright; beginners tend to lean the body backwards in this movement as a result of not relaxing the small of the back and tucking under (see following note).
- **Relax the hips** as you sit backwards; start to pull in the pelvic floor and the lower abdominal muscles, whilst tucking the tailbone/coccyx under.
- **'Opening':** This is an 'opening' movement.

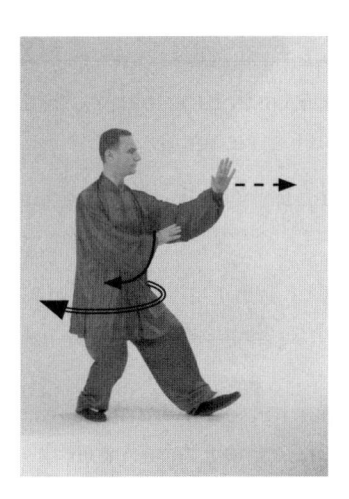

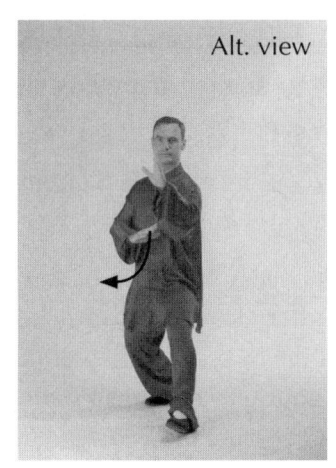

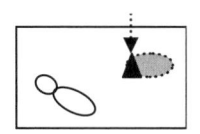

Alt. view

BRIEF 3
Rotate arms with palms inwards; place heel.

DETAILS
Turn the centreline back towards 10.00.

As you do so, lower the elbows so that the left and right palms rotate to face inwards (thumb-sides up), so that the left palm faces to the right, and the right palm faces to the left.

Lift the left foot and move it into the centreline with the toes raised and the knee slightly bent.

The eyes look to 9.00.

Centre back.

NOTES

- **The left wrist** is at shoulder-height.

- **The positioning of the hands:** There is some scope for variation here. The 'textbook' version is that the right palm is approximately opposite the left elbow crease, and the fingers of the right hand point at the right wrist. A triangle is therefore formed (left elbow to right palm to left wrist).

    It is not unusual to see the right hand in a variety of different positions though, either below or above the level of the left elbow. It is not important so long as the 'feel' of the movement is retained (see note below).

- **The distance between the hands** (as looked at from 9.00 down the 'channel' of the arms) is the width of an adult arm.

- **The left arm** shouldn't be over-extended; the left elbow is bent to approximately 135°.

- **Sink the shoulders** and very slightly hyper-extend them, thereby connecting the shoulders to the elbows (the 'Bow of the Arms'; see pp.347–8).

- **The 'feel' of the movement** is of locking or breaking an opponent's arm between your hands – your left hand on the opponent's right elbow, and your right hand on his right wrist. It is therefore a feeling of squeezing the limb between your arms (see 'The distance between the hands' above). The squeezing is achieved by sinking the elbows, compressing the palms, and 'closing' from the centre, *not* by pushing your elbows together.

- **Body angle:** The body will finish with the centreline turned slightly to your right (9.30/10.00).

- **Body posture:** The back should either be upright or leaning very slightly forwards; beginners often lean backwards on this position because of tightening the small of the back.

    Pull in the pelvic floor and the lower abdominal muscles, and tuck the tailbone/coccyx under; raise the crown of the head, releasing the back of the neck.

- **'Closing':** This is a 'closed' movement.

FORM 6: CURVE BACK ARMS ON BOTH SIDES (REPULSE MONKEY ON BOTH SIDES) (STEP BACK AND CURL THE ARMS) (LEFT AND RIGHT)

左右倒卷肱 (Zuǒyòu Dàojuǎngōng)

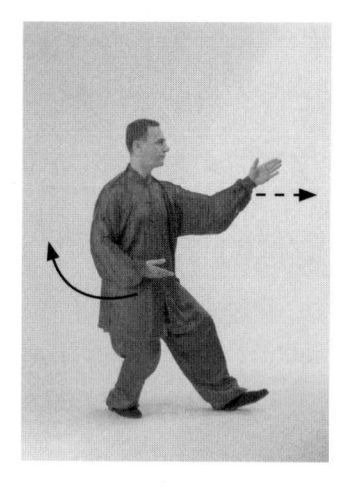

BRIEF 1
Turn body to the right, and open the arms, turning the palms up; look right.

DETAILS
Turn your hips to the right, simultaneously circling your right hand out sideways. Then continue to raise it in an arc to approximately 1.00 with the right palm up.

Extend the left arm towards 9.00 turning the palm upwards.

The arms are opened to about 120°.

The eyes look towards your right hand initially, but then turn back to look towards the left hand.

Centre right.

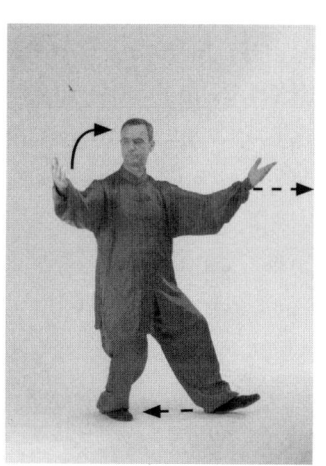

NOTES

- **Method of the right arm movement:**
  1. Moving from Play the Pipa, turn the hips and let the right forearm move outwards towards 1.00 keeping it approximately parallel to the ground, and the palm turning upwards. The left thigh will finish approximately between the two opened arms.

2. At this stage, there is a feeling of almost a pivotal point between the right hip and the right elbow (but see below also).

3. Then, leading the movement with the fingertips, push the right arm out to approximately 1.00 extending it so that the hand reaches shoulder-height.

4. **Coordination with the hips:** The right arm movement should be coordinated with the turn of the hips/centre to the right, i.e. make sure

that the right elbow coordinates with the right hip. There is therefore a sense of the turning hip controlling the movement of the elbow.

5. The shoulder should not feel as though the arm is opening to *behind* you.
Beginners often pull the arm back to 3.00 (behind the line of the shoulders), thereby lifting the right shoulder-blade, and possibly the right shoulder itself.

- **Coordination of the left arm:** The left arm turns palm upwards. Extend the arm; there is a feeling of extending your fingertips to 9.00 with the turn of the waist to the right.
  Work the left hips with the left elbow, i.e. the hip rotates 'forwards' and takes the elbow with it.

- **Coordination of the elbows/arm rotation:** Feel the inwards (downwards) rotation of both elbows working together.

- **Coordinate the elbows and the knees:** They should feel connected, as though they are working together.

- **The knees spiral** outwards as you open the arms.

- **'Opening':** This is an 'open' movement, but note that, as the arms lift, the elbows are starting to rotate downwards and inwards (feel the rotation of the elbows working together – see above); the body is therefore in the process of preparing to 'close', whilst the legs are in the process of 'opening' (see the note directly above).

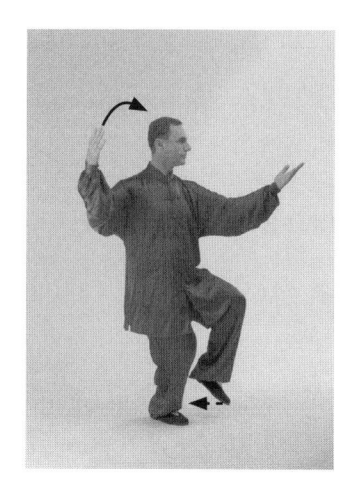

DESCRIPTION OF THE YANG TÀIJÍ 24-STEP SHORT FORM

BRIEF 2
Fold arm; foot in.

DETAILS
Sinking your right elbow, fold it so that the right hand moves towards the midline of the body at about throat height.
　　Draw your left foot back towards the right foot.
　　Your left hand (palm up) starts to move back with the turn of the hips.
　　Your eyes continue to look towards 9.00.
　　Centre right.

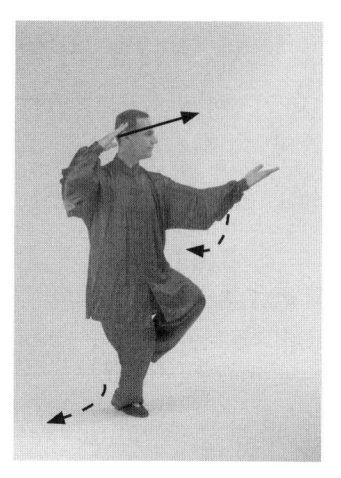

NOTES

- **'Curling' the arm:** Dropping the right elbow towards the right hip will also help to relax the right shoulder. It will also help the right arm to move correctly with the turn of the body.
　　Think of folding the right hand towards the centreline.

- **The left arm:** Leave the left arm still pointing to 9.00, but relax the arm so that the elbow sinks and rotates downwards.

- **Angle of body:** The centre is still turned to the right as you both fold the right arm and bring the left foot back. However, because the foot is moving backwards, the hips will begin to rotate back to the left; the body is therefore in the process of starting the turn to the left.

- **Coordination:** Work the right knee, right hip and right elbow together.

- **Sink further into the right foot** as the right elbow folds.

- **The left foot:** It is the turn of the hips that begin to rotate to the left side that causes the left foot to draw in.

- **'Closing':** The body is now in the process of 'closing'.

THE YANG TAIJI 24-STEP SHORT FORM

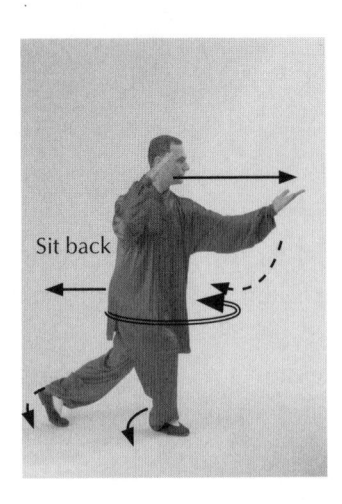

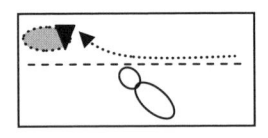

BRIEF 3
Foot behind; no weight on it.

DETAILS
Place the left toes behind you to 3.00; there should be no weight on them.

The eyes look to 9.00.

Centre still right but starting to turn back to 9.00.

NOTES

- **Placing the foot behind:** The weight should stay on the front foot; beginners often make the mistake of shifting it on to the rear foot at this stage.

- **Stepping:** Use the turn of the hips to place the left foot, *simultaneously sinking* as you step.

    Avoid 'scissor' stepping: Step directly backwards, be careful not to place your left foot directly behind your right foot, this puts the pelvis in the wrong position, twists the body incorrectly, and makes the balance unstable.

- **The right wrist** should be relaxed; the palm of the hand faces downwards at about 45°. Beginners tend to tense the wrist and keep the fingers lifted and pointing upwards.

- **Close the centre and chest:** There is a feeling of the elbows pressing towards each other, or rotating inwards.

- **Connections of the joints:** The hips are rotating to the left as the left foot moves behind you; retain the feeling of the hips, upper body, and elbows working together.

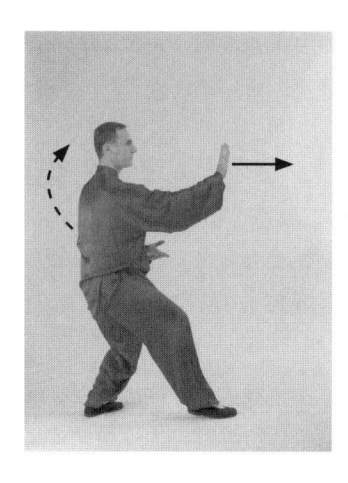

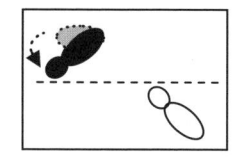

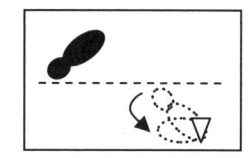

DESCRIPTION OF THE YANG TÀIJÍ 24-STEP SHORT FORM

Brief 4
Push and pull; adjust the front foot.

Details
Your left palm draws back to finish ahead of your left hip with the palm up.

Your right palm pushes away to 9.00, with the wrist at shoulder-height – the tip of the index-finger directly between your centreline and 9.00.

Adjust the right foot pivoting on the *toes* (i.e. the heel will move outwards), but leave the right heel slightly off the ground.

The eyes look to 9.00.

Centre left and back.

Notes

- **Moving into the position:** During the push/pull, the hands will pass quite close to each other – one virtually above the other.

- **Coordination of the movement:** The hands should work together with the shift of the weight so that all movement starts and finishes together. The transfer of weight on to the left foot only completes at the end of the movement – in other words, avoid sitting back too quickly so that the hands end up working independently.

  Coordination of the joints: Concentrate on the turning of the hips during the movement and notice how their turning controls the movements of the elbows.

- **Final weight percentages:** Leave a small amount of weight (20–30%) on the ball of the front foot.

- **Body angle:** The centreline will be slightly turned to the left (about 15°) at the end of the movement.

- **Left hand position:** Beginners often have the hand at the waist in the wrong position. The left palm is not as far back as the *side* of the hip, nor is it in the middle of your body in front of your navel; it finishes at the midpoint between these two places (the 'front/side' of the waist).

If it is incorrectly placed, the left elbow will finish behind the line of your back, which is mechanically weak as it over-stretches the front of the shoulder, and pulls the left scapula inwards towards the spine.

Resting against the body or not: It is easier to teach beginners to rest the left hand against the body. In fact the hand should finish 3–4 inches (7–10 cm) away from the 'front/side' of the waist.

The left arm: Make sure that the arm is completely relaxed and that there is a small space under the armpit; the elbow should not therefore be too close to the body. (The arm position has been described as 'carrying a carpet under your arm'.)

- **'Closed':** The body is 'closed' in this posture. Tuck the tailbone/coccyx under, releasing the small of the back and the back of the neck, and gently pull up/in the lower abdominal muscles.

Moving into Repulse Monkey 2

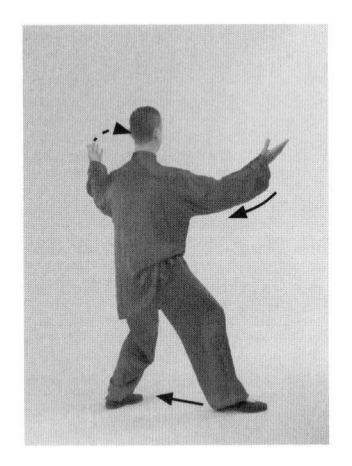

BRIEF 1
Open the arms, turning the left palm up; look left.

DETAILS
As you turn your centreline towards your left knee, open your left forearm out to your left side and then lift it to about 5.00, so that the arms are opened to about 120°.

The right hand extends towards 9.00, the palm turning upwards.

The eyes look towards your left hand initially, but then turn back to look towards the right hand.

Centre left.

NOTES

- **Method of the right arm movement:**

  1. From the previous movement, as you turn the hips, let the left forearm move outwards towards 5.00, keeping it approximately parallel to the ground, and the palm turning upwards. The right thigh will finish approximately between the two opened arms.

  2. At this stage, there is a feeling of almost a pivotal point between the left hip and the left elbow (but see below also).

  3. Then, leading the movement with the fingertips, push the left arm out to approximately 5.00 extending it so that the hand reaches shoulder-height.

  4. **Coordination with the hips:** The left arm movement should be coordinated with the turn of the hips/centre to the left, i.e. make sure that the left elbow coordinates with the left hip. There is therefore a sense of the turning hip controlling the movement of the elbow.

  5. The shoulder should not feel as though the arm is opening to *behind* you.
     Beginners often pull the arm back to 3.00 (behind the line of the shoulders), thereby lifting the left shoulder-blade, and possibly the left shoulder itself.

- **Coordination of the right arm:** The right arm turns palm upwards. Extend the arm; there is a feeling of extending your fingertips to 9.00 with the turn of the waist to the left.

  Work the right hips with the right elbow, i.e. the hip rotates 'forwards' and takes the elbow with it.

- **Coordination of the elbows/arm rotation:** Feel the inwards (downwards) rotation of both elbows working together.

- **Coordinate the elbows and the knees:** They should feel connected, as though they are working together.

- **The knees spiral** outwards as you open the arms.

- **'Opening':** This is an 'open' movement, but note that, as the arms lift, the elbows are starting to rotate downwards and inwards (feel the rotation of the elbows working together – see above); the body is therefore in the process of preparing to 'close', whilst the legs are in the process of 'opening' (see the note directly above).

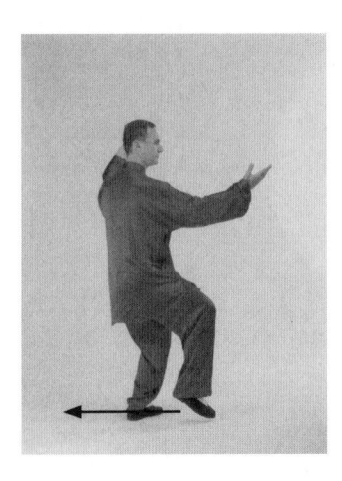

BRIEF 2
Fold arm; foot in.

DETAILS
Sinking your left elbow, fold it so that the left hand moves towards the midline of the body at about throat height.
    Draw your right foot back towards the left foot.
    Your right hand (palm up) starts to move back with the turn of the hips.
    Your eyes continue to look towards 9.00.
    Centre left.

NOTES

- **'Curling' the arm:** Dropping the left elbow towards the left hip will also help to relax the left shoulder. It will also help the left arm to move correctly with the turn of the body.
  Think of folding the left hand towards the centreline.

- **The right arm:** Leave the right arm still pointing to 9.00, but relax the arm so that the elbow sinks and rotates downwards.

- **Angle of body:** The centre is still turned to the left as you both fold the left arm and bring the right foot back. However, because the foot is moving backwards, the hips will begin to rotate back to the right; the body is therefore in the process of starting the turn to the right.

- **Coordination:** Work the left knee, left hip and left elbow together.

- **Sink further into the left foot** as the left elbow folds.

- **The right foot:** It is the turn of the hips that begin to rotate to the right side that causes the right foot to draw in.

- **'Closing':** The body is now in the process of 'closing'.

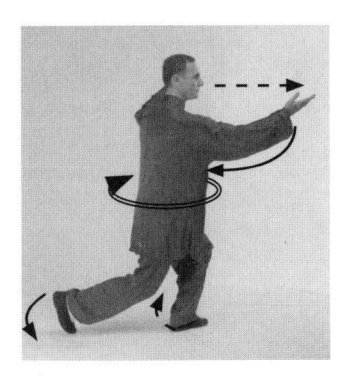

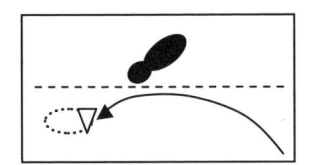

DESCRIPTION OF THE YANG TÀIJÍ 24-STEP SHORT FORM

BRIEF 3
Foot behind; no weight on it.

DETAILS

Place the right toes behind you to 3.00; there should be no weight on them.

The eyes look to 9.00.

Centre still left but starting to turn back to 9.00.

NOTES

- **Placing the foot behind:** The weight should stay on the front foot; beginners often make the mistake of shifting it on to the rear foot at this stage.

- **Stepping:** Use the turn of the hips to place the right foot, *simultaneously sinking* as you step.

  Avoid 'scissor' stepping: Step directly backwards, be careful not to place your right foot directly behind your left foot, this puts the pelvis in the wrong position, twists the body incorrectly, and makes the balance unstable.

- **The left wrist** should be relaxed; the palm of the hand faces downwards at about 45°. Beginners tend to tense the wrist and keep the fingers lifted and pointing upwards.

- **Close the centre and chest:** There is a feeling of the elbows pressing towards each other, or rotating inwards.

- **Connections of the joints:** The hips are rotating to the right as the right foot moves behind you; retain the feeling of the hips, upper body, and elbows working together.

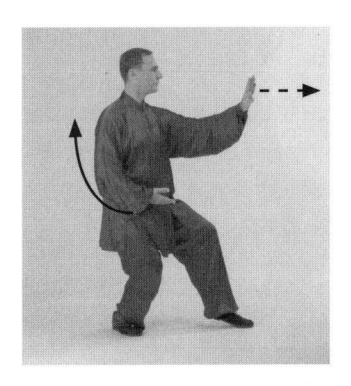

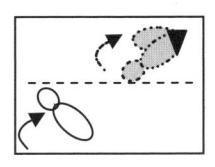

BRIEF 4
Push and pull; adjust the front foot.

DETAILS

Your right palm draws back to finish ahead of your right hip with the palm up.

Your left palm pushes away to 9.00, with the wrist at shoulder-height – the tip of the index-finger directly between your centreline and 9.00.

Adjust the left foot pivoting on the *toes* (i.e. the heel will move outwards), but leave the left heel slightly off the ground.

The eyes look to 9.00.

Centre right and back.

Notes

- **Moving into the position:** During the push/pull, the hands will pass quite close to each other – one virtually above the other.

- **Coordination of the movement:** The hands should work together with the shift of the weight so that all movement starts and finishes together. The transfer of weight on to the right foot only completes at the end of the movement – in other words, avoid sitting back too quickly so that the hands end up working independently.

   Coordination of the joints: Concentrate on the turning of the hips during the movement and notice how their turning controls the movements of the elbows.

- **Final weight percentages:** Leave a small amount of weight (20–30%) on the ball of the front foot.

- **Body angle:** The centreline will be slightly turned to the right (about 15°) at the end of the movement.

- **Right hand position:** Beginners often have the hand at the waist in the wrong position. The right palm is not as far back as the *side* of the hip, nor is it in the middle of your body in front of your navel; it finishes at the midpoint between these two places (the 'front/side' of the waist).

   If it is incorrectly placed, the right elbow will finish behind the line of your back, which is mechanically weak as it over-stretches the front of the shoulder, and pulls the right scapula inwards towards the spine.

   Resting against the body or not: It is easier to teach beginners to rest the right hand against the body. In fact the hand should finish 3–4 inches (7–10 cm) away from the 'front/side' of the waist.

   The right arm: Make sure that the arm is completely relaxed and that there is a small space under the armpit; the elbow should not therefore be too close to the body. (The arm position has been described as 'carrying a carpet under your arm'.)

- **'Closed':** The body is 'closed' in this posture. Tuck the tailbone/coccyx under, releasing the small of the back and the back of the neck, and gently pull up/in the lower abdominal muscles.

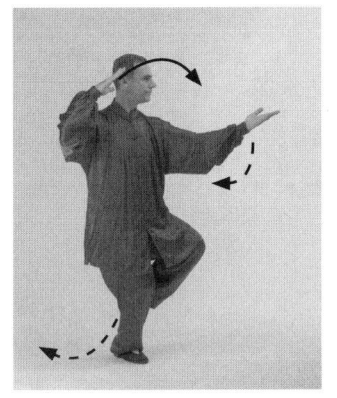

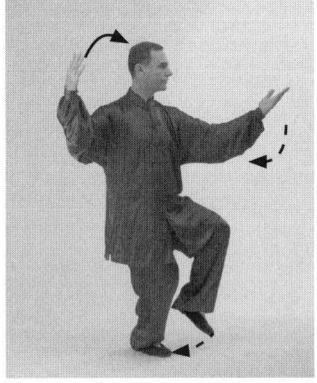

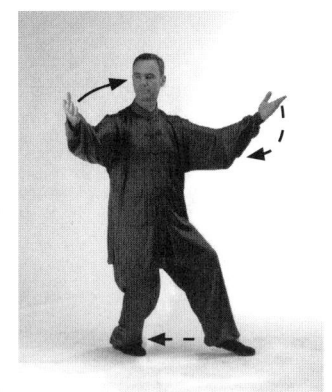

Moving into Repulse Monkey 3

As Repulse Monkey 1 (pp.129–134) but the right hand doesn't need to move down to the right hip first, prior to moving out to the right side.

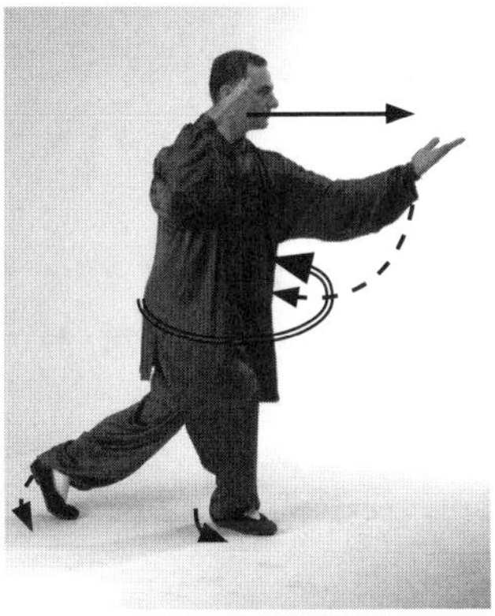

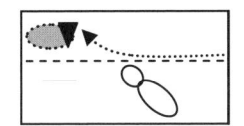

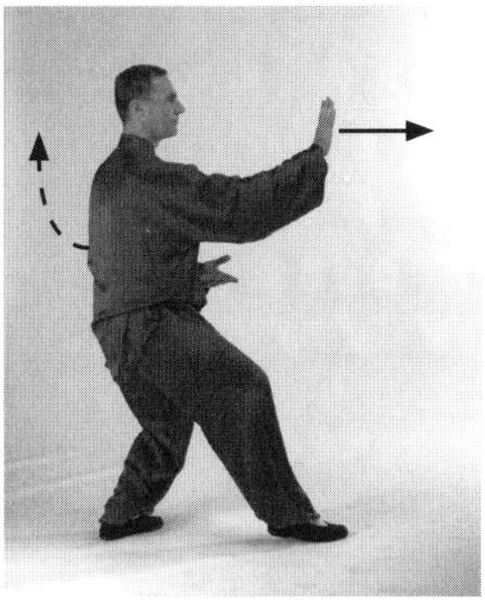

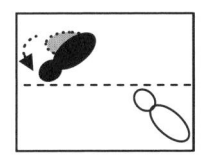

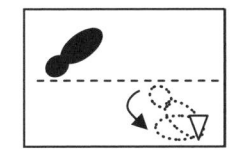

Moving into Repulse Monkey 4

As Repulse Monkey 2 on pp.134–9.

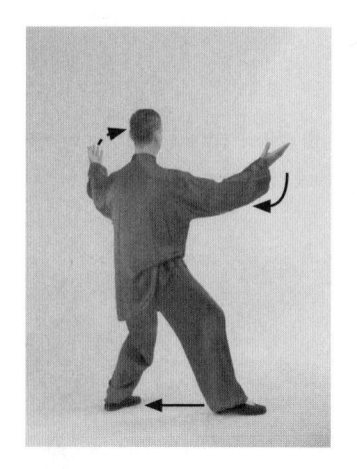

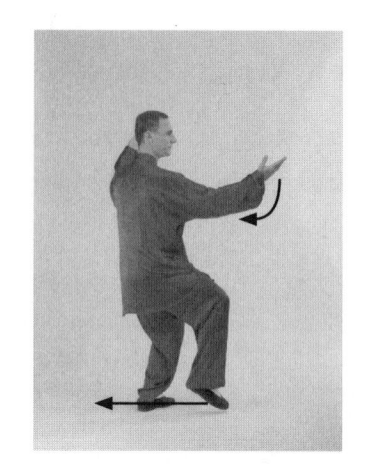

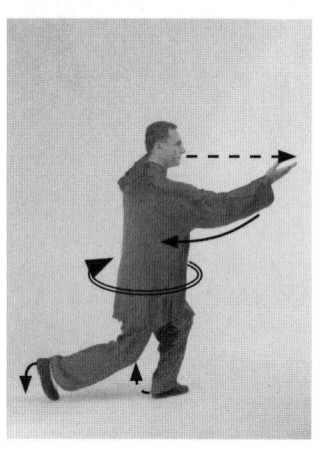

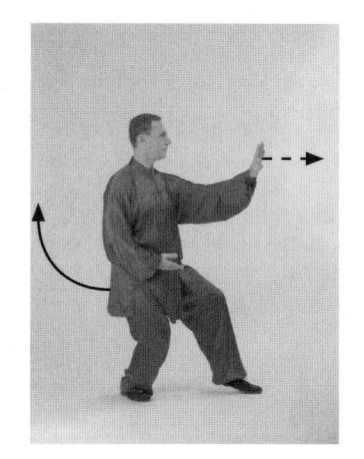

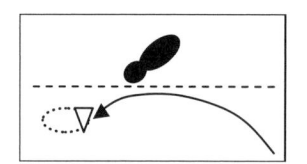

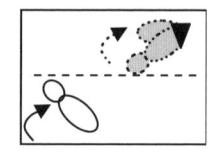

SECTION 3

(2 MOVEMENTS)

7. **Grasp the Bird's (Sparrow's/Peacock's) Tail (Left Style)**
   左揽雀尾 (Zuǒ Lǎnquèwěi)

8. **Grasp the Bird's (Sparrow's/Peacock's) Tail (Right Style)**
   右揽雀尾 (Yòu Lǎnquèwěi)

FORM 7 : GRASP THE BIRD'S (SPARROW'S/PEACOCK'S) TAIL (LEFT STYLE)

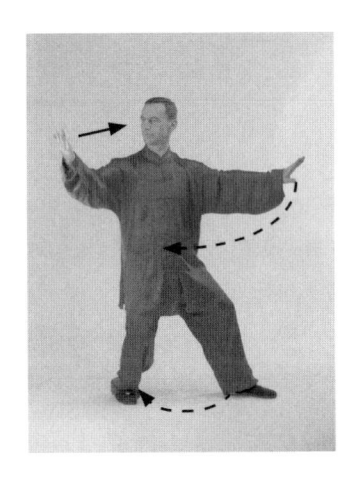

左揽雀尾 (Zuǒ Lǎnquèwěi)

BRIEF 1
Open the arms; palms down (but see Notes below).

DETAILS
Turn the centre to the right, and open your right arm out to 1.00/1.30, the right palm facing down.

As you do this, extend the fingers of the left hand towards 9.00, also with the palm down.

Turn your head to look to the right beyond your hand.

Centre right.

NOTES

- **The arms (beginner):** It's not obligatory to open the arms with the right palm facing down, the arms can be opened with right palm up, but for beginners it is useful to use the 'both hands palms down' method as it differentiates this movement from the opening movement of Repulse Monkey.

  As in Repulse Monkey, avoid the right arm opening too far behind you.

- **Advanced:** See Notes on p.143 for a more advanced method.

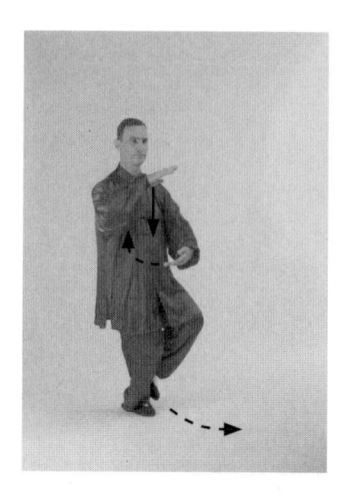

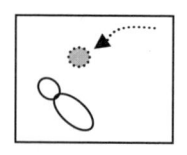

BRIEF 2
Circle arms; left foot in.

DETAILS

Circle the hands anti-clockwise: the right elbow bends, the forearm folding inwards towards your centreline with palm still down.

The left arm lowers and then starts to lift with palm up below the right hand.

The left foot draws into the right foot.

The body faces 10.30.

The eyes look over the right hand.

NOTES

- **The left toes:**

  - Beginners can lightly touch the ground, but for others the toes shouldn't touch the floor.

  - Because of the overall intention of the movements from the end of Repulse Monkey to Péng, some teachers (for martial reasons) do not bring the left foot completely back beside the right foot.

  - Whichever particular method you choose to follow, both agree that the left foot should be emptied of all weight so that the left hip can relax. The ankle should be loose.

- **The left arm** sinks, initially with the left elbow leading, but because of the turn of the body to the right (to 12.00), there is also a feeling of the arm just dropping to protect the lower front of the body.

  The fingertips will lead the inwards movement of the left hand as the left foot draws in; this is the start of the 'closing' movement (see 'Closing' on the following page).

- **Coordinate:**

  - the sinking of the left arm with the shift of weight

  - the release of the left leg with the drawing inwards of the left wrist.

- **'Holding the ball'**: There are many schools that teach that there is a 'hold the ball' posture here. This is fine for beginners as it gives an approximate shape of the arms, but there is no static 'ball' posture here as such.

- **Closing:** As the arms begin to circle anti-clockwise, the body begins a process of compressing, the elbows moving together and the chest closing. The ball symbolizes the moment between 'open' and 'closed' arms, but is not a feature in itself.

- **The arms in Briefs 1 and 2 (more advanced):** The feeling behind this part of the movement is as follows:

  - **Brief 1:**

    As the body turns to the right, the left arm gently pushes to 9.00 with the turn to the hips to the front (this continues the direction of energy of the left hand push in the final movement of the last Repulse Monkey).

    The right arm (with the right elbow and right hip working together) moves out sideways without dropping – the hand swinging outwards with the palm upwards.

  - **Brief 2:**

    The left arm then sinks with the left elbow (and then the wrist) leading, and with the palm facing downwards; the right hand rises and circles inwards.

    There should be a sense of opposition in direction of the two hands, the left palm lowering, and the right palm rising; this is the start of the 'closing' of the arms taking place.

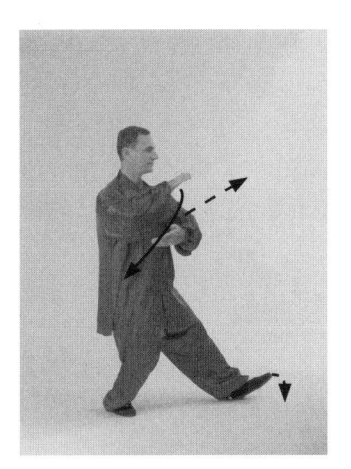

BRIEF 3
Turn back towards 9.00; place left heel.

DETAILS
Turn the body towards 9.00, and step ahead to 9.00 with the left foot. This is not a wide stance, and should be about one fist wide.

At the same time, the left hand starts to circle upwards and away from you.

The right hand starts to push downwards (see Notes on the following page).
The eyes follow the turn of the centreline.
Centre left.

NOTES

- **The step:** This is not a wide Bow Stance; only step about 4 inches (10 cm) wide (see also 'The stance' note on the following page).
- **The body starts to turn** back to the left.
- **The arms:** At this point there is a 'closing' or compression of the body and upper limbs.
  - The fingertips of the lower left hand start to rise (whilst the body is starting to turn back to the left).
  - The rising left fingertips pass close to the right elbow, almost as though the left hand is wiping the right elbow. This continues the line of energy of the left hand which is a rising anti-clockwise circle.
  - The right elbow/forearm starts to sink (whilst the body is starting to turn back to the left).
  - The right hand starts to push downwards within the curve of the left arm.
  - There is a feeling of the elbows closing together; the left elbow rising, and the right elbow sinking.
- **The lower body:** The pelvis/tailbone/coccyx is tucked under, and the lower abdominals are pulled in – a pelvic rotation.
- **The feeling of Péng:** As you turn the body back to 9.00 again, there's a feeling of expansion between the left arm and the centre – your centre going backwards, but the left arm going the opposite way.
- **Testing the movement:** This tests Briefs 2 and 3.
  Working with a partner who is standing at approximately 9.00, ask him to place his hands on your left wrist and left elbow and to push your arm gently towards the centre of your body (or towards 3.00).

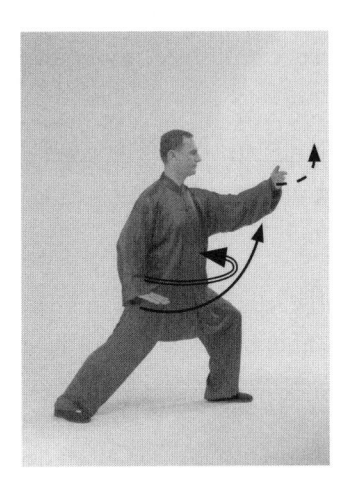

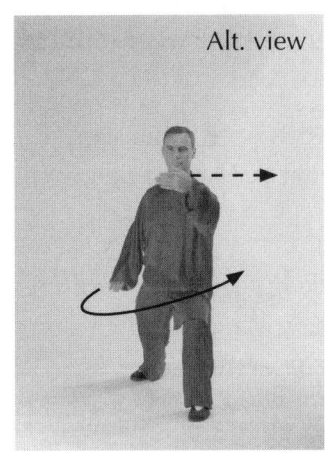

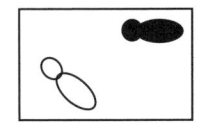

BRIEF 4
Single-hand Péng 掤. Weight forwards; right palm pushes down; left wrist to throat height facing you.

DETAILS

Transfer the weight on to the left foot.

Raise the left hand so that it is circled in front of you with the palm facing you at mouth-height, and the wrist approximately at the height of your shoulder.

Your right hand pushes down by the side of your body with the palm down, the fingers facing towards 9.00, and the thumb edge of the hand about 10 cm from the body.

The eyes look to 9.00.

Centre forwards.

NOTES

- **The stance:**

  - The width of the step should be the equivalent of one fist (4 inches, or 10 cm).

  - The stance should not be as wide as in Parting the Wild Horse's Mane, or Brush Knee and Twist Step.

    There are three reasons for this:

    1. The energy of Péng is directly forwards to 9.00 (unlike Parting the Wild Horse's Mane, where the energy is diagonal).

    2. The pelvis is at a different angle to both Parting the Wild Horse's Mane and Brush Knee and Twist Step.

    3. The hand and foot of the same side are forwards, i.e. in this case it is the left side (unlike Brush Knee and Twist Step which are *opposite* hand and foot).

The narrower stance therefore allows you to push straight ahead off the back foot – the energy of the push isn't split by a wider gap between the two feet.

- **The centreline** and the pelvis are turned approximately 15° to your right, whereas in Parting the Wild Horse's Mane, they are turned to approximately 30–45°.

- **The left arm:**
  - **The arm** is 'rounded'; the palm doesn't turn upwards as it does in Parting the Wild Horse's Mane. Beginners understandably tend to confuse the hand positions of the two postures.
  - **The forearm** is angled to approximately 45°.
  - **The energy** is in the forearm.
  - **The left wrist** is ahead of the centreline of the body, but because the body is turned slightly to the right (see note above), the wrist will appear to be ahead of the right shoulder when looked at from 9.00. This puts the energy of the movement into the forearm.
  - **The left wrist** is approximately at shoulder-height.
    If you are pushing someone towards 9.00 and your arm is too low, you would have to lift the arm upwards as you pushed; this would be hard work and mechanically inefficient. The same applies if your arm is too high – someone pushing on your forearm would be creating the effect of a bridge that raises in the middle; the energy would be forced upwards rather than directly ahead.

- **The right hand:**
  - The right hand pushes down to the floor, whilst the left wrist expands away from you; this creates the connection across the bow of the arms.
  - The right hand push is predominantly downwards, but also slightly backwards which means that, whilst the left arm is working with the left leg, the right arm is therefore working with the right leg.
    Don't pull the right hand too far backwards; you need to feel the bow around the shoulders to find the right place, but when looked at from the side, it will be somewhere between the thighs slightly towards the rear leg.
  - The push downwards should be gentle and continuous.

- **Testing the entire movement of Péng:** To get the feeling of Péng it helps to work with a partner.

Start from Repulse Monkey and, as you start to lower your left arm, have a partner put his hands on your left elbow and wrist and gently but consistently and firmly push towards you. You should experience a deflection of your push to your left, a lifting of your push (by which time your energy will have dissipated), and a return of your energy towards yourself.

In order to make this work correctly, it is important that you maintain a feeling of Péng in your left arm, and do not allow it to collapse. Good coordination of body and left arm is essential!

Note that there is a diagonal and vertical rotational circle created by the left arm, not only a vertical one.

- **'Open'**: This is an 'open' movement.

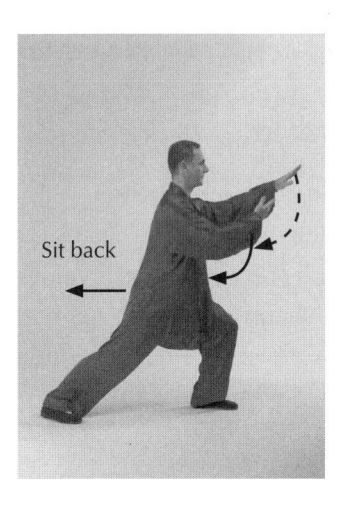

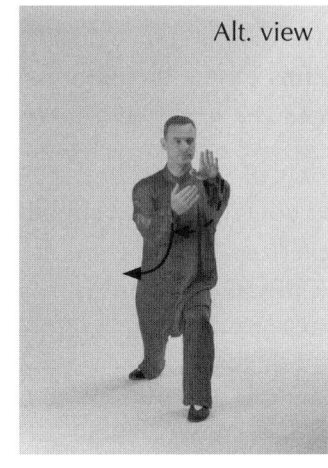

Brief 5

Turn the body left; turn left hand; circle the right hand upwards turning it.

Details

Turn your waist towards your left knee, allowing the hands to move slightly to the left with the turn.

The left hand turns palm down and moves to approximately 8.00 with the turn of the waist.

The right hand (initially with the palm downwards) circles away from you and upwards to the height of your left elbow, the palm gradually turning to face upwards. It rises to opposite the left elbow, with the fingers pointing at the left wrist.

The eyes follow the left hand.

Centre left.

Notes

- **This move is the start of Lǚ 捋.**

- **Turn the waist** only to the left, not the hips; turning the hips will cause the rear leg to collapse.

The right knee: As you turn to the left, release the right knee so that it bends outwards very slightly.

As you turn the body, sink into the left foot.

- **The arm movements:** Beginners tend to attempt to move the arms independently to the left, rather than relying on the turn of the waist to do the work for them. This results in over-twisting of the body to the left.

  As you turn to the left, maintain a 'mental' connection between the left elbow and the left knee (or hip). Doing so will alter the way that the left arm operates.

- **The right hand** is lifted to the height of the left elbow because, in application, this measures the length of an adult forearm – i.e. your left palm would be under an opponent's right elbow, and your right palm would be holding his right wrist.

  The turning of the palms can be thought of as an opponent's arm that you are holding being twisted and rotated clockwise (from your perspective).

- **The right hand's change of energy:** In the previous movement (Péng) the right hand was pushing downwards and slightly backwards.

  Rather than just reversing the direction in which the right hand is moving, convert the backwards and downwards push by turning it into a small anti-clockwise circle; this changes into the lifting of the movement described above and connects the movements with no break in the 'thread' of the energy.

- **'Closing':** This is the start of a 'closing' movement.

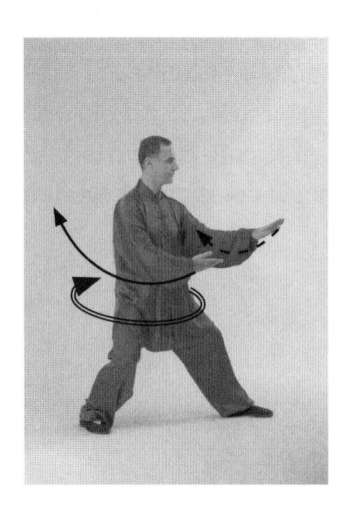

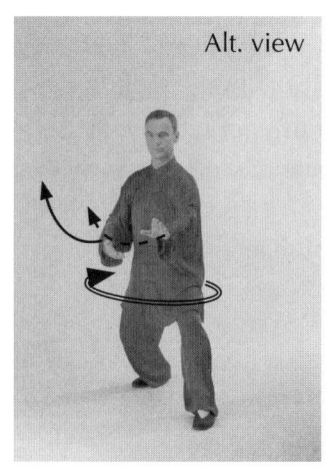

Alt. view

BRIEF 6
Lǚ 捋 (roll back). Lower the hands; turn the body taking the hands out to the rear diagonal.

DETAILS
Sit back on to the right foot and lower the hands approximately to the height of your

waist (with left hand palm down, and right hand palm up); as you do so gradually turn the body towards the 10.30 corner.

As you continue to turn the waist, the arms extend outwards to approximately 1.00/1.30 with the left hand now starting to lift in front of your abdomen (the palm facing your body) and the right arm extending well out to the side (with the palm partly turned upwards).

Centre back and right.

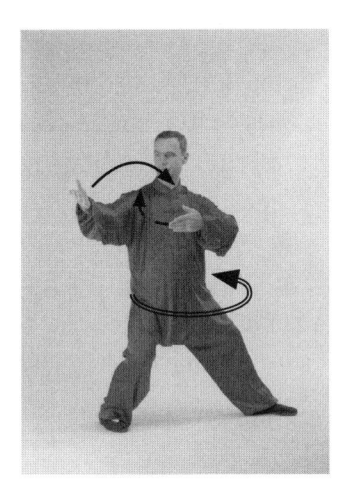

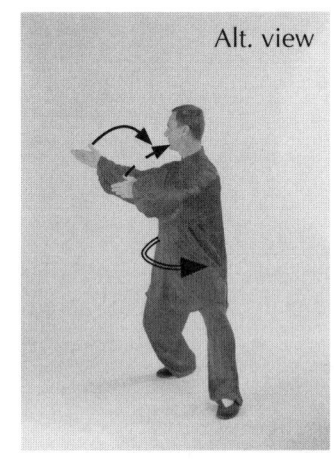

NOTES

- **The distance between your hands:** This should be the same as in the previous two movements, i.e. your right palm should still be level with your left elbow.

- **Lowering the arms** should happen by sinking both elbows.

- **Connection between the hips and elbows:** It is particularly useful in this movement to feel a connection between the hips and the elbows as you sit back and turn. Use the turn of the waist to make the arms move to your right side.

- **The left foot** should remain flat as you sit back; beginners tend to lift the toes.

- **The left knee** should stay in alignment with the left toes as you sit back; avoid its collapsing inwards, particularly at the end of the movement.

- **The knees:** Feel the 'opening' of the knees as you turn.

- **The posture:** The body should be upright, the coccyx tucked under, and the lower abdominal muscles gently pulled inwards.

- **'Closing':** This is a 'closed' movement.

- **Lǔ 捋 finishes** with the arms out sideways and the body turned, in other words, before the energy starts to move forwards again.

THE YANG TÀIJÍ 24-STEP SHORT FORM

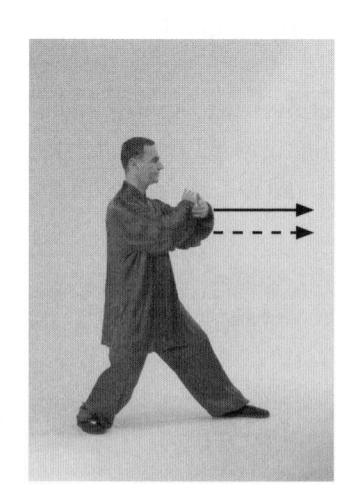

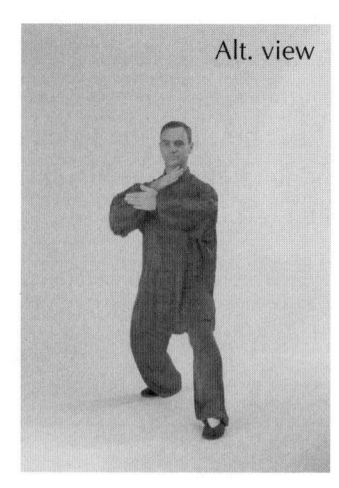

Alt. view

BRIEF 7
Body turns back to 9.00; bring heels of palms together.

DETAILS
As the body turns back to 9.00 again, the left palm continues to rise up the centreline of your body to chest height.

The right arm folds at the elbow, the hand moving inwards towards the left wrist with the palm facing away from you (but see 'Refinement' note on p.151) in front of the chest.

The heels of both palms meet together as you finish squaring the body to 9.00.

The weight remains on the right foot.

The eyes watch the right hand as it circles out to the side, and they then turn to look back to 9.00.

Centre left and backwards.

NOTES

- **This is the start of Jǐ** 挤.

- **The right shoulder** must be relaxed and sunk as you 'circle' the arm.

- **Body/arm connection:** The circling of the arms is controlled by the turning of the waist and hips; avoid an independent arm movement.

- **The left toes** should remain on the ground.

- **'Jǐ'** 挤 is very similar to a 'supported' Péng (see notes on Péng 掤, Lǚ 捋, Jǐ 挤, Àn 按 on pp.156–8).

    It is often performed with a space between the hands, so that there is a feeling of 'squeezing' something between the palms. But it is often performed with the hands touching. In the Yang Tàijì 24-Step Short Form this can be with either the right fingers or the heel of the right hand on the left wrist crease, and it can even be performed with the right *forearm* on the inside of the left forearm (rather than on the wrist).

The main feature of these latter ways of doing the hand connection is that the inside hand is supporting the outside hand (either wrist or forearm); the power is focused at this point, and therefore the point is strengthened by the other hand.

- **The arms** are not parallel to the ground; the elbows are slightly lower that the wrists (but see 'Refinement' note below).
- **The weight** should remain predominantly on the right foot; beginners often move the weight on to the left foot too early.
- **See 'Refinement' note below** for further detail.
- **'Closing':** As you sit back into the right foot, pull your lower abdominal muscles in, allowing the tailbone/coccyx to tuck under.

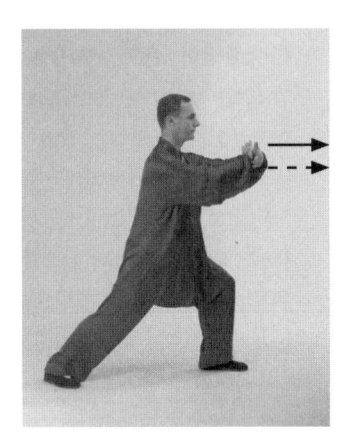

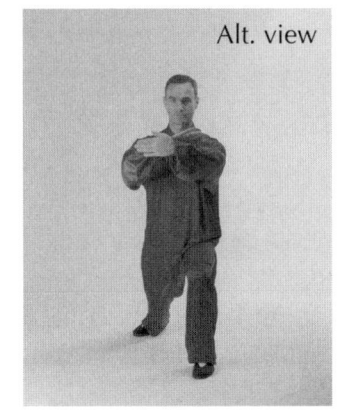

Alt. view

BRIEF 8
Jǐ 挤 (press/squeeze). Weight forwards; extend connected hands.

DETAILS
Press forwards with both hands, shifting the weight on to the left foot.
The eyes continue to look to 9.00.
Centre forwards.

NOTES

- **Refinement** to the 'circling' of the arms: When you circle the arm around to connect it to the left forearm/wrist (Brief 7), connect it with the palm turned to face your left shoulder or even to face your chest.
  The right elbow should be sunk so that the forearm is at approximately 45° (or possibly even more vertical).

Refinement to the 'press': As you press forwards, lift the right elbow and simultaneously rotate the right palm to face away from you to 9.00.

THE YANG TÀIJÍ 24-STEP SHORT FORM

- **Testing:** To test this movement with a partner, ask him to push continuously on your left arm with a gentle but firm force as you move from about halfway through Briefs 5 to 8. The push should be directly towards your body. This way you can feel the Péng energy of the movement together with the right hand support of Jǐ.

- **'Opening':** This is an 'open' movement.

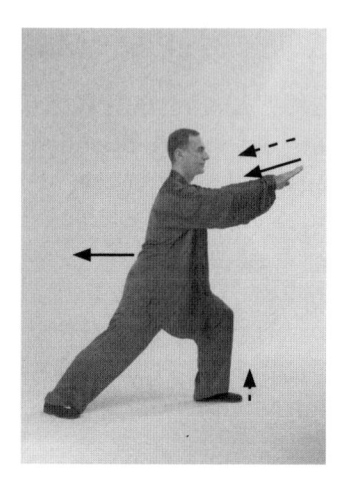

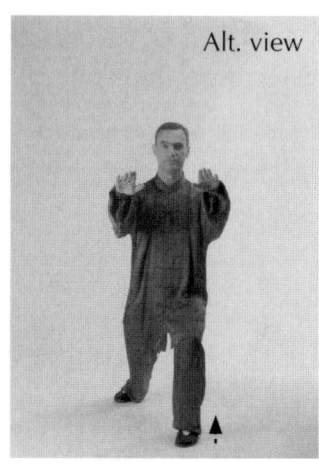

Alt. view

BRIEF 9
Weight continues forwards; 'wipe' and separate the hands.

DETAILS
Continue the weight fractionally further on to the left foot, the palms rotating so that they begin to turn downwards (still crossed at the wrists – the right hand will therefore be on top of the left hand). Without stopping, separate the hands to a shoulder's width by passing the right hand over the back of the left hand 'wipe'.

The eyes continue to look to 9.00.

NOTES

- **This movement is still a part of Jǐ.** The arms should feel almost like a follow-through in a tennis stroke. Move a fraction more weight forwards, and gently **press the front foot into the ground**, almost like a brake.

- **Separating the hands:** Beginners often separate the hands too early, so for the purposes of teaching, I give the 'hand separation' its own movement number.

    The idea of 'wiping' the hands is not important but helps beginners to separate their hands.

    The left hand gradually rotates palm down which connects Jǐ to the next movement.

- **This is where Jǐ 挤 finishes:** The hands have separated, the energy has not yet started to withdraw, but has dissipated.

- **Variation:** Some practitioners prefer to begin shifting the weight backwards at this point (my own personal preference). The backwards push off the left foot causes the separation of the hands in the same way that, when trying to shake sauce out of a bottle, you have to pull the bottle backwards to make it come out.

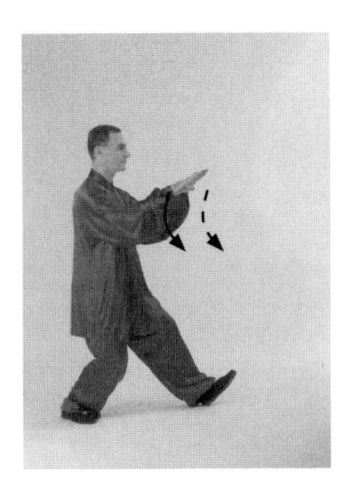

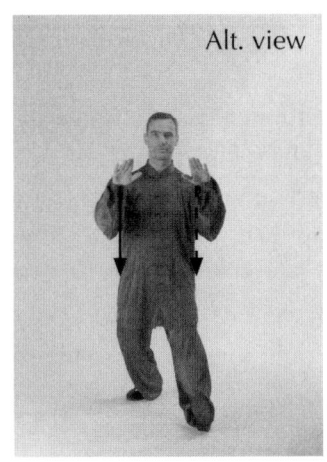

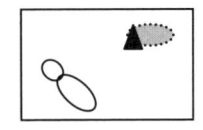

Alt. view

BRIEF 10
Sit back; hands towards shoulders; left toes up.

DETAILS
Sit back on to the right foot drawing the hands back at shoulder-height; start to sink the elbows as the hands come closer to your shoulders/upper chest.
   Lift the toes of the left foot.
   The eyes continue to look to 9.00.
   Centre backwards.

NOTES

- **Àn 按 (push downwards):** This entire part of the movement (Briefs 10–12) is usually referred to as Àn 按 although, strictly speaking, Àn means a *downwards* push, and Tuī 推 is a push *ahead/forwards*.

- **Coordination of the joints:** The bending of the right knee should work together with the bending of the elbows.

- **'Closing':** Continuing from Jǐ, the 'closing' begins as the energy now starts to withdraw.

THE YANG TÀIJÍ 24-STEP SHORT FORM

As you sit back on to the right foot, bending the knee, start to pull your lower abdominal muscles in, allowing the tailbone/coccyx to begin tucking under.

This and the following movements involve the 'closing' of the body, almost a 'contraction' of the chest, and the sinking of the elbows is part of this. So as you sit back, be aware of the gradual contraction of the elbows, which not only lower towards the floor, but also contract by bending.

Variation

- **Variation:** Some practitioners like to rotate the body slightly to the right at this point. As with all variations, it depends entirely upon the use of the movement (application) as to whether you do or do not.

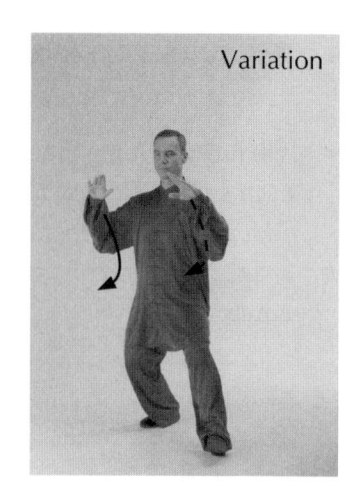

From the point of view of comfort, I personally think that turning the body is better for the right knee because the right hip is able to relax more, but there isn't much in it!

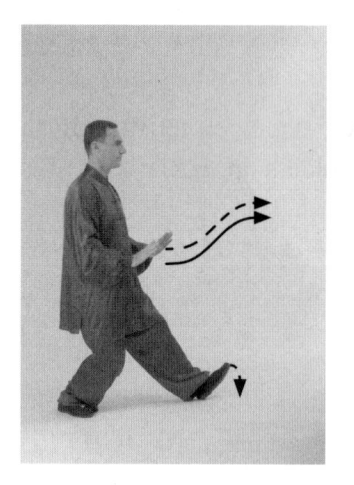

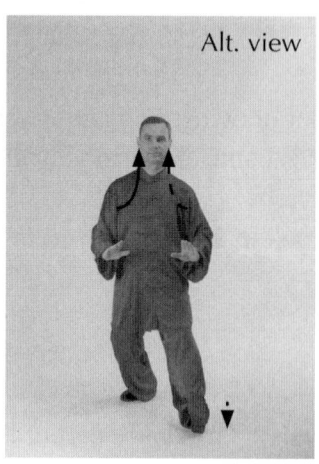

Alt. view

BRIEF 11
Àn 按 (push downwards). Complete the sitting back; hands down to abdomen/waist.

DETAILS
Sink the elbows, circling and lowering the hands from in front of the shoulders/upper chest to the height of your abdomen/waist.

Left toes are still up.
The eyes continue to look to 9.00.
Centre backwards.

Notes

- **This movement is Àn 按 (push downwards)**.
- **The hands:**
  - **Method:** Sink the *elbows* to lower the hands.
  - **Height:** Beginners tend to take the hands too low to the *hips*, rather than the waist.
  - **Angle:** The fingers should be slightly lifted; the feeling/awareness should be in the palms.
- **Connections:** There should be a feeling of relaxing the shoulders into the hips.
- **'Close':** Tuck the tailbone/coccyx well under, 'close' completely, but keep the neck relaxed.
- **Variation** continuing the rotation of body: As you sink the body into the back foot (lowering the hands), the body finishes the slight turn to the right.

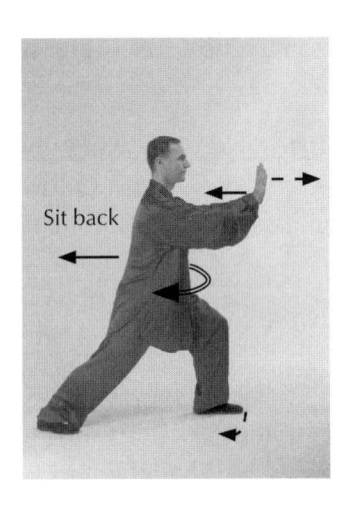

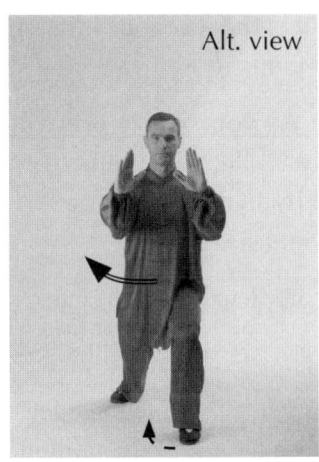

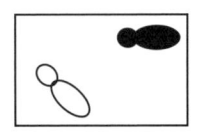

Brief 12
Weight forwards; double handed push.

Details
Place the left toes and move the weight into a left Bow Stance as you push towards 9.00 with both palms.
The eyes still look to 9.00.
Centre forwards.

Notes

- **Tuī 推 (push ahead):** Although this movement is part of the previous movement, strictly speaking this is Tuī (meaning push ahead), rather than Àn (the previous *downwards* pushing movement).

- **The push**, starting from the waist, is initially diagonally upwards, but then curves for a forwards push. It is not an upwards-diagonal push; there is a feel of lifting then pushing away.

  The palms will be slightly rounded at the end of the move, as though pushing a large ball (pushing with the hypothenar eminences).

  The hands finish with the wrists at the height of your shoulders; the palms will be a shoulder's width apart.

- **Relax the shoulders:** Beginners tend to lift the shoulders when pushing; keep them relaxed and sunk.

- **Sink the elbows** as you push, thereby closing the chest.

- **Connections of the joints:** When pushing, be aware of:

  - the right leg and arms working together, i.e. moving in opposite directions to each other from the centre ('Every action has an equal and opposite reaction'.)
  - the hips working with the elbows
  - the straightening out of the rear knee joint in the same ratio as the straightening of the elbow joints.

- **Energy up the spine:** As you sink into the hips (particularly relaxing the right hip), bring energy up the spine to between the shoulder blades (allow the spine to flex), slightly hyper-extending the shoulders forwards throughout the push (but without lifting them).

- **Sink the hips** as you complete the push, particularly the right hip.

- **Spiral the knees** outwards as you complete the push.

- **Neck and tailbone:** As you complete the push, release the neck and allow it to lengthen as you release the tip of the tailbone/coccyx allowing it to drop.

Péng 掤, Lǔ 捋, Jǐ 挤, Àn 按

Forms 7 and 8 contain four of the eight 'energies' of tàijí (Péng 掤, Lǔ 捋, Jǐ 挤, Àn 按), the other four being:

1. Cǎi 采 (pick/pluck/collect/gather) – refers to grasping or pulling with the fingers.
2. Liè 挒 (often translated as split/twist/rend, or even as 'using the wrist') – refers to the use of the forearm and wrist to strike.

3. Zhǒu 肘 (elbow) – refers to the use of the elbow to block or strike.

4. Kào 靠 (lean on/against/support) – refers to the use of the shoulder (front or back of) or the top of the upper arm at shoulder-height to block or strike.

Note that these four 'energies' also refer to different parts of the arm from fingers to shoulders, or vice versa.

Péng 掤

Péng 掤 is often translated as 'ward off', as in warding off an attack, but there is also a quality of springiness about Péng rather like pushing against an aerobics ball and feeling it bouncing back; Péng therefore contains the idea or quality of resilience and expansiveness.

The energy of Péng can be directed to any part of the body but, in the case of the movement above, it is directed into the upper arm and forearm.

The other quality that Péng has is that of 'sensing' or what is referred to by the Chinese as 'listening energy' – tīngjìng (听劲).

'Listening' means that you use your arm something like an insect might use its antennae. Being in contact with your partner/opponent, you sense the direction, strength and intention of his movements; at the same time the resilient quality of your arm acts like a shield in front of you, but a shield that can also be used in attack to propel your opponent backwards with the back of your forearm.

Péng energy should be the foundation of all eight energies.

This could be referred to as an 'open' movement.

Lǚ 捋

Lǚ 捋 is often referred to as 'roll back'.

It is both a 'listening' energy and a 'following' energy with the additional function of directing or redirecting an opponent's energy.

An example might be of a batsman in a game of cricket who, instead of hitting the ball directly back at the bowler, angles his bat so that the ball glances off to left or right, hardly disturbing the original direction of the ball but enough to keep him safe.

In application it can be used to hold an opponent's wrist and elbow and to rotate the body so that the opponent's energy is re-directed from his original intention and his balance is upset.

There should not be any 'pull' involved as this changes the energy to Cǎi 采, whilst a downwards push changes the energy to Àn 按. I mention this because you often see Lǚ practised with a partner as a mixture of Àn and Cǎi.

This could be called a 'closed' movement'.

157

Jǐ 挤

Jǐ 挤 is usually translated as 'press'.

In the Form it is a reversal of energy after Lǚ; the opponent's energy has been brought forwards and to the side, and is forced then to withdraw.

As in all of these movements, there is 'listening' involved as you follow the opponent's retreating energy and use the back of the wrist to drive him backwards. In Jǐ though, the back of the wrist is supported by the other hand; it is this hand (pushing on the inside of your wrist) which, along with the rear leg and the turning hip (the right hip in the case of the Jǐ described above), provides most of the power in the movement.

In this form Jǐ is performed with the inside hand on the wrist, but Jǐ can also be seen (e.g. in Pushing Hands) with the inside hand on the elbow or the forearm.

Jǐ is like a supported Péng. In Péng the body is slightly sideways on, and therefore the energy tends to be more in the region of the upper arm/elbow/forearm. But in Jǐ the body is more square-on and the energy tends to be in the wrist. The other arm therefore is brought in to assist.

This is an 'opening' movement.

Àn 按

Àn 按 means 'push down', but in the Yang Tàijí 24-Step Short Form and many other forms it usually refers to the whole of the last movement including the push ahead at the end – which really is Tuī 推.

As always there is 'listening' involved in the movement as you sit back, following an opponent's push towards you and then redirecting it downwards before pushing back towards him and completing the circle.

The intention of using Àn is to cause an opponent's energy to want to rise which makes upsetting his balance much easier.

In application, Àn is often performed by 'pulling' the opponent towards you first – drawing him in (this makes him want to retreat), then by pushing him down (Àn, which makes him want to rise up…so his energy now wants to go back *and* rise up), and then by pushing him in the direction that his energy is asking to go (backwards and upwards). Strictly speaking the pulling towards you is not Àn, it is Cǎi 采, but the overall movement is usually referred to as Àn. As an application it is extremely effective.

This is a 'closed' movement.

FORM 8 : GRASP THE BIRD'S (SPARROW'S/PEACOCK'S) TAIL (RIGHT STYLE)

右揽雀尾 (Yòu Lǎnquèwěi)

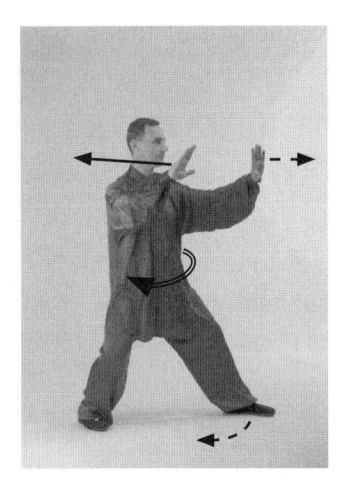

BRIEF 1
Transition. Sit back on to the right foot; turn to 12.00; open the arms.

DETAILS
Move the weight back on to the right foot.

Lift the left toes slightly off the floor, and, as you turn towards 12.00, pivot your left foot on the heel so that the toes point to 12.00.

At the same time, open the right arm towards 1.30.

As you open the right arm, feel as though you are pushing the left arm out in approximately the 9.00 direction; it *will* also begin to move towards 12.00 with the turn of the body, but will not come around as far as the right hand.

The fingertips of both hands stay slightly lifted, but this is a horizontal arm movement.

The eyes follow the right hand.

Centre right.

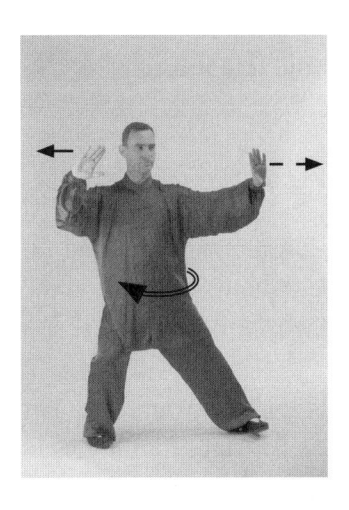

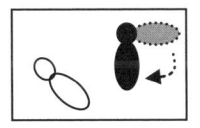

NOTES

- **The left hand:** There is a feeling of continuing the energy of the left hand's previous movement. In other words, the left hand was pushing to 9.00, and should continue to do so as you sit back and turn (as you continue the push, relax the wrist). However, at the same time the body is turning, and therefore the left arm also needs to start to move around towards 12.00.

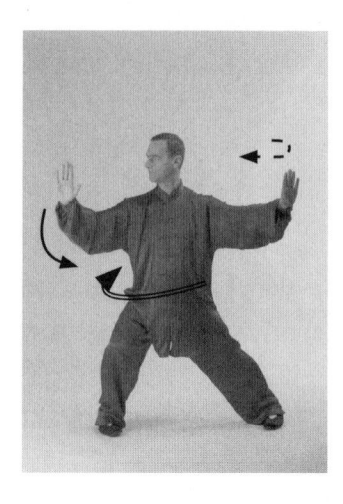

There are therefore three aspects to feel as you perform this movement:

1. The continuation of the left hand energy as you turn.

2. The separation or widening of the arms – the 'opening' of the upper body.

3. The connection of the left arm to the left leg (or left elbow to left knee).

- **The right hand** can arc very slightly upwards and then downwards back to the same height.

  The palm of the right hand faces away from you during the turn, and there is a feeling of the elbow leading the arm.

Expand the outside edge of the hand (the hypothenar eminence) as the hand moves around.

- **Sitting back and turning:**

  - Sink the right hip and let the knees 'open' by spiralling both of them outwards slightly.

  - It is the hip that turns the left foot.

  - As you sit back and turn, pull the lower abdominal muscles gently in, and allow the tailbone/coccyx to tuck under.

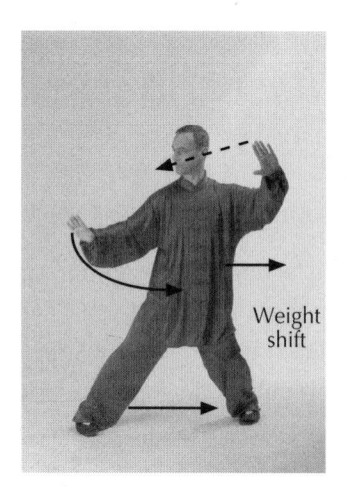

BRIEF 2
Sit back; sink right hand; fold left arm.

DETAILS
Sit back on to the left foot.

As you sit back, the left arm swings around towards 12.00 (parallel to the ground) and folds at the elbow, the hand moving in front of the chest with the palm down.

Simultaneously, the right hand lowers ahead of the right thigh, and then, as the right foot draws in beside the left foot, the palm turns up and the hand finishes in front of the hips.

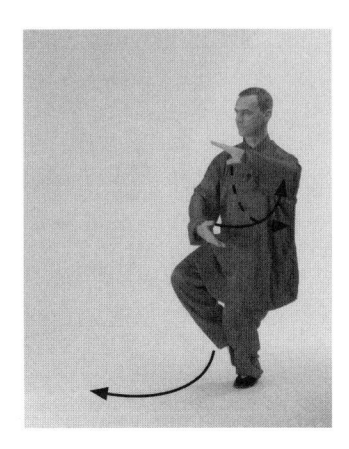

DESCRIPTION OF THE YANG TÀIJÍ 24-STEP SHORT FORM

Together therefore the arms have a feel of circling clockwise.

The body faces approximately 12.00/1.00.

The eyes now look over the left hand.

Centre right.

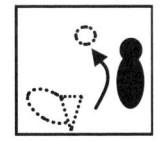

NOTES

- **The left hand** movement is the hardest to feel correctly; it's important to relinquish control of the arm almost allowing momentum to do all the work.

  When bending the elbow, there is a sensation of walking into your own forearm.

  The right arm sinks, initially with the right elbow leading, but because of the turn of the body to the left (to 12.00), there is also a feeling of the arm just dropping to protect the lower front of the body (see 'Testing the movement' on p.164).

  The fingertips will lead the inwards movement of the right hand as the right foot draws in; this is the start of the 'closing' movement (see 'Closing' on p.162).

  Coordinate:

  - the sinking of the right arm with the shift of weight
  - the bending of the left elbow and left knee
  - the release of the right leg with the drawing inwards of the right wrist.

- **The right toes:**

  - Beginners can lightly touch the ground, but for others the toes shouldn't touch the floor.
  - Because of the overall intention of the movement (from the end of Form 7 to Péng), some teachers (for martial reasons) do not bring the right foot completely back beside the left foot. They would argue that the energy-movement/direction of this entire rotation (Briefs 1 and 2) is one of

rotating to the right, and therefore bringing the right foot all the way back breaks this energy.

- Whichever particular method you choose to follow, all agree that the right foot should be emptied of all weight so that the right hip can relax. The ankle should be loose.

- **The turning of the body:** Briefs 1 and 2 are a continuous turn from left (9.00) to right (3.00).

- **Posture:** Avoid leaning.

- **The arms in Briefs 1 and 2 (more advanced):** The feeling behind this part of the movement is as follows:

  - **Brief 1:**

    As the body turns to the right, the left arm gently continues to push to 9.00 as the hips turn to the front (this continues the direction of energy of the left hand push in the final movement of Form 7: Àn).

    The right arm (with the right elbow and right hip working together) circles out sideways without dropping – the hand swinging outwards with the palm turned diagonally downwards.

  - **Brief 2:**

    The right arm then sinks with the right elbow (and then the wrist) leading, and with the palm facing downwards; the left hand folds, the wrist circling inwards.

    The right palm is therefore lowering, and the left palm folding; this is the start of the 'closing' of the arms taking place.

- **'Closing':** This is the start of the 'closing' movement (see also 'Holding the ball' below).

- **'Holding the ball':** There are many schools that teach that there is a 'hold the ball' posture here. This is fine for beginners as it gives an approximate shape of the arms, but there is no static 'ball' posture here as such.

- **Closing:** As the arms begin to circle clockwise, the body begins a process of compressing, the elbows moving together and the chest closing. The ball symbolizes the moment between 'open' and 'closed' of the arms, but is not a feature in itself.

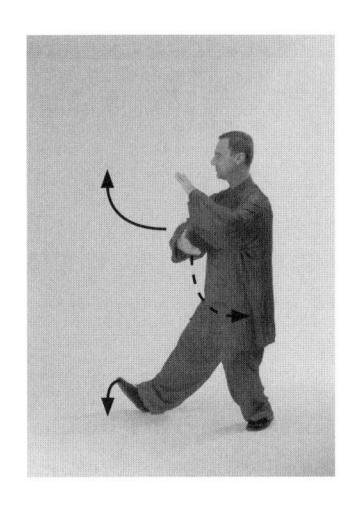

Brief 3

Turn back towards 3.00; place right heel.

Details

Turn the body towards 3.00, and step ahead to 3.00 with the right foot. This is not a wide stance, and should be about one fist wide.

At the same time, the right hand starts to circle upwards and away from you.

The left hand starts to push downwards (see Notes below).

The eyes follow the turn of the centreline.

Centre right.

Notes

- **The step:** This is not a wide Bow Stance; only step about 4 inches (10 cm) wide (see also 'The stance' note on p.145).

    Beginners tend not to step far enough around with the right foot.

- **The body starts to turn** back to the right.

- **The arms:** At this point there is a 'closing' or compression of the body and upper limbs.

    - The fingertips of the lower right hand start to rise (whilst the body is starting to turn back to the right).

    - The rising right fingertips pass close to the left elbow, almost as though the right hand is wiping the left elbow. This continues the line of energy of the right hand which is a rising clockwise circle.

    - The left elbow/forearm starts to sink (whilst the body is starting to turn back to the right).

    - The left hand starts to push downwards within the curve of the right arm.

    - There is a feeling of the elbows closing together; the right elbow rising, and the left elbow sinking.

- **The lower body:** The pelvis/tailbone/coccyx is tucked under, and the lower abdominals are pulled in – a pelvic rotation.

- **The feeling of Péng:** As you turn the body back to 3.00 again, there's a feeling of expansion between the right arm and the centre – your centre going backwards, but the right arm going the opposite way.

- **Testing the movement:** This tests Briefs 2 and 3.

    Working with a partner who is standing at approximately 3.00, ask him to place his hands on your right wrist and right elbow and to push your arm gently towards the centre of your body (or towards 9.00).

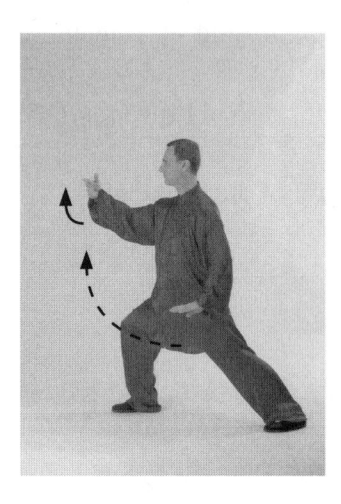

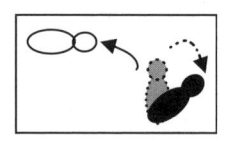

BRIEF 4

Single-hand Péng 掤. Weight forwards; left palm pushes down; right wrist to throat height facing you.

DETAILS

Transfer the weight on to the right foot.

Raise the right hand so that it is circled in front of you with the palm facing you at mouth-height, and the wrist approximately at the height of your shoulder.

Your left hand pushes down by the side of your body with the palm down, the fingers facing towards 3.00, and the thumb edge of the hand about 10 cm from the body.

The eyes look to 3.00.

Centre forwards.

NOTES

- As for Form 7 (Brief 4) on p.145.

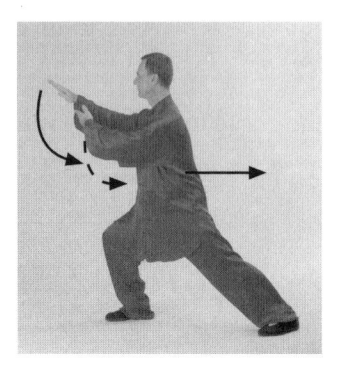

BRIEF 5

Turn the body right; turn right hand; circle the left hand upwards turning it.

DETAILS

Turn your waist towards your right knee, allowing the hands to move slightly to the right with the turn.

The right hand turns palm down and moves to approximately 4.00 with the turn of the waist.

The left hand (initially with the palm downwards) circles away from you and upwards to the height of your right elbow, the palm gradually turning to face upwards. It rises to opposite the right elbow, with the fingers pointing at the right wrist.

The eyes follow the right hand.

Centre right.

NOTES

- As for Form 7 (Brief 5) on p.147.

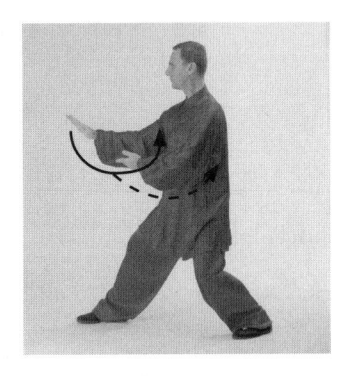

BRIEF 6

Lǚ 捋 (roll back). Lower the hands; turn the body taking the hands out to the rear diagonal.

DETAILS

Sit back on to the left foot and lower the hands approximately to the height of your waist (with right hand palm down, and left hand palm up); as you do so gradually turn the body towards the 1.30 corner.

As you continue to turn the waist, the arms extend outwards to approximately 10.00/11.00 with the right hand now starting to lift in front of your abdomen (the palm facing your body) and the left arm extending well out to the side (with the palm partly turned upwards).

Centre back and left.

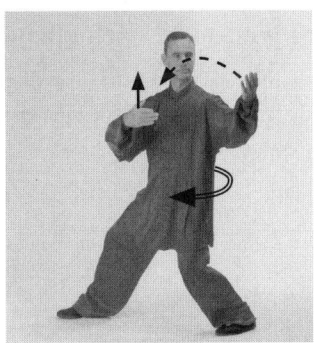

NOTES

- As for Form 7 (Brief 6) on p.149.

THE YANG TÀIJÍ 24-STEP SHORT FORM

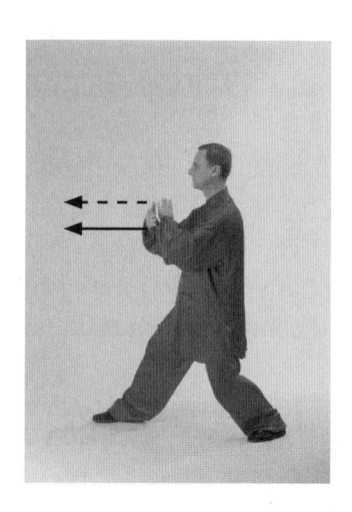

BRIEF 7

Body turns back to 3.00; bring heels of palms together.

DETAILS

As the body turns back to 3.00 again, the right palm continues to rise up the centreline of your body to chest height.

The left arm folds at the elbow, the hand moving inwards towards the right wrist with the palm facing away from you (but see 'Variation' below) in front of the chest.

The heels of both palms meet together as you finish squaring the body to 3.00.

The weight remains on the left foot.

The eyes watch the left hand as it circles out to the side, and they then turn to look back to 3.00.

Centre right and backwards.

NOTES

- As for Form 7 (Brief 7) on p.150, but note the variation below.

- **Variation:** There is a refinement both to the way that you circle the arms and to the way that the 'press' is performed:

  When you circle the arm around to connect it to the right forearm/wrist, connect it with the palm turned *down* or even facing you, and the left elbow sunk so that the forearm is at approximately 45° (or possibly even fractionally less). As you press forwards, the lifting of the left elbow is achieved by turning the palm to 3.00 as you press.

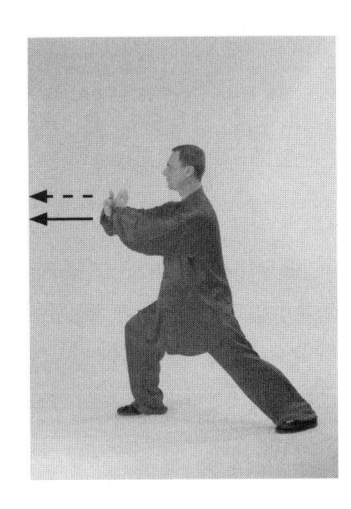

Brief 8

Jǐ 挤 (press/squeeze). Weight forwards; extend connected hands.

Details

Press forwards with both hands, shifting the weight on to the right foot.

    The eyes continue to look to 3.00.
    Centre forwards.

Notes

- As for Form 7 (Brief 8) on p.151.

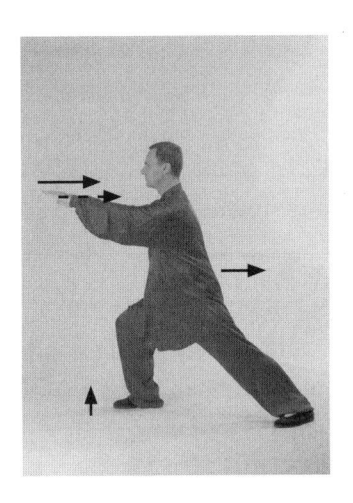

Brief 9

Weight continues forwards; 'wipe' and separate the hands.

Details

Continue the weight fractionally further on to the right foot, the palms rotating so that they begin to turn downwards (still crossed at the wrists – the left hand will therefore be on top of the right hand). Without stopping, separate the hands to a shoulder's width by passing the left hand over the back of the right hand.

    The eyes continue to look to 3.00.

Notes

- As for Form 7 (Brief 9) on p.152.

Brief 10

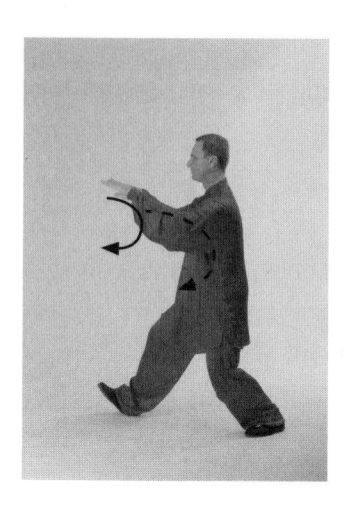

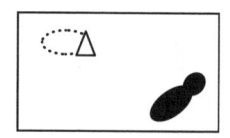

Sit back; hands towards shoulders; right toes up.

Details

Sit back on to the left foot drawing the hands back at shoulder-height; start to sink the elbows as the hands come closer to your shoulders/upper chest.
　　Lift the toes of the right foot.
　　The eyes continue to look to 3.00.
　　Centre backwards.

Notes

- As for Form 7 (Brief 10) on p.153.

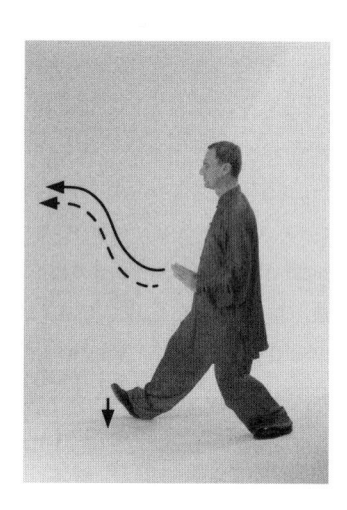

Brief 11

Àn 按 (push downwards). Complete the sitting back; hands down to abdomen/waist.

Details

Sink the elbows, circling and lowering the hands from in front of the shoulders/upper chest to the height of your abdomen/waist.
　　The eyes continue to look to 3.00.
　　Centre backwards.

Notes

- As for Form 7 (Brief 11) on p.155.

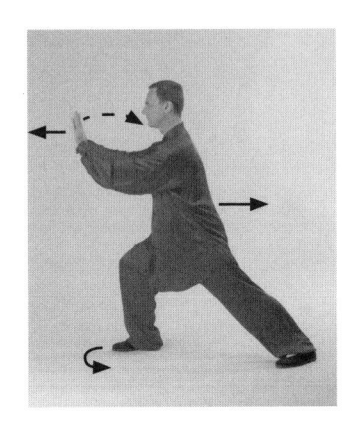

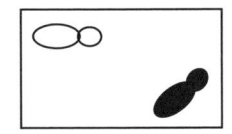

DESCRIPTION OF THE YANG TÀIJÍ 24-STEP SHORT FORM

BRIEF 12
Weight forwards; double handed push.

DETAILS
Place the right toes and move the weight into a right Bow Stance as you push towards 3.00 with both palms.
    The eyes still look to 3.00.
    Centre forwards.

NOTES

- As for Form 7 (Brief 12) on p.155.
- **Variation** using the turn of the body: See photographs below.

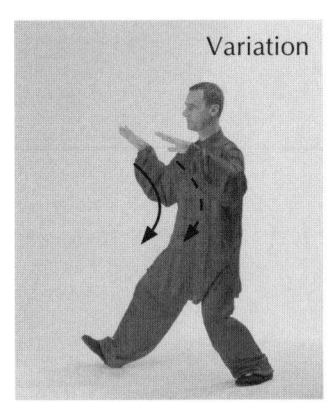

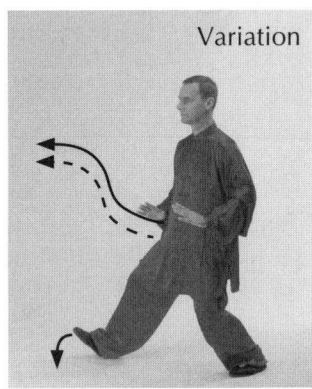

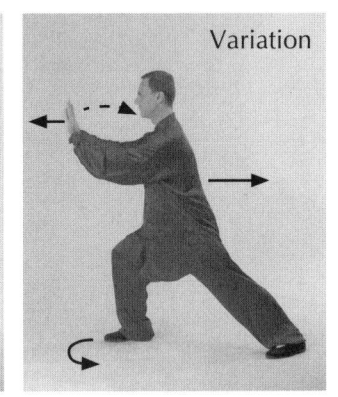

SECTION 4

(3 MOVEMENTS)

9. **Single Whip (Single Biān)**
   单鞭 (Dānbiān)

10. **Wave Hands Like Clouds (Wave/Move the Hands Like Clouds)**
    云手 (Yúnshǒu)

11. **Single Whip (Single Biān)**
    单鞭 (Dānbiān)

FORM 9: SINGLE WHIP (SINGLE BIĀN)

单鞭 (Dānbiān)

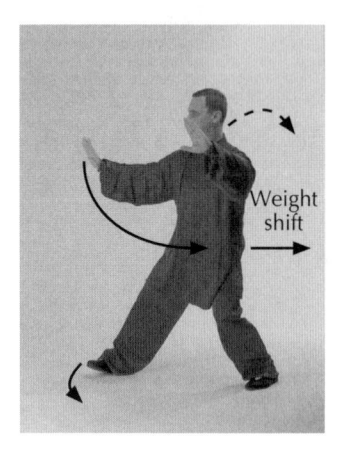

BRIEF 1
Start to sit back on to the left foot; begin to lower right arm.

DETAILS
Start to move the weight back on to the left foot – enough to raise the right toes slightly.
  Begin to lower the right hand.
  The eyes follow the left hand.

NOTES

- **Sitting back:** Sit back just enough to free the right toes so that you are able to turn them.
  As you sit back, tuck the pelvis under, drawing in the lower abdominal muscles.
  Keep the body upright.

- **The right arm:**

  - First of all briefly continue the direction of energy of the previous movement, i.e. to 3.00.

  - Then lower the right arm by sinking the right elbow (feel the weight of your own elbow).

  - Coordinate the lowering of the right arm with the transference of weight.

- **Variation:** Some practitioners turn the left palm outwards during this movement, others turn the palm to face inwards (see 'Variation' at end of Brief 2, pp.172–3).

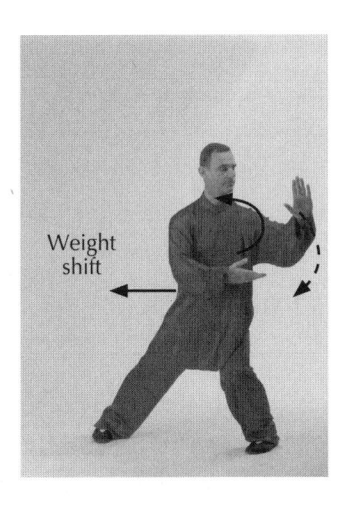

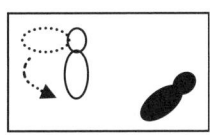

BRIEF 2
Continue to sit back as you turn the hips; right arm sinks and turns with the body; turn your right toes.

DETAILS
Turn your hips towards 12.00, turning your right toes to face 12.00.

As you turn your hips and waist, your right palm will move to the left approximately to the height of your hips/thighs.

The left hand moves across your front at throat height with the palm still turned away from you (but see 'Variation' on pp.172–3).
By the end of the move your upper body is facing 11.00.
The eyes follow the left hand throughout the turn.
Centre left.

NOTES

- **Turning the right toes:**

  - Use the turn of the hips to turn the toes.

  - The right toes should be turned to 12.00. Beginners tend not to turn the toes enough; this causes a problem in the final movement.

- **The left knee:** Keep the left knee over the left toes; if the hip (Kuà) isn't relaxed, or is locked, it will want to turn out beyond the toes.
- **Posture:** Keep the hips/tailbone/coccyx tucked under as you turn; because you are pigeon-toed, it will be tempting to stick the bottom out.
- **The movement of the arms** comes from the turn of the waist; avoid moving the arms independently.
- **Method of lowering the right arm:**
  - Use the turn of the hips to move the right arm (as well as the right toes).
  - The lowering of the right arm is done by first sinking the elbow, then the wrist, and then finally by dropping the fingertips; there is a feeling of the tips of the fingers leading the right hand only at the end – particularly as the hand starts to lift in the movement that follows.
  - Keep the right hand fairly close to the body, and the arm very relaxed.
- **The left arm:**
  - The left elbow shouldn't drop any further as you turn from the right side (1.30) to the left side (11.00). Keep the forearm at approximately 45°.
  - As you reach the left 11.00 'corner', allow the left elbow to relax and sink.
  - If using the 'palm inwards' variation (see 'Variation' below), begin to turn the left palm outwards as you arrive at the 11.00 'corner' – coordinate this with the sinking of the left elbow, and extending of the arm (see note immediately above).
- **Centreline:** At the end of the movement, the centreline of the body will be approximately between the two hands (i.e. if you are standing at 11.00 and looking at someone in this position, his centreline will be facing you (although this does depend upon the flexibility of his waist) and his hands will be on either side of that centreline).
- **'Closing':** There should be a feeling of the chest closing as you arrive at the left corner. Notice how the elbows are starting to move together.
- **Variation:** Some practitioners turn the left palm outwards during this movement, others turn the palm to face inwards.

    Both have advantages/disadvantages; if you are defending a push/strike from 1.00 using your left forearm/elbow, the palm turned inwards is better as there is more of a feeling of 'Péng' formed in the arm; this is also true if you are feeling the movement as a pull from 3.00.

However, if you want more power in a deflection to an attack from, say, 11.00 (i.e. slightly to your left and behind you), then the palm away method is better.

It all depends on where you want to place the energy in the arm at any specific time.

- **Testing:** It's easy to feel the difference when testing the movement with a partner.
  - Have your partner stand at 1.00 and push your left elbow and forearm with both hands.
  - Then try with your partner gently pulling your arm from 3.00.
  - Then try with your partner gently pushing your left elbow from 1.00.

    In all cases, try both methods, i.e. with the palm turned inwards and then outwards.

    My personal preference is to have the palm facing inwards as it's easier to relax the shoulder.

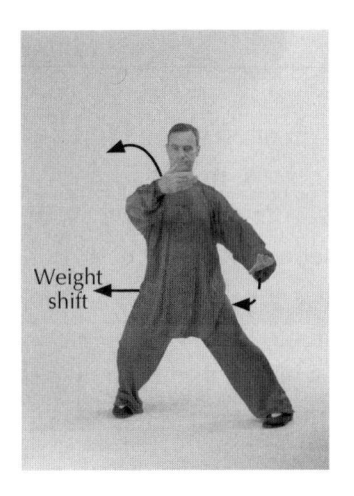

BRIEF 3
Change hands; weight central (temporarily).

DETAILS
'Change hands' (in this text) means that the left hand, having been the higher of the two at shoulder-height, now drops, and the right hand rises. At the same time the weight starts to shift back on to the right foot.

The rising hand (the right hand) lifts up the front of the body, opposite the buttons or zipper of your jacket (the midline). It lifts to throat-height (with palm facing you).

At the same time, the left hand has a feeling of almost pushing away to the left diagonal whilst the left arm sinks to approximately 45° on your left side.

Simultaneously, the weight starts to shift back on to the right foot to approximately 50/50 between the two feet.

THE YANG TÀIJÍ 24-STEP SHORT FORM

The eyes stay at the same height and then start to follow the right hand as it reaches shoulder-height.

NOTES

- **The left arm:**
  - Continue to turn the left palm away.
  - To lower the left arm, feel the weight of the left elbow sinking.
  - Coordinate the sinking of the arm with the transfer of weight.
- **The right hand:** The fingertips lead the right hand upwards, rather than the palm or wrist.
- **The hips/pelvis/tailbone/coccyx** should be tucked under throughout.
- **The feet** do not move but you can start to free the left foot.

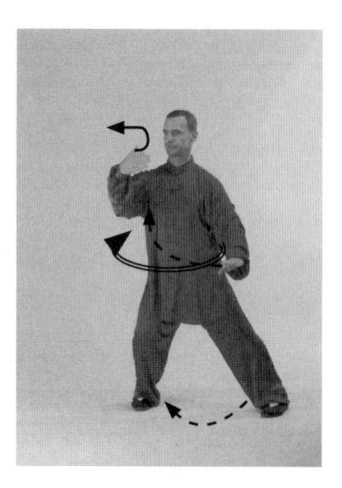

BRIEF 4

Weight on the right foot; hands move to the right side.

DETAILS

Continue to move the weight on to the right foot.
  As you do so, turn your waist towards 1.00.
  The right hand moves to the right corner with the turn of the waist, the palm starting to rotate outwards as your hand reaches the 1.00 corner – but not as yet completely rotated.
  Your left hand moves with the turn of the waist towards the right side of your body at waist/pelvis height.
  The eyes look beyond the right hand.

NOTES

- **The movement of the arms** comes from the turn of the *waist*; avoid moving the arms independently.
- **Method of lowering the left arm:**
  - Use the turn of the hips to move the left arm.

- The lowering of the left arm is done by first sinking the elbow, then the wrist, and then finally by dropping the fingertips; there is a feeling of the tips of the fingers leading the left hand only at the end – particularly as the hand starts to lift in the movement that follows.

- Keep the left hand fairly close to the body, and the arm very relaxed.

- **The right arm:**

  - The right elbow shouldn't drop any further as you turn from the left side (11.00) to the right side (1.30). Keep the forearm at approximately 45°.

  - As you reach the left 1.00 'corner', allow the right elbow to relax and sink, simultaneously starting to rotate the palm outwards.

- **Centreline:** At the end of the movement, the centreline of the body will be approximately between the two hands (i.e. if you are standing at 12.00/1.00 and looking at someone in this position, his centreline will be facing you (although this does depend upon the flexibility of his waist) and his hands will be on either side of that centreline).

- **'Closing':** There should be a feeling of the chest closing as you arrive at the right corner. Notice how the elbows are starting to move together.

- **Waist and hip turn:**

  - In Brief 2 the hips moved the arms; in this movement the hips have very little movement but the waist has more control over the movement of the arms.

  - Keep the hips/tailbone/coccyx tucked under as you turn the waist.

- **The left foot:** As you turn the waist towards 1.00 free the left heel allowing it to move inwards as needed.

THE YANG TÀIJÍ 24-STEP SHORT FORM

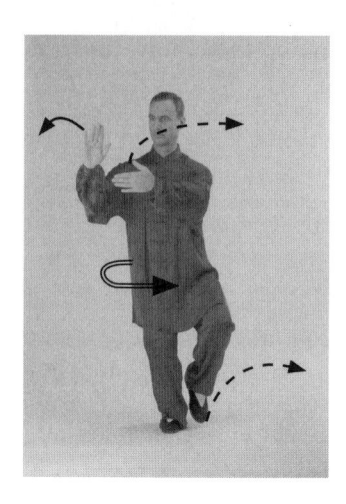

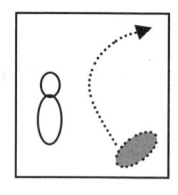

Brief 5
Left hand rises; left foot in; push right hand.

Details
Raise the left hand up your shirt-buttons/zipper (midline) to approximately heart height with the left palm facing you.

Simultaneously the right palm, still facing the corner, extends towards 1.00.

Draw the left foot into the right foot in a T-step (but see Notes below).

The eyes look along the right arm.

Notes

- **Coordination:**

  - The outwards rotation of the right palm coordinates with the sinking of the right elbow, and the extension of the right arm.

  - Feel the rising left elbow and left knee working together.

- **The left hand:**

  - The fingertips lead the hand upwards, rather than the palm or wrist.

  - When lifting the left arm avoid over-lifting the elbow.

- **The shoulders** should be relaxed.

- **The hips** start to turn to the left.

- **The left foot:** It isn't essential to bring the left foot completely into the right ankle, but for beginners it is good practice to do so.

  The reason for not doing so is that your energetic intention is to 9.00. That this is weakened by bringing the foot in is easily felt if a partner gently pushes your left upper arm/shoulder as you do Briefs 4 to 6.

- **The body 'closes'** prior to the 'opening' in the movement that follows. Pull in the lower abdominal muscles; sink the elbows, rotating them slightly inwards.

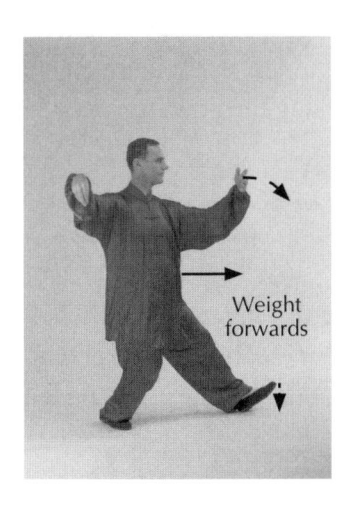

BRIEF 6
Bunch and hook; left hand rises; left heel steps.

DETAILS
Bunch the fingers and thumb of the right palm together, and hook the bunched fingers downwards bending at the wrist into a 'crane's beak'.
  Lift the left fingertips a little higher.
  Place the left heel towards 9.00, widening your step.
  The body turns further to your left (the left arm therefore moving leftwards also).
  Eyes follow the direction of the left hand.

NOTES

- **The left hand:** Sink the left elbow as you raise the left hand, but maintain a feeling of Péng in the arm.

  Coordination: Feel the left elbow and left knee working together.

- **The right wrist** remains at shoulder-height.

- **Crane's beak:**

  - The fingers of the right hand should be bunched together so that the tips of the fingers and thumb are together. The fingers should be firmly pulled back towards the elbow, stretching the back of the wrist.

  - In application the bunching and hooking of the right hand should be done during the next movement (as you move the weight on to the left foot). If it is done at this point, the application is not so effective – the grasp of the opponent's right arm (the bunch and hook) and the left arm/body strike should be almost simultaneous.

- **Stepping:**

  - **Width of step:** Although you are stepping to 9.00, the stance needs to be widened to somewhere between 4–8 inches (10–20 cm) wide. Therefore when stepping, it might feel a little like a diagonal step to 7.30, because of trying to widen the stance.

- **The right knee:** Keep the right knee over the right toes; beginners tend to let the knee collapse inwards. It is preferable to feel as though you are stepping with the thigh, i.e. as though you are using the thigh to open the leg, rather than lifting the foot out sideways.

- **'Opening':** The legs are 'opening' at this point.

- **The hips/pelvis/tailbone/coccyx** should stay tucked under as you step.

• **The overall energy of the movement:** The feeling of energy from Briefs 3 to 7 is to 9.00. Although you move to the 1.00 'corner' at Brief 4, you should think *through* the movement to Brief 6. This has a considerable effect on the feel in performance.

• **Relax:** Beginners tend to tense the upper body at this point.

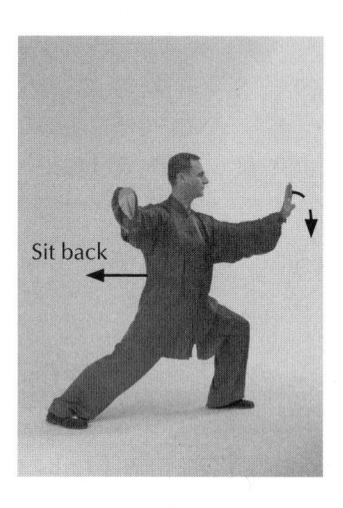

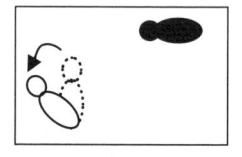

BRIEF 7
Single Whip 单鞭 (Dānbiān).
Weight forwards; left palm to 9.00.

DETAILS
Transfer the weight to the left foot to form a left Bow Stance facing 9.00 and slip the rear heel.

Simultaneously arc the left palm up and over turning the left palm to face 9.00.

The right arm, still with the hand in the crane's beak, remains pointing to 1.00.

The eyes look beyond the left fingertips.

NOTES

• **The left toes** point to 9.00.

• **Slip the rear heel** using the hips to do so.

• **The stance** should be about two fists, 8 inches (20 cm) wide.

• **Angle of body:**

  • The centreline of the body will face approximately 11.00, i.e. at the midpoint between the directions of the arms (which are at 9.00 and 1.00), or at about 45° to the right.

- Because the body is turned to the right, the right arm will not point directly at 12.00, but more towards 1.00. Beginners tend to pull the arm even further back (to 2.00 or 3.00) which lifts both the right scapula and shoulder.
- **The 'feel' of the movement** is of the body trying to slip sideways through a narrow opening.

  There is also a feel of Kào 靠 (shoulder strike) for the left side of the body in the movement.
- **The left hand** gradually rotates palm away as the arm arcs over to 9.00 (but see 'Variations' below).
- **Variations:** There are a number of ways of moving the left arm.
  - Some extend the arm (palm still facing inwards) whilst keeping it parallel to the ground throughout (moving it with the turn of the body). As their arm reaches 9.00, they drop the elbow and turn their palm away.
  - Others turn the body with the arm 'fixed' so it doesn't extend at all; then, as the back of the hand reaches 9.00, they turn the palm to 9.00 and extend the palm outwards in that direction.
  - The **'textbook' version**, and also my personal preference, is to circle the hand upwards so that the fingers go to the height of the top of the head (or higher) and then lower it at the end of the arc so that the tip of the index finger is directly ahead of the tip of the nose (i.e. the same as wrist and shoulder being the same height).

    This latter version makes sense in that 1) it completes the circle begun by the arm in Brief 1, and 2) is part of a circle that continues in the movements that follow.

    It also makes sense from the point of generating power in an application.
- **The left arm:** As you arrive in the posture, the left arm uses 'Àn' – pushing downwards. Feel as though it is not only the hand, but also the elbow and the upper arm pushing down.
- **Height of wrists:** The wrists should finish at the height of the shoulders (although you often see the right wrist held higher – incorrectly in my view).

  An alternative way of looking at the left hand is that the tip of the left finger should be at the height of the tip of your nose.

THE YANG TÀIJÍ 24-STEP SHORT FORM

- **'Open' the knees:** As you arrive in the posture spiral the knees outwards, opening the knees over the toes.

- **Coordinate:**
  - the sinking of both elbows
  - the extension of both arms.

- **The 'feel' of the arms** in the final posture is of the elbows sinking, the arms moving in towards each other, whilst both hands simultaneously push outwards (the right hand still in the crane's beak).

- **Connections:** The elbows and knees should be working together – the knees spiralling outwards, and elbows spiralling inwards.

- **Testing the posture:** Hold the posture and a partner holds your left wrist and pushes directly at your body, and then does the same with the right wrist.

FORM 10: CLOUD HANDS (WAVE/MOVE THE HANDS LIKE CLOUDS)

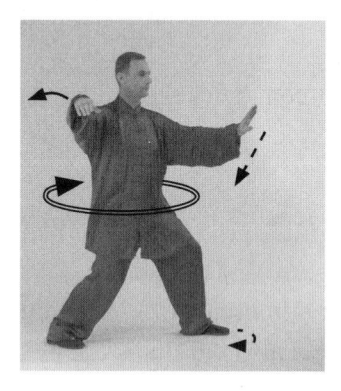

云手 (Yúnshŏu)

BRIEF 1A
Begin to sit back; lower the left hand.

DETAILS
Start to sit back on to your right foot and lower your left hand.

NOTES

- **The left arm:** Sink the elbow to lower it.
- **The right arm:** Relax the right elbow without lowering the arm.

- **Coordinate:**
  - the sinking left arm and the shifting of the weight
  - the left arm and left leg
  - the bending right knee and right elbow
  - feel the elbows working together.

- **'Closing':**
  - **The centre:** Tuck the tailbone/coccyx under.
  - **The upper body:** As the elbows gradually begin to move towards each other, the upper body also starts to close.

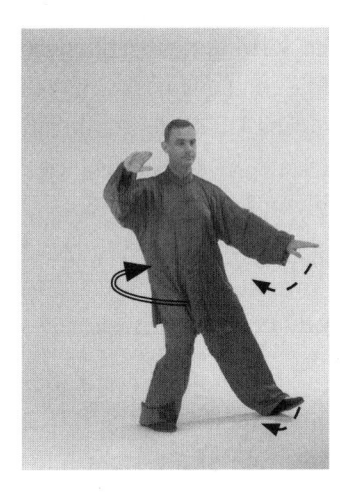

BRIEF 1B

Turn hips to the right; left hand moves right with turn of hips; turn left toes.

DETAILS

With the turn of the hips to the right, the left hand moves to your right.

At the same time, the turn of the hips pivots your left foot 90° on the heel, so that it points to 12.00.

By the end of the move both arms are pointing approximately towards 12.30/1.00.

The right hand has opened, the palm also facing 12.30/1.00.

The left hand is in the process of rising, the palm turned slightly upwards.

The eyes look beyond the right hand.

Because of the angle of the right foot (which continues to point to 10.30), the hips are turned to approximately 11.00 (or further depending upon the flexibility of the practitioner).

The body (waist upwards) is turned towards 12.30/1.00.

This will be referred to as 'corner 1'.

THE YANG TÀIJÍ 24-STEP SHORT FORM

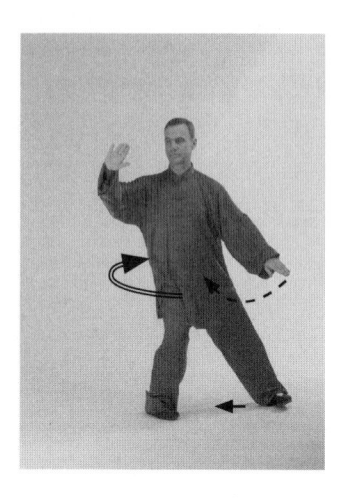

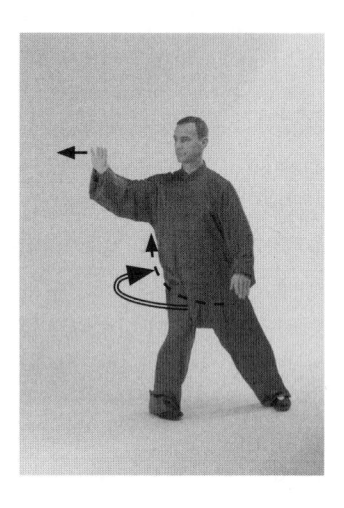

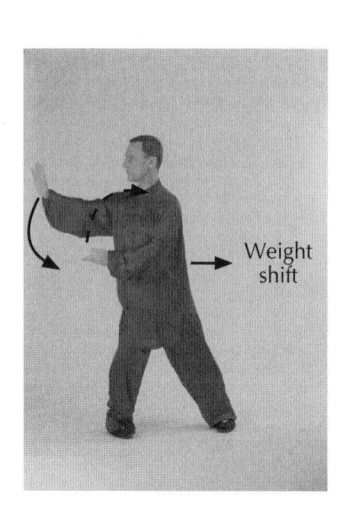

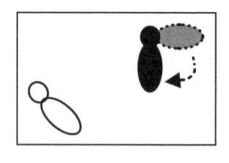

NOTES

- **Turning the left toes:** Use the turn of the hips to move the left toes.

- **Angle of feet:** Because the right foot hasn't moved, the feet will be slightly 'pigeon-toed' at the end of the move.

- **The hands:**

  - As the right hand opens, sink the elbow further; at the same time, the left palm rises.

  - Although it is predominantly the turn of the waist that moves the left hand (the hips are involved to a certain extent), lead the movement with the fingertips (this applies to all lower hand movements in Cloud Hands). This can best be felt if someone hooks his arm through yours as you turn your body, so you have a feeling of pulling him around to your other side – in this case your right side.

- **The tail-bone/coccyx:** Tuck the tail-bone/coccyx firmly under, pulling in the lower abdominal muscles. Because of the angle of the right foot, the right hip/buttock will 'stick out' if not consciously relaxed.

- **The waist** should turn further towards the right 'corner' – beyond the amount that the hips have turned.

- **Turning the body to the right:** Because of the angle of the right foot, the body will be more restricted when turning to the right than in later Cloud Hands 'right corners'.

- **'Closing':** This is the 'Yin' part of the movement; the body is 'closing'.

182

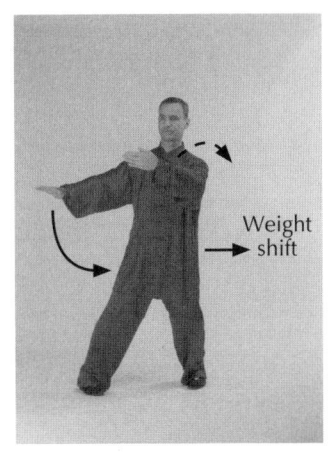

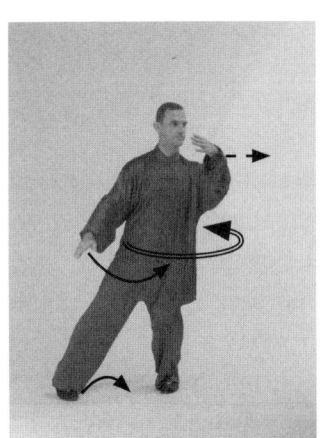

BRIEF 2
Moving into corner 2; change hands; transfer your weight to corner 2.

DETAILS
'Change your hands' by sinking your right elbow/wrist/hand, whilst simultaneously continuing to raise your left hand up the centreline of the body (the left palm will end up facing you at mouth height).

As this happens, move the weight on to your left foot.

As you continue to shift the weight, turn your upper body to your left.

Your left hand, with wrist at throat height, moves across to the left corner with the turn of the body – the palm starting to turn away as it reaches the corner.

Your right hand moves across to your left side with the turn of the body.

This is 'corner 2'.

The eyes follow the turn of the body, i.e. they look to the left corner beyond the left hand.

NOTES

- **The left hand:** The lifting of the left hand comes from the upper arm; but also sink the left shoulder at the same time.

- **The right hand:** Although it is the turn of the waist that moves the right hand, lead the hand movement with the fingertips.

- **The movement of the hands:** It is the turn of the upper body that makes the hands appear to move but, actually, relative to the body, they virtually don't move at all.

- **Coordinate** the sinking/lifting of the right/left arms with the shifting of the weight. There should be a feeling of the arms and legs working together.

- **Angle of pelvis:** Because of the angle of the right foot, the pelvis will be turned slightly to the left corner.

THE YANG TÀIJÍ 24-STEP SHORT FORM

- **The coccyx/tailbone** should be tucked under throughout.
- **The waist:** Turn the upper body from the waist, avoid twisting the hips to the corner.
- **The knees** have a feeling of 'opening' or separating.
- **'Open':** This is the 'Yang' part of the movement; this movement is an 'open' one.

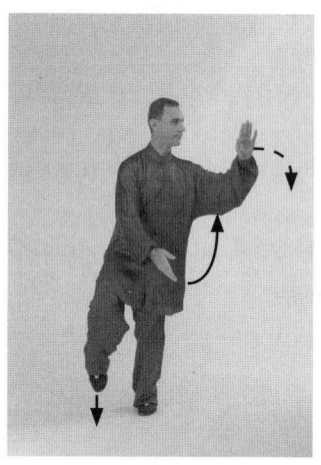

BRIEF 3A

Change your hands; draw the right foot in; weight to middle.

DETAILS

'Change your hands' by sinking your left elbow/wrist/hand, whilst simultaneously continuing to raise your right hand up the centreline of the body (the right palm will end up facing you at mouth height).

As this happens, lift your right foot in alongside your left foot (about one fist's distance between the feet – see note on 'Connections' below).

The eyes follow the upper hand.

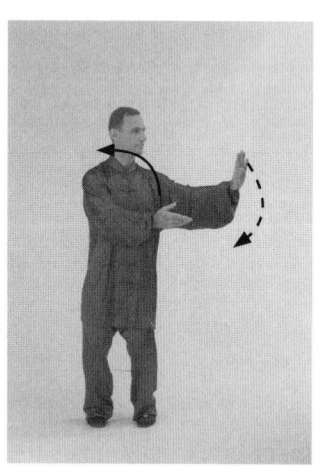

NOTES

- **Connections:**
    - There is a connection between the right leg and the sinking left arm; the two need to work together; the 'feel' is that the sinking arm brings the right foot in – alongside the left foot.

        (Alternatively you could look at it as though the rising right hand is bringing the foot in – the right elbow and right knee working together. It's not too important which

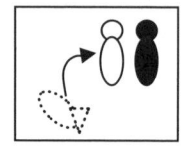

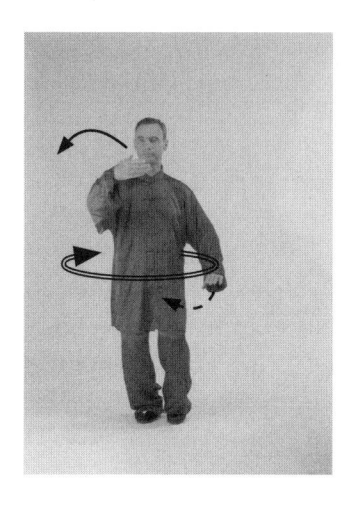

DESCRIPTION OF THE YANG TÀIJÍ 24-STEP SHORT FORM

way you view it; what is important is that the upper and lower are coordinated.)

- **Method of foot movement:** In addition to the above, feel the connection between the sinking of the left hand and the transfer of the weight. Sinking the left hand helps to fully transfer the weight on to the left foot enabling the right foot to move.

- **The feet** should now be parallel with the toes pointing to 12.00.

- **Distance between the feet:** When the right foot has stepped inwards, the gap is 4–8 inches (20–30 cm) wide.

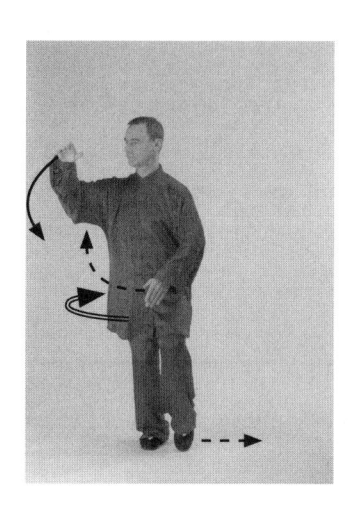

BRIEF 3B
Moving into corner 3; turn right.

DETAILS
Transfer your weight on to your right foot, turning your body to your right.
With the turn of the waist to the right, the left hand moves to the right (at pelvis/waist height).
The right hand, at throat height, passes across to your right with the turn of the body, the palm turned away by the time it has reached the 1.30 corner.
The eyes follow the right hand.

NOTES

- **The feet** do not move.

- **The pelvis** is square to 12.00; the upper torso has turned to 1.00, turning from the waist.

- **The coccyx/tailbone** is tucked under.

- **The weight** is firmly on the right foot.

- **'Closing':** This is the 'Yin' part of the movement; the body is 'closing'.

185

THE YANG TÀIJÍ 24-STEP SHORT FORM

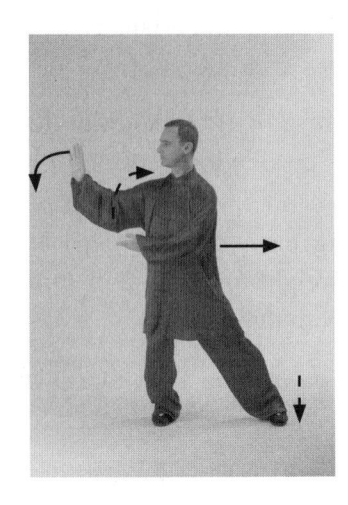

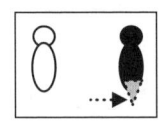

BRIEF 4A
Change hands; left foot step.

DETAILS

'Change your hands' by sinking your right elbow/wrist/hand, whilst simultaneously continuing to raise your left hand up the centreline of the body (the left palm will end up facing you at approximately mouth height).

Step sideways to 9.00 with the left toes without placing the left heel.

By the end of the move both arms will be between your centreline and 1.00.

The waist is turned towards 1.00 ('corner 3').

The eyes look beyond the right hand.

NOTES

- **Step with the left toes:** Traditional Yang 108-Step Form steps with the heel; the modern forms tend to step with the toes. The main advantage when teaching beginners is that it stops them from putting any weight on to the left foot, i.e. from transferring the weight too early.

- **Connections:**

    - There is a connection between the left leg and the sinking right arm; the two need to work together; the 'feel' is that the sinking arm causes the left foot to step out.

        (Alternatively you could look at it as though the rising left hand is working with the sideways step of the left foot – the left elbow and left knee working contrary to each other. It's not too important which way you view it; what is important is that the upper and lower are coordinated.)

    - **Method of foot movement:** In addition to the above, feel the connection between the sinking of the right hand and the transfer of the weight. Sinking the right hand helps to fully transfer the weight on to the right foot enabling the left foot to move.

- **Number of steps:** This is the first step out of two sideways steps with the left foot.

- **The pelvis** is square to 12.00.
- **The coccyx/tailbone** should be tucked under.

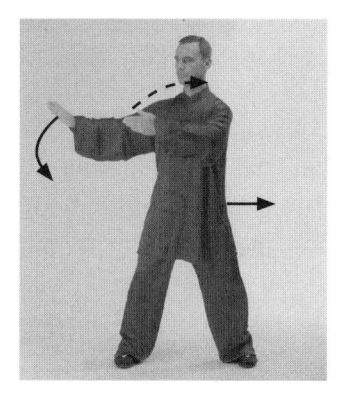

BRIEF 4B

Moving into corner 4; transfer your weight to the left foot.

DETAILS

Place the left heel on the ground with the toes pointing to 12.00, and move the weight back on to the left foot.

There is no foot movement between these two corners.

The eyes look beyond the left hand.

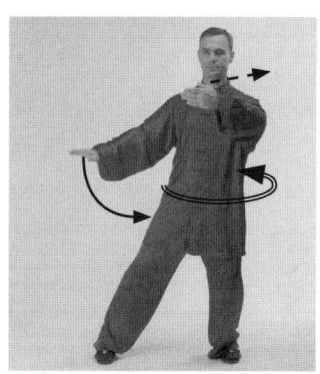

NOTES

- **The feet** are parallel.
- **The pelvis** is square to 12.00; the upper torso has turned to 11.00, turning from the waist.
- **The coccyx/tailbone** should be tucked under.
- **The knees** have a feeling of 'opening' or separating.
- **'Opening':** This is the 'Yang' part of the movement; this is an 'open' movement.

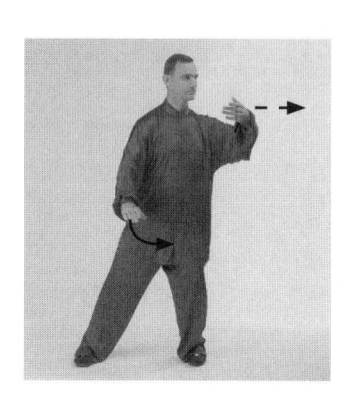

THE YANG TÀIJÍ 24-STEP SHORT FORM

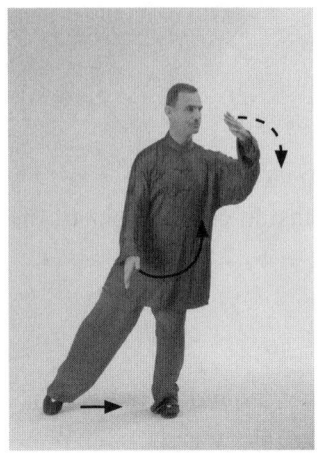

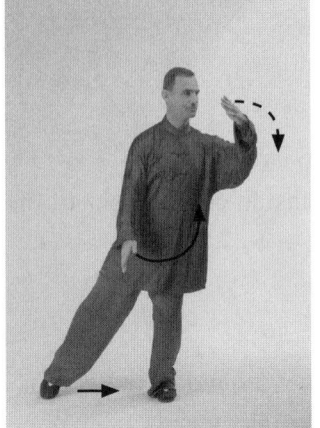

Brief 5a

Change your hands; draw the right foot in; weight to middle.

Details

'Change your hands' by sinking your left elbow/wrist/hand, whilst simultaneously continuing to raise your right hand up the centreline of the body (the right palm will end up facing you at mouth height).

As this happens, lift your right foot in alongside your left foot.

The eyes follow the upper hand.

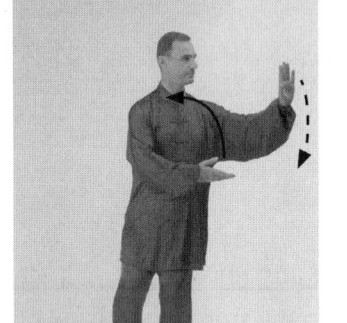

Notes

- As for Brief 3a on p.184.

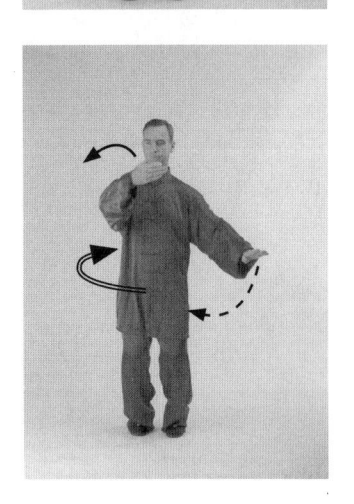

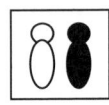

188

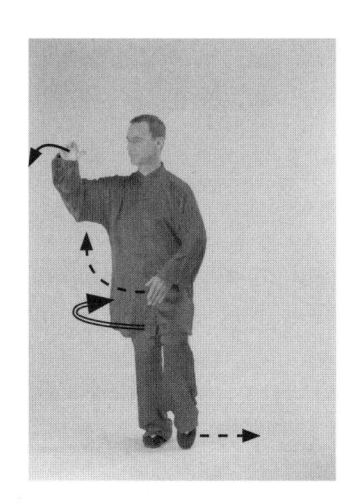

BRIEF 5B
Moving into corner 5; turn right.

DETAILS
Transfer your weight on to your right foot, turning your body to your right.

With the turn of the waist to the right, the left hand moves to the right (at pelvis/waist height).

The right hand, at throat height, passes across to your right with the turn of the body, the palm turned away by the time it has reached the 1.30 corner.

The eyes follow the right hand.

NOTES

- As for Brief 3b on p.185.

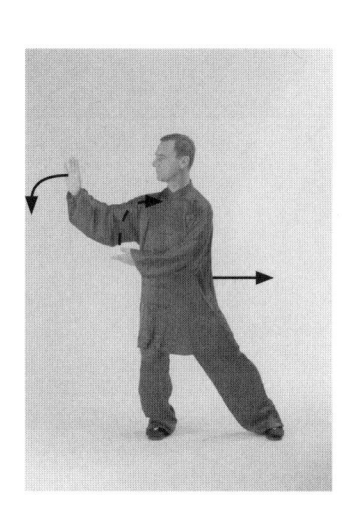

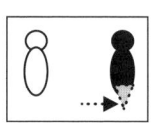

BRIEF 6A
Change hands; left foot step.

DETAILS
'Change your hands' by sinking your right elbow/ wrist/hand, whilst simultaneously continuing to raise your left hand up the centreline of the body (the left palm will end up facing you at approximately mouth height).

Step sideways to 9.00 with the left toes without placing the left heel.

By the end of the move both arms will be between your centreline and 1.00.

The waist is turned towards 1.00 ('corner 5').

The eyes look beyond the right hand.

NOTES

- As for Brief 4a on p.186.

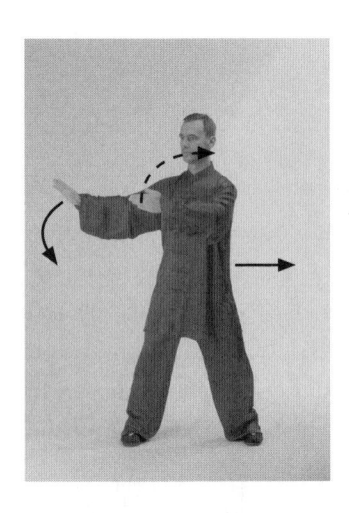

BRIEF 6B

Moving into corner 6; transfer your weight to the left foot.

DETAILS

Place the left heel on the ground with the toes pointing to 12.00, and move the weight back towards the left foot.

There is no foot movement between these two corners.

The eyes look beyond the left hand.

NOTES

- As for Brief 4b on p.187.

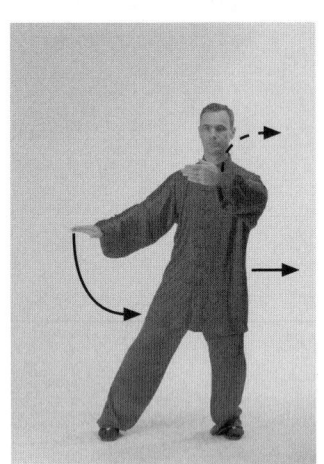

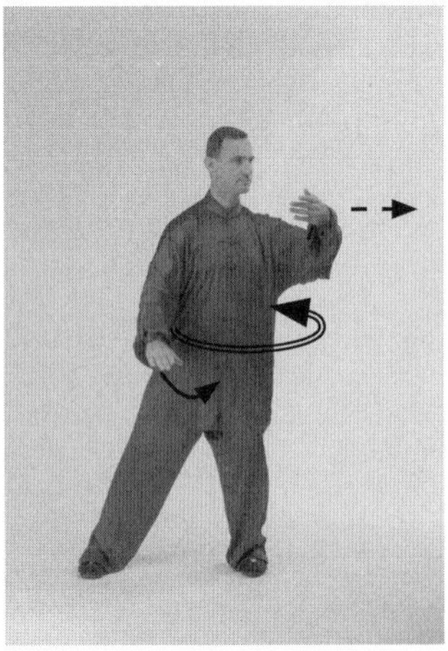

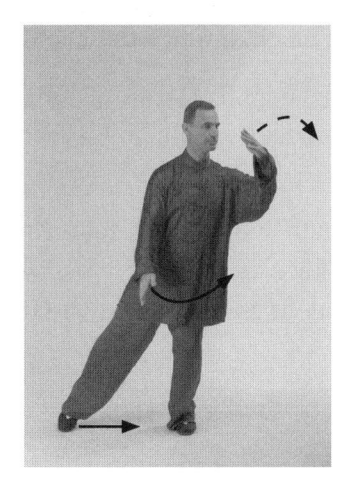

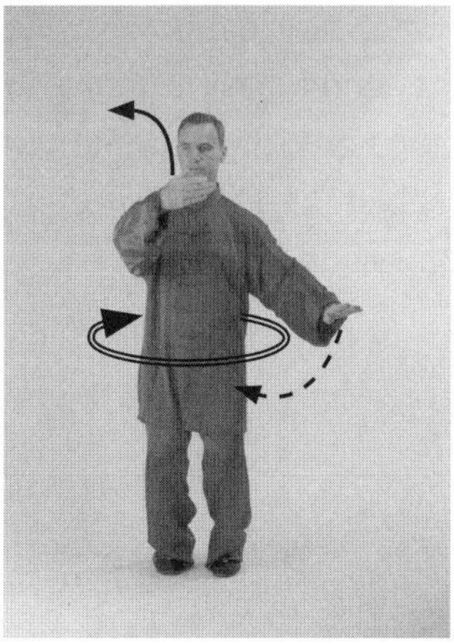

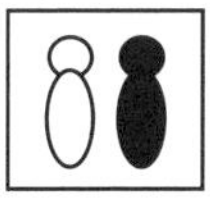

DESCRIPTION OF THE YANG TÀIJÍ 24-STEP SHORT FORM

BRIEF 7
Change your hands; draw the right foot in; weight to middle.

DETAILS
'Change your hands' by sinking your left elbow/wrist/hand, whilst simultaneously continuing to raise your right hand up the centreline of the body (the right palm will end up facing you at mouth height).

As this happens, lift your right foot in alongside your left foot, and then transfer your weight to between your feet.

The eyes follow the upper hand.

NOTES

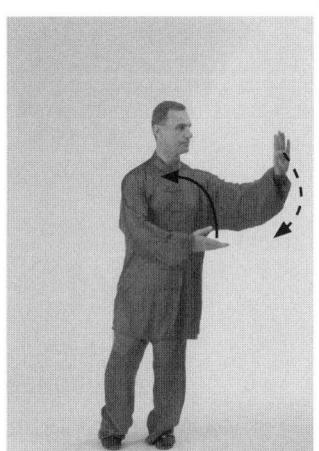

- As for Brief 3a on p.184.

GENERAL POINTS WHEN PERFORMING CLOUD HANDS

- **Body/arm coordination:** The arms don't move independently; the turning of the upper body (from the waist upwards), together with both the shifting of the weight from one foot to the other, and the side stepping makes the arms move.

- **The hips** stay square to 12.00.

- **The stance** is Kāibù 开步 followed by Xiǎokāibù = 小开步. Xiǎo means 'small', so when the feet come together it's a 'small' Kàibù 开步, 'Open Stance'.

- **Stepping method:** When stepping use the concept of 'point, rise; point, fall' and 'rise gently, fall gently' (see p.57).

- **Posture:** Keep the body upright when stepping sideways; avoid 'rocking' the body from left foot to right foot in order to lift and place the foot.

- **Height of body:** The body-centre stays at the same height throughout; avoid 'bobbing' up and down.
- **The feet:** Keep the feet parallel whether stepping inwards with the right foot or outwards with the left foot.
- **The knees:** Keep the knees over the toes throughout Cloud Hands. In other words, when stepping sideways, don't let the right knee collapse inwards towards the left knee; the legs should retain the feeling of an 'upside-down-U' throughout the stepping sequence.

FORM 11: SINGLE WHIP (SINGLE BIĀN)

单鞭 (Dānbiān)

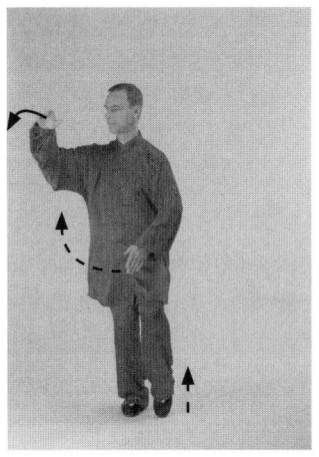

Brief 1
Moving into corner 7; turn right.

Details
Transfer your weight on to your right foot, turning your body to your right.

With the turn of the waist to the right, the left hand moves to the right (at pelvis/waist height).

The right hand, at throat height, passes across to your right with the turn of the body, the palm turned away by the time it has reached the 1.30 corner.

The eyes follow the right hand.

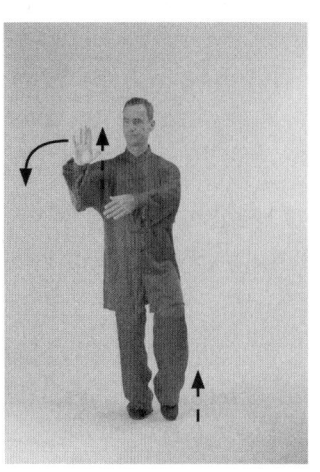

Notes
- As for Brief 3b on p.185.

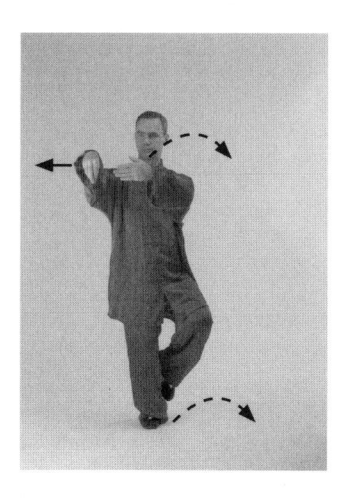

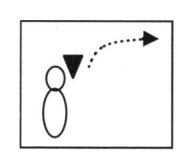

DESCRIPTION OF THE YANG TÀIJÍ 24-STEP SHORT FORM

BRIEF 2
Extend right palm; left hand rises.

DETAILS

This time, instead of pushing *down* with the right hand, extend the right arm by pushing the palm outwards to approximately 1.00, keeping it parallel to the ground.

At the same time, lift the left arm to chest height, with the palm facing your body.

Simultaneously lift the left heel.

The eyes continue to look to 1.00.

NOTES

- **Lifting the left hand:** The fingertips lead the left hand upwards, rather than the palm or wrist. Avoid over-lifting the elbow.

- **Coordination:** Feel the rising **left elbow** and **left knee** working together.

- **The shoulders** should both be relaxed.

- **The hips** start to turn to the left.

- **The weight:** Sink further into the right foot.

- **The coccyx/tailbone** should be tucked under; feel as though you are 'hanging' the sacrum.

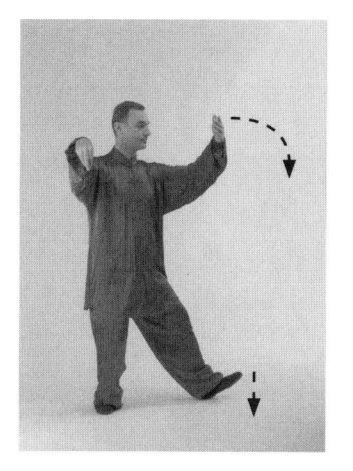

BRIEF 3

Bunch and hook (crane's beak); left hand rises; left heel steps.

DETAILS

Bunch the fingers and thumb of the right palm together, and hook the bunched fingers downwards bending at the wrist into a 'crane's beak'.

Lift the left fingertips higher (the continuation of the left arm circle).

193

THE YANG TÀIJÍ 24-STEP SHORT FORM

Step sideways to 9.00 with the left *heel* widening your step.

The body turns further to your left (the left arm therefore moving leftwards also).

Eyes follow the direction of the left hand.

NOTES

- As for Form 9 (Brief 6) on p.177.

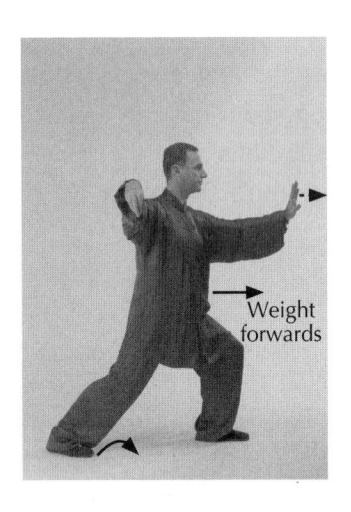

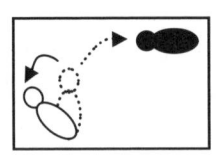

BRIEF 4
Single Whip 单鞭 (Dānbiān).

DETAILS

Complete the transfer of the weight to the left foot to Form a left Bow Stance facing 9.00 and slip the rear heel.

Simultaneously arc the left palm up and over turning the left palm to face 9.00.

The right arm, still with the hand in the crane's beak, remains pointing to 1.00.

The eyes look beyond the left fingertips to 9.00.

NOTES

- As for Form 9 (Brief 7) on p.178.

SECTION 5

(4 MOVEMENTS)

Two are about footwork, one focuses on the palm, and one on the fist.

12. **High Pat on Horse (Pat Horse from on High) (Gauge the Height of the Horse) (Strike the Face with the Palm)**
    高探马 (Gāotànmǎ)

13. **Kick with Right Heel (Separate Right Foot)**
    右蹬脚 (Yòu Dēngjiǎo)

14. **Strike (Opponent's) Ears with Both Fists**
    双峰贯耳 (Shuāngfēng Guàn'ěr)

15. **Turn and Kick with Left Heel (Separate Left Foot)**
    转身左蹬脚 (Zhuǎnshēn Zuǒ Dēngjiǎo)

FORM 12: HIGH PAT ON HORSE (PAT HORSE FROM ON HIGH) (GAUGE THE HEIGHT OF THE HORSE) (STRIKE THE FACE WITH THE PALM)

高探马 (Gāotànmǎ)

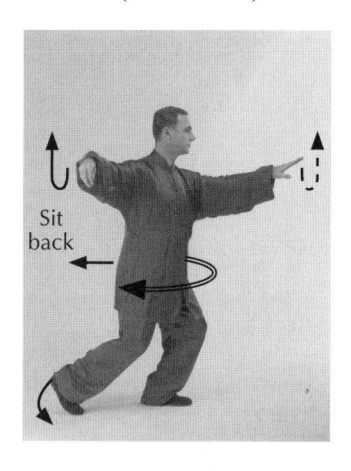

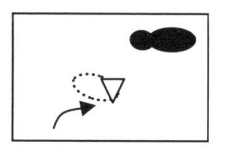

BRIEF 1
Half a pace forwards.

DETAILS
Move the weight over the front foot bringing the right toes half a pace forwards towards the left heel.

Relax the wrists and the right fingers. The hands open at this point (so that both palms face the ground) and then start to rotate palms upwards.

The eyes continue to look beyond the left fingertips.

NOTES

- **Turn of hip:** Use a slight turn of the right hip to 9.00 in order to bring the right toes forwards.

- **The right arm:** Because of the turn of the hip, the right arm will also move towards 12.00.

- **The right foot half-step:** Usually the right foot is only brought in *half* a pace towards 9.00, so it will not move as far forwards as the left heel. This is a little like a Sun style tàijí step.

  Avoid collapsing the right knee inwards as you bring the foot in.

- **The left palm** has a feeling of pushing forwards slightly to 9.00 as you move the weight on to the left foot.

- **'Closing':** The turning upwards of the palms is the start of the 'closing' of the arms; therefore feel both elbows starting to rotate downwards/inwards.

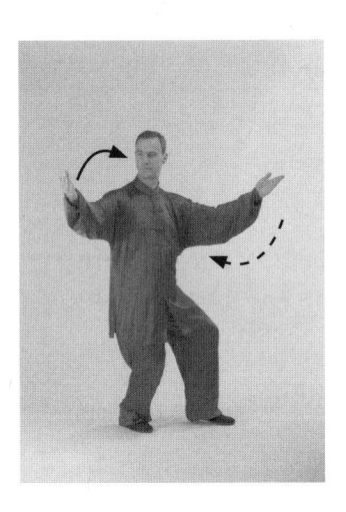

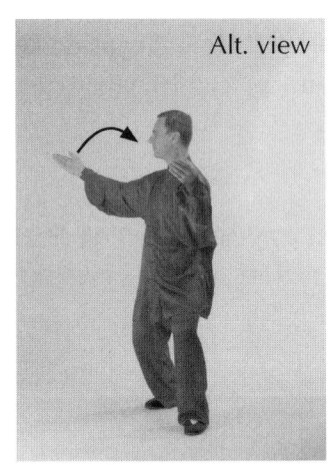

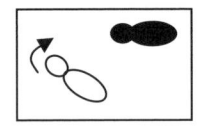

BRIEF 2
Sit back; fold the right arm; the eyes look towards your right hand, and then back to 9.00.

DETAILS

As you sit back on to the right foot, turn your centreline to your right, adjusting the right heel so that the foot points towards 10.30.

The right hand bends at the elbow, the wrist moving towards the centreline at shoulder-height – see 'The right arm' note on the following page.

The eyes look towards your right hand, and then follow the right hand as it moves back towards the body.

Notes

- **Beginner's left arm method:**
  Leave the left hand where it is – pointing to 9.00 with the palm upwards.

- **Turning the centre to the right** is important as it affects the movement of the arms in the more advanced method of 'circling' the arms (see 'Variation - left arm' on the following page).

- **The right arm:**

  - When you 'fold' the right arm, sink the elbow; otherwise the shoulder tends to lift.

  - The arm can move into a position almost vertical in front of your chest with the palm facing 6.00 (i.e. the little finger edge pointing to 9.00).

  - When folding the right arm, think of folding the hand towards the centreline, as in both Brush Knee and Twist Step (Form 4), and Repulse Monkey (Form 6).

- **Continuing to 'close':**

  - The elbows starting to move together is the upper body closing further; feel the contraction of the elbows as they move inwards towards each other.

  - The torso is also 'closing' as you sit back on to the right foot, tucking the coccyx/tailbone under and gently pulling in the lower abdominal muscles.

  - Coordinate torso and arms: The 'closing' comes from the dāntián and not from the upper body alone.

- **The left foot** does not have to move at this stage.

- **The knees** spiral 'open'; open both Kuà.

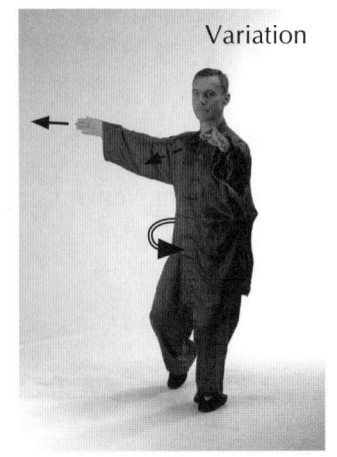

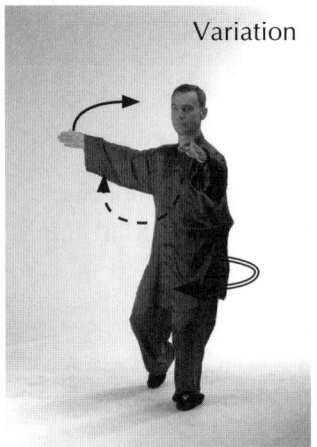

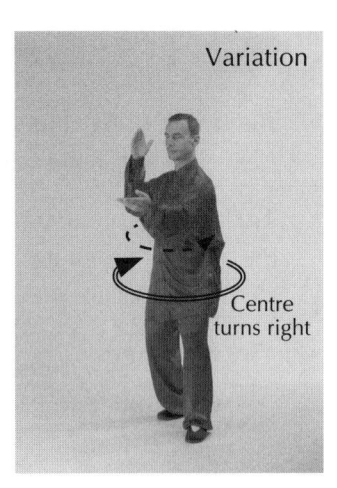

- **Variation – left arm:**

    As the centreline is in the process of turning to the right, this means that the left arm will not be left pointing to 9.00 but will start to circle (horizontally) towards 10.00/11.00. Make sure that the centreline of the body is midway between the two arms.

    When this happens, there is a feeling of the elbows starting to move together (see Notes on the previous page).

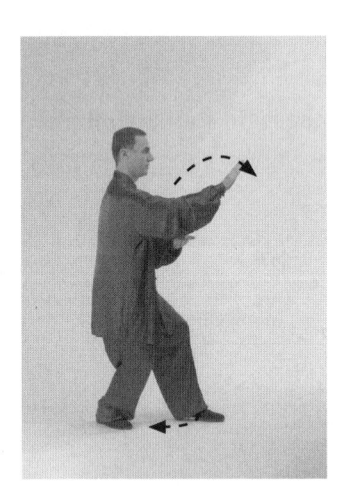

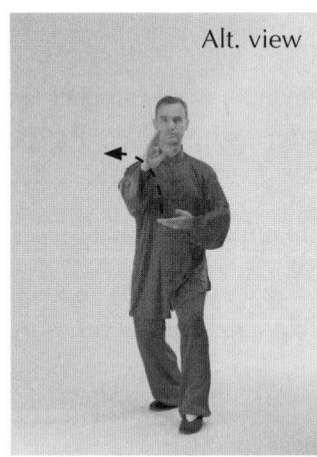

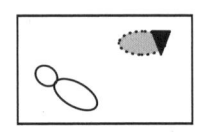

BRIEF 3
Push/pull; adjust left toes into centreline if necessary.

DETAILS
Push the little finger edge of your right hand towards 9.00 (the right fingers fairly vertical) and then turn the palm to face away as you complete the movement (but see note 'The right hand' on the following page).

The left hand continues its horizontal circle to finish palm up to the left of, and just below the level of, your right elbow, and directly ahead of your centreline (i.e. between your body and 9.00).

As the hands arrive in their final position, move your left toes into the centreline (without bringing them back towards the right foot first) in an Empty Stance – the heel off the ground (but see note 'The left toes' below).

The hips are square to 9.00, the waist has turned slightly to the left (the centreline towards 8.00) and the weight is still on the right foot.

The eyes look beyond the right hand (see note below).

NOTES

- **The right hand:** The vertical little finger edge (the hypothenar eminence) pushes towards 9.00, but the palm turns away towards the end of the push. This has the effect of moving the push out to 10.00, which creates a smooth transition into Form 13. (See 'Variation' photo to the right.)

  Variation

- **Height of the right hand:** Bearing in mind that the alternative name for this Form is 'Strike the Face with the Palm', the right hand is therefore fractionally higher than in Repulse Monkey.

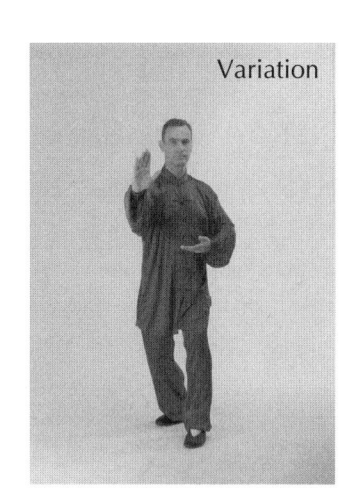

- **The left hand:** As the shoulders turn slightly to your left, the left hand will automatically move backwards. Be conscious of a small anti-clockwise circle with this hand which makes the connection to the next movement.

- **The left toes:** It is not essential to move them. Whether you do or not depends upon the width of your stance. What is important though is the *ability* to move them – i.e. there should be very little weight on them.

- **The eyes:** Because the push will move out to 10.00 (see 'The right hand' above), the eyes will follow the right hand.

- **Hips/upper body angles:** The hips are square to 9.00, but the waist is turned slightly to the left. There is a slight feeling in this posture of an archer drawing a bow.

- **Comparison to Repulse Monkey:** This posture has a very similar feel to Repulse Monkey 2 and 4. The main differences are 1) the position of the

THE YANG TÀIJÍ 24-STEP SHORT FORM

left hand (being ahead of the centreline of the body in this Form, rather than ahead of the left or right hip in Repulse Monkey), and 2) the opposite foot to the hand is forwards (in Repulse Monkey the foot and hand on the same side are both forwards).

- **The coccyx/tailbone** should be tucked well under; the lower abdominals should be pulled in, i.e. close the centre and sink into the right foot.

FORM 13: KICK WITH RIGHT HEEL (SEPARATE RIGHT FOOT)

右蹬脚 (Yòu Dēngjiǎo)

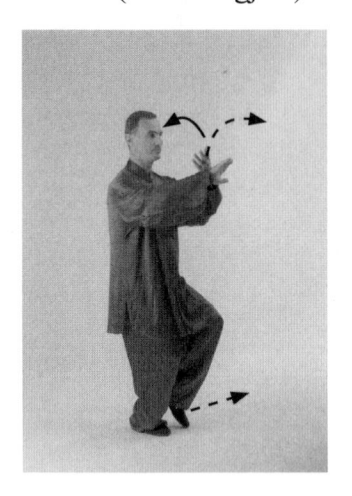

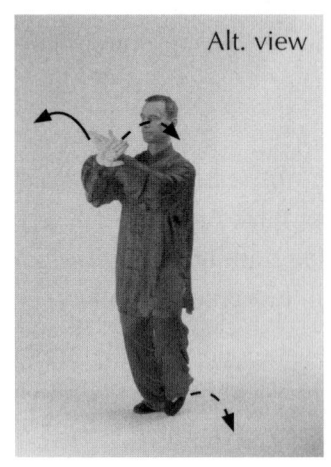

BRIEF 1
Relax right wrist; slide left palm over the top; left foot in towards the right foot.

DETAILS
Turn your left hip to the right so that your centreline turns towards 10.00/10.30 where you have just been kicking.

The right arm changes angle from being vertical to almost horizontal; i.e. push down with the right hand, but don't lower the elbow too far.

Slide your left hand, with palm up, over the right wrist so that the backs of the wrists touch. Aim the fingertips towards 10.00/10.30.

Start to raise the left foot prior to stepping.

At the end of this part of the move, the backs of your wrists are crossed.

The eyes look beyond the left fingertips to 10.00/10.30.

NOTES

- **Turning the hips:** It is the turn of the hips/centre to the right that moves the left arm and hand; feel a connection between the left hip and the left elbow.

- **The crossing of the hands:**

    The left hand: When sliding the left wrist over the right wrist, there should be a feeling of the fingers of the left hand leading as though to strike to an opponent's throat at 10.00/10.30. In other words, keep some direction and intention in the movement.

    The right hand: In application the alteration of angle of the right arm can be a push downwards.

- **Left foot variations:** Some practitioners do not bring the left foot into the right ankle, but they just free the foot so that there is no weight on it. (This is my personal preference, and this is followed in the next move by stepping directly to 8.00 or 9.00.)

    Whether you do or don't bring the foot in depends entirely upon the way that you are using the application – in other words, is someone's foot in the way or not that causes you to step around it?

    What *is* important is that the foot is completely 'free' so that either option is available. For example see the photo above.

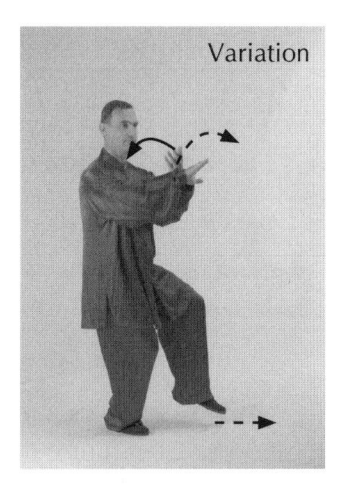

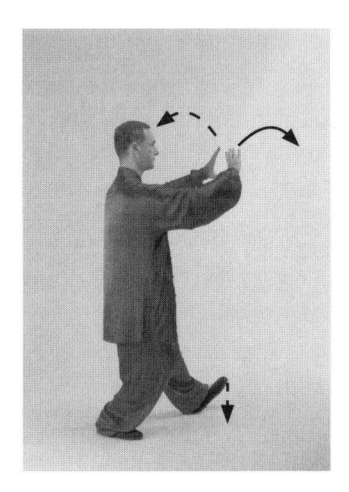

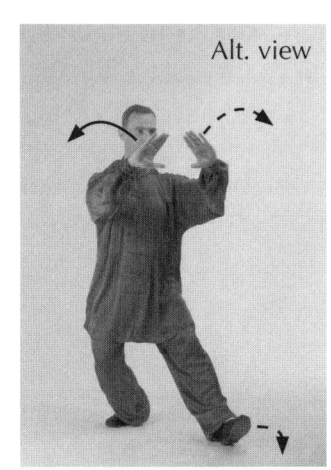

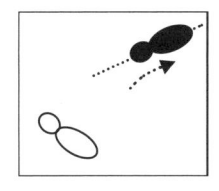

Variation

Alt. view

BRIEF 2
Place the left foot; start to lift hands and turn the left palm.

Details

Keeping the weight on your left foot, turn the body left and place your left heel to about 8.00 with the toes raised.

The crossed hands move around to 8.00 with the turn of the body; the hands lift to face height and begin to rotate and separate, the left palm to face away (with the wrists still crossed at throat height).

Keep the weight on the right foot.

The eyes follow the left hand.

Notes

- **There are a number of problems with this movement:**

  - **Posture:** Be careful that you don't tilt the pelvis as you turn.

  - **Balance** can be an issue on the turn. This is helped if you are aware of your posture and tuck your tailbone under as you turn, sinking slightly further into the right foot.

  - **Turn-out:** This movement is very difficult for those practitioners without good turn-out. It requires a turn-out of the thighs of 90° (something that most people, whether beginners or experienced, find difficult); inevitably, the backside sticks out, the right knee collapses inwards, and the balance becomes a major issue.

- **Variation using a different angle of body:** Some practitioners like to keep the body/chest turned to 10.00 as they step to 8.00.

  The advantage of this method is that it eradicates almost all of the above problems.

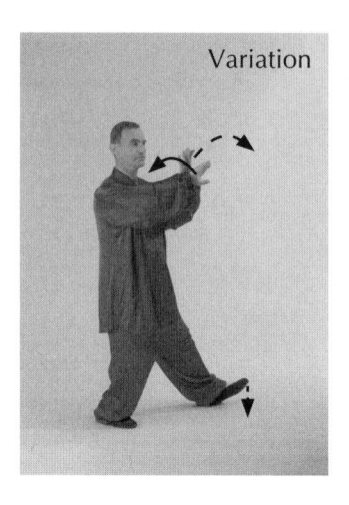

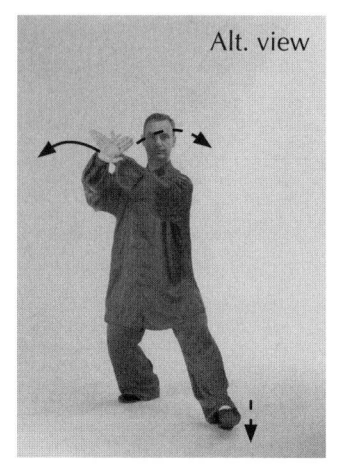

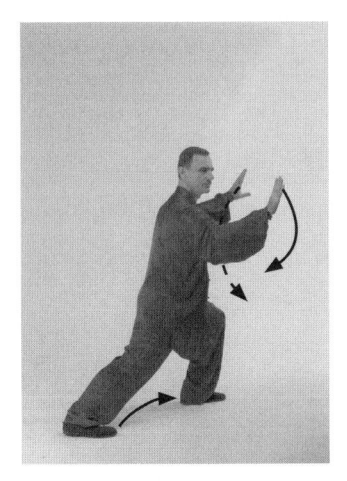

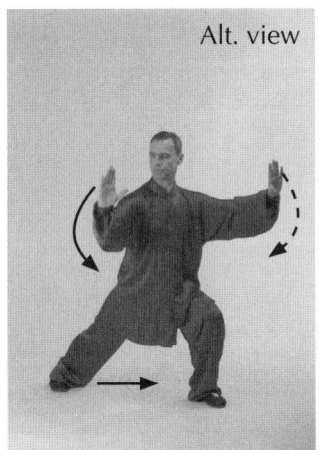

DESCRIPTION OF THE YANG TÀIJÍ 24-STEP SHORT FORM

Alt. view

BRIEF 3
Weight forwards; arms open equally to either side.

DETAILS
Place the left toes pointing at 7.30/8.00 (but also see 'Variations' on p.204), and move your weight on to your left foot (moving into a Bow Stance).

Keeping the centreline facing 7.30/8.00, arc your arms slightly upwards and then outwards and back downwards to shoulder height (the arms to 6.00 – left arm, and 10.00 – right arm, approximately). Sink your weight into your left foot as the arms open to parallel to the ground.

Finish the movement with the eyes looking beyond your right hand.

NOTES

- **The left foot:** The correct angle of the foot when placing the left toes determines the difficulty of the kick that follows. If you place the toes to 8.00 (rather than to 7.30), it makes the kick slightly easier in that the pelvis doesn't have to open as wide.

  With this method you can slip your rear heel as your weight transfers to your left foot.

- **The arms:**

Opening the arms: The 'arcing' of the hands/arms shouldn't be too excessive. There is a feeling of pushing the fingertips upwards as you separate them; the fingertips shouldn't lift much above the head. As you open the arms, gradually rotate the palms so that, by the time that the arms are open, the palms have turned outwards.

Compare the circling of the left arm as you move into the final posture of Single Whip, the arm movement of which is identical in feel but with only a 'single' arm.

Applications:

- This can be used as a shoulder-barge (Kào) with the front of the right shoulder (the area of the anterior deltoid muscle).

- The right arm could be thought of as blocking a strike from 10.00.

The open arm position: Beginners find it very difficult to get the feel of the arm position.

The arms should be slightly forwards of the body with the wrists turned outwards at shoulder-height, and most importantly the elbows should be sunk. The fingertips will be lifted, the hand as vertical as possible (therefore the thumb side of the wrist flexed inwards), and the little finger edge of the hand will be furthest from the body.

Body/arms relationship: There should be symmetry between the two arms; the centreline of the body should not point more towards the right arm than the left arm. This is a mistake that beginners often make.

- **Sinking the elbows** will help to relax the shoulders.

- **'Opening':** Over all this is an 'open' position.

- **Variations:**

    1. (Alteration of foot and body angle):

        Step to 7.30, but turn the toes to *9.00*.

        Keep the body facing *10.00/10.30* as you open the arms (the arms to 9.30 – left arm, and 1.00 – right arm, approximately). (See photos on the right of page.)

        Application: This is using the movement as an *upper back* shoulder-barge (Kào) to the 7.30 direction.

        Finish the movement with the eyes looking beyond your right hand.

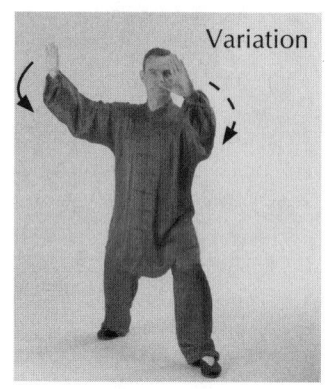

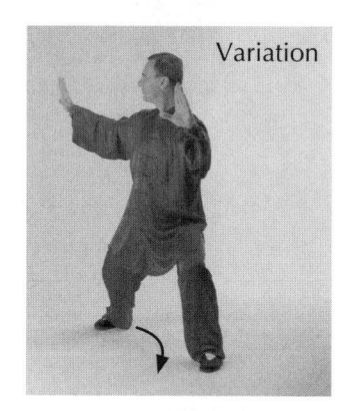

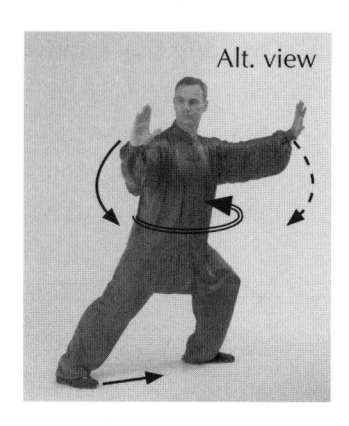

Moving into the next movement: As the weight transfers over the left foot, turn the body to 9.00.

2. (Almost the same as the original description above, but with a slight variation of foot angle):

   Step to 7.30, but turn the toes to *8.00/9.00*.
   Immediately turn the body to 9.00 as you shift the weight forwards on to the left foot. (See photos on p.204.)

   Application: This uses the application 'Kào' to 9.00 using the *front* of the right shoulder.

Comments: My personal preference is for Variation 1. It is martially strong, and seems to have greater practical function than the opening of the arms with the body facing either 7.30 or 9.00 – where a push to the right hand of the practitioner would easily unbalance him.

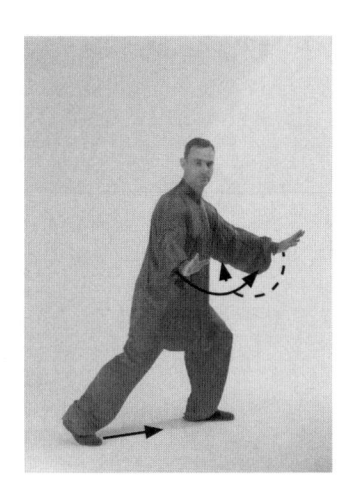

BRIEF 4
Cross hands low; right foot in.

DETAILS
Whichever version you use, turn your centreline to 9.00.

As you do so, continue to circle your hands downwards to cross them at waist height (see Notes below for more details of the hand position).

Simultaneously free your right heel and draw your right foot towards your left foot so that the foot arrives close to the left ankle as the hands cross.

The eyes can either stay facing the 10.00 corner, or can turn to look back to the 7.30/8.00 corner.

NOTES

- **Method of lowering the arms:** Sink the elbows first, gradually rotating them inwards. Continue to rotate them inwards as you sink the wrists, and then lead the fingertips inwards to cross at the wrists. The energy should be in the forearms.

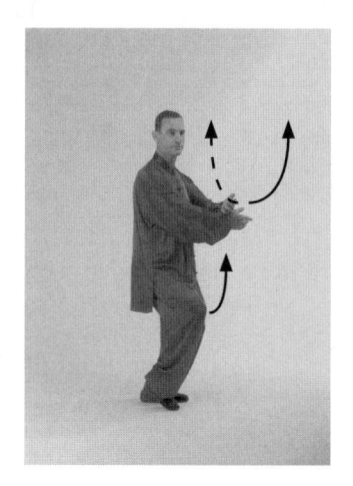

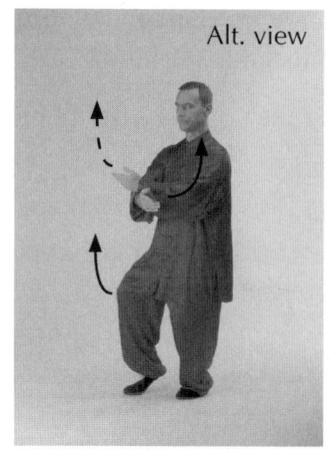

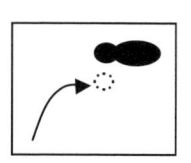

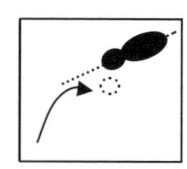

- **The crossing of the hands** causes beginners a few problems. When crossing them in the lower position, hold the right palm in front of your abdomen, and then place the left wrist against the thumb side (radial side) of your right wrist (the left hand will therefore appear to be on top of, or inside the right hand). The palms are not facing the body, nor are they facing the ceiling, they are somewhere in between.

    Do not hold the hands too close to the body; they should be about 8 inches (20 cm) ahead of the waist.

- **The crossed arms:** Keep a space under the armpits – in other words, don't drop the elbows too much – the elbows shouldn't be against the sides of the chest.

- **The left leg** should be bent.

- **The right foot:** Beginners can rest the toes on the floor alongside the left foot.

- **Posture:** Keep the body upright; avoid leaning forwards.

- **The head:** The eyes should be level; avoid dropping the head and looking down – because the hands are dropping, beginners often drop the head at this point.

- **The pelvis** should be relaxed and sunk; gently pull in the lower abdominal muscles, allowing the coccyx/tailbone to tuck under.

- **'Closing':** This is a 'closed' position. Coordinate the upper and the lower. Notice how the elbows and knees work together, in particular the right elbow and right knee.

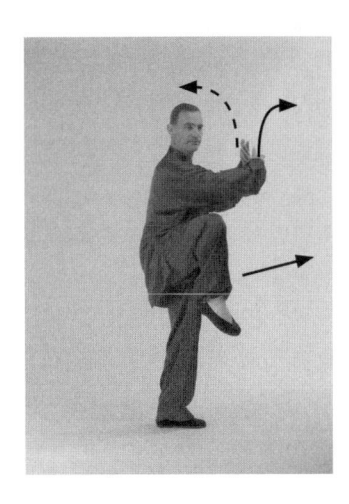

BRIEF 5
Stand up; lift hands and knee.

DETAILS
As you straighten the left leg, raise the right knee.

Lift the crossed hands upwards to in front of your throat. The hands rise up your centreline so that the wrists reach the same height as your shoulders with the right hand on the outside (furthest away from you); the palms should be facing you.

The eyes look between the hands.

NOTES

- **Lifting the hands:** The lifting of the arms and right knee is a little like a puppeteer lifting a puppet's limb – feel as though the elbows are lifting the knee. Keep the hands approximately 4–8 inches (10–20 cm) away from the body as you lift. The knee opens out to point at 10.00/10.30 as it rises.

- **Lift the hands** leading with the fingertips.

- **Pull in the lower abdominal muscles** as you lift the knee; apart from anything else, it helps the raising of the knee by tucking the buttocks under.

- **Variation:** Some practitioners don't lift the knee all the way up at this stage; they make the final lift of the knee as they separate the hands in the next movement.

Comments: This is not a variation that I personally use as I feel that it breaks the connection between the upper and the lower body – the elbows and knees no longer working together in unison.

Brief 6a
Start to separate hands; turn palms; lift the right toes.

Details
Push the fingertips upwards to begin the separation of the hands. As the hands separate, gradually start to turn your palms to face outwards.

Raise your right knee higher (without extending the leg yet) and lift the toes. The eyes start to look towards your right.

Notes

- **Lifting the knee** as high as possible before the kick makes a surprising difference to the height of the kick.
- **The shoulders** should be sunk.
- **Align the right elbow and right knee.**
- **Sink/relax your pelvis** and continue to pull in the lower abdominal muscles as you lift the knee.
- **'Opening':** The body is starting to 'open'.
- **Separation of the arms:** The opening of the arms has the same feel to the movement of the left arm and hand when moving into the final posture of Single Whip (see also note 'Opening the arms' on the following page).

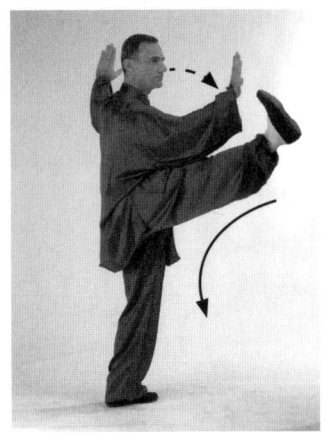

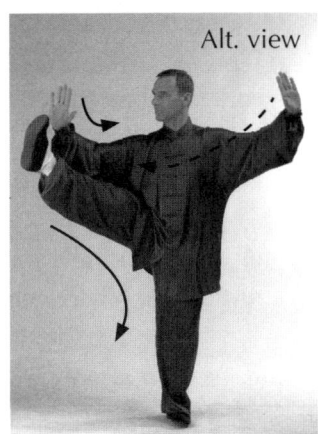

DESCRIPTION OF THE YANG TÀIJÍ 24-STEP SHORT FORM

BRIEF 6B
Open arms and kick.

DETAILS
Continue to separate the arms, arcing them upwards and then outwards, and then downwards so that the wrists arrive at shoulder height.

The right calf extends and kicks with the heel to 10.00/10.30.

The hands arrive in position on either side of you as the kick is completed.

The eyes look in the direction of the kick.

Alt. view

NOTES

- **Dēngjiǎo 蹬脚 (heel kick):** Standing in relaxed fashion on the supporting leg which is slightly bent, raise the other leg bent at the knee, hooking the foot back. With the heel as the power point, slowly press the leg out, extending it naturally with the foot above waist height.

- **The shoulders:** Keep them relaxed – most beginners lift the shoulders when kicking (see note on 'Balance' on the following page).

- **Opening the arms:** The 'arcing' of the hands/arms shouldn't be too exaggerated. There is a feeling of pushing the fingertips upwards as you separate them; the fingertips shouldn't lift much above the head. As you open the arms gradually rotate the palms so that, by the time that the arms are open, the palms have turned outwards.

  Compare the circling of the left arm as you move into the final posture of Single Whip; this arm movement is identical in feel but with only a 'single' arm.

The open arm position: Beginners find it very difficult to get the feel of the arm position.

The arms should be slightly forwards of the body with the wrists turned outwards at shoulder-height, and most importantly the elbows should be sunk. The fingertips will be lifted, the hand as vertical as possible (therefore

209

the thumb side of the wrist flexed inwards), and the little finger edge of the hand will be furthest from the body.

Body/arms relationship: There should be symmetry between the two arms; the centreline of the body should not point more towards the right arm than the left arm. This is a mistake that beginners often make.

- **The right arm** should be on the same line as the right leg.

- **The supporting leg** (on which you are standing) should be straight, neither bent forwards at the knee, nor locked backwards at the knee. Just relax it by relaxing the pelvis and left hip.

- **Timing of kick and arms:** The kick should be timed with the completion of the opening of the arms.

- **The kick** doesn't have to be high. Beginners, and even some experienced practitioners, seem to feel that it is necessary to kick as high as they can at the expense of every other muscle in the body, so they end up leaning backwards and usually losing their balance.

  From a martial point of view, it is much more effective to kick low, for example to an opponent's knee, than higher where the foot can easily be caught.

  If you do want to practise kicking higher, lift the knee as high as you can before extending the calf.

- **The kick and the right hip:** When kicking, the right hip should be relaxed; many practitioners lift it because they are trying to lift the leg with the wrong muscles. Sink the right buttock and gently pull in the lower abdominal muscles; use the pelvic tilt (under-turn of the pelvis) to create the kick. Doing this connects the legs together, enabling the power of one to be supported by the other. Lifting the right hip breaks both the muscular and energetic connection between the legs, as though you are trying to lift one away from the other and use it independently.

- **Balance** can be a problem. This is usually caused by two things, 1) the locking of the pelvis which destabilizes the core of the body, and 2) the lifting of the shoulders as the kick is made, i.e. the qi is lifted.

  It is therefore essential (not only for the balance to be maintained but also for the kick to be effective) that both the upper and lower body are relaxed, the elbows sunk, and that you concentrate on sinking into the foot on which you are standing.

  A good 'trick' that works well is to press the supporting foot downwards as you simultaneously kick outwards.

FORM 14: STRIKE (OPPONENT'S) EARS WITH BOTH FISTS

双峰贯耳 (Shuāngfēng Guàn'ěr)

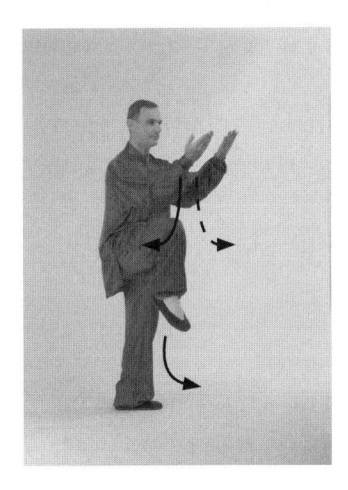

BRIEF 1A
Relax right calf; hands to 10.00/10.30 with palms up; start to bend left knee.

DETAILS
Relax the right calf, but leave the knee raised.
Begin to sink into your left foot by bending the left knee.
Circle the left hand around towards 10.00/10.30, gradually turning both palms to face upwards at shoulder-height.
The eyes look between the hands.

NOTES

- **The hips:** Bring the hips around to face 10.00/10.30. This is important because it correctly gauges the width of the step in Brief 2.

- **The arms** are well extended, a distance of approximately the width of your head between the hands.

- **'Closing':** The body starts to 'close', the elbows rotating inwards, the centre sinking, the tailbone gently tucking under. Both this movement and the one that follows are a continuous process of 'closing'.

  - From the previous movement with the arms open for the kick, there is a gradual inwards rolling of the elbows as the left hand circles around to the 10.00/10.30 corner. The 'closing' of the chest/upper body is easily felt as the elbows move towards each other.

  - At the same time, the dāntián is folding, the leg on which you are standing is beginning to bend; the closing of the lower part of the body is completed in the next movement.

Brief 1b
Continue to bend left knee; lower hands to thighs; begin to extend the right heel.

Details
Continue to bend your left knee, and start to place your right heel towards 10/10.30.

Lower the backs of the hands towards your upper thighs. As the hands arrive in position, they can either be made into loose fists or left as open palms on either side of the hips.

The eyes continue to look in the direction of 10.00/10.30.

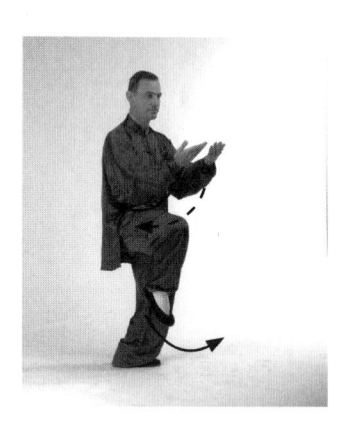

Notes
- **The coordination of the arms and the body** is achieved by feeling the elbows being drawn downwards as a result of the sinking of the hips.

- **Hand position:** Sink the hands towards the upper part of the thighs. Some practitioners take them to the sides of the waist; this is not a method that I personally like as it 1) disconnects the shoulder joints, pulling the shoulders backwards, and 2) the elbows are disconnected from the hips, the elbows moving behind the body.

- **The coccyx/tailbone** should be tucked under, the pelvis relaxed.

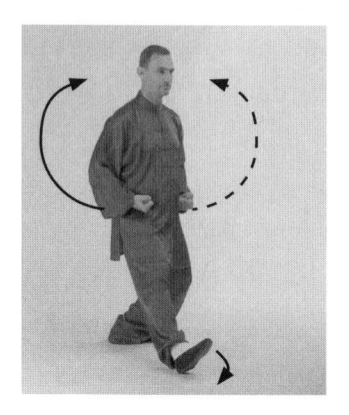

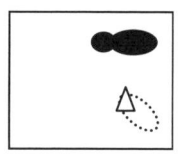

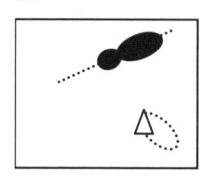

Brief 2
Extend the right foot stepping with the heel; weight forwards; circle fists sideways; strike ears with fists.

DESCRIPTION OF THE YANG TÀIJÍ 24-STEP SHORT FORM

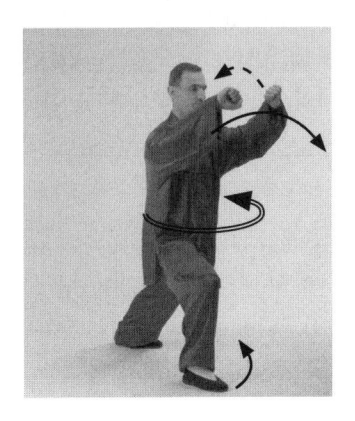

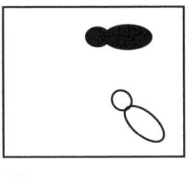

Details

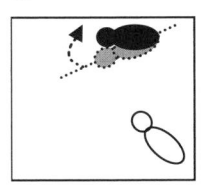

Start to move your weight on to your right foot, the toes pointing to 10.00/10.30. (See the 'Footprints' note below on the options for the placing of the left foot.)

As you do so, circle the fists out on either side of you and, as you continue to shift the weight forwards, the fists continue to rise to the height of your eyes/ears with the palms facing outwards.

At the end of the move, the distance between your fists should be the width of your head.

The eyes look between the fists at the end of the movement.

Notes

- **Footprints:** The variation on the angle of the left foot is determined by how you placed the left foot when stepping in Form 13 (Kick with Right Heel). See pp.201–4 for the placing of the left foot in Form 13.

- **Width of step:** Because the hips are squared to the 10.00/10.30 corner, the step should be a comfortable one that accomodates the width of your hips.

- **Direction of strike:** The right foot and the strike can be to either 10.00 or 10.30.

- **The shoulders:** The final posture of this movement can cause beginners some problems. They quite often find it difficult to lift the fists to eye/ear height whilst simultaneously relaxing the shoulders.

- **Forming the fists:** If the hands are not already in fists, form the fists as you shift the weight forwards.

- **Final arm position:** In the final posture, the elbows should be lower than the wrists. Think of this as a strike to the centre of the head from *underneath* the ears, rather than to either side of the head.

- **Coordination:** Use the coordination of the entire body to drive the fists forwards. This means that you feel the hips being moved forwards by the driving influence of the rear foot pressing into the ground, and as the hips move forwards, the elbows are also propelled forwards.

- **Variations for striking with fists:**

    1. Some practitioners (as they begin to shift their weight forwards on to the right foot) move the arms out sideways with the palms of the fists twisting backwards. The *backs* of the fists therefore lead forwards to the 10.00/10.30 corner before moving together (to a head's width apart).

    2. Some practitioners (as they begin to shift their weight forwards on to the right foot) keep the elbows close to the hips (retaining the feeling of connection between the elbows and the hips) and separate their fists sideways with the palms of the fists still upwards. As the weight shifts forwards, the arms will spiral so that the palms twist outwards.

    Comments: Of the two variations above, my personal preference is for the latter. I feel that there is very little power generated by the former, whereas in the latter it can easily be felt that considerable power is transferred to the fists. The rotation of both arm and centre adds power to the movement; like drilling, it has the power to penetrate.

    Testing: It is easy to do a comparative test of the two striking methods:

    1. Variation 1 above: Have a partner push on the backs of the wrists as you do the striking movement, and

    2. Variation 2 above: Have a partner push on the front of the fists as you do the striking movement.

    The rotating punches: If using the latter of the two striking variations above, this is the first of two spiralling or rotating punches in the 24-Step Form.

- **Generating the power in the punch:** Moving away from the 24-Step Form for a second, if you have your fist (with palm turned upwards) by your hip, and you punch directly ahead whilst simultaneously turning the hips and rotating the palm to face downwards, you have the correct feeling for this movement.

    In the 24-Step Form, all that is necessary is to do the same spiralling movement whilst simultaneously circling the left and right punches out sideways.

- **The eyes (options):** There are a few options for the head/eyes here, although all versions finish with the eyes looking between the fists. You can either look straight to the 10.00/10.30 corner throughout the movement, or you can look to the left or right as you move the weight forwards.

  Looking to left or right: The reason for this is that one fist will be predominant (left or right); you therefore focus on that particular fist. So if (for example) you are focusing on your left fist, the body will turn fractionally to the left as you start to make the punch (the eyes therefore briefly following), and will then turn back to 10.00/10.30 as you complete the punch.

FORM 15: TURN AND KICK WITH LEFT HEEL (SEPARATE LEFT FOOT)

转身左蹬脚 (Zhuǎnshēn Zuǒ Dēngjiǎo)

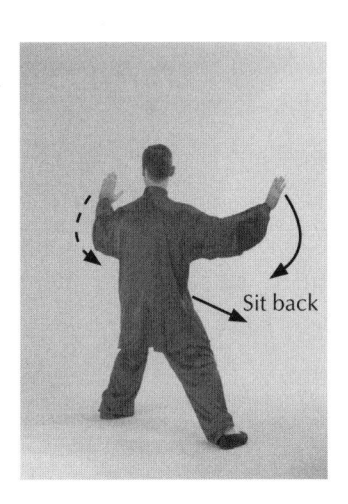

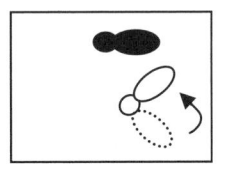

Brief 1
Sit back and open your palms; turn to the left and open your arms.

Details
Move the weight on to the left foot and, as you turn your hips to the left, pivot your right toes inwards (pivoting on the heel) to point as far around towards 7.30 as you can manage.

As you do so, open your fists into palms facing away from you, and separate the arms to either side of you.

The left hand opens to approximately 6.00, and the right hand opens to approximately 10.00.

The eyes follow and look through the left hand.

Notes

- **Shifting weight on to the left foot:** The weight transfer should be just enough to turn the right toes.

Avoiding sticking the pelvis out: As you begin to move the weight on to the left foot, lift the left heel fractionally inwards. This eradicates the awkward pelvic position which makes the practitioner stick his backside out.

The turn of the right toes to 7.30 is important because the correct positioning of this foot determines 1) how easy it will be to do the kick at the end of this movement, and 2) how easy it will be to perform the following movement (Snake Creeps Down).

Some people are flexible enough to be able to turn the right foot even further around towards 6.00. This makes the kick easier, but makes Snake Creeps Down harder; the ideal angle therefore is 7.30.

- **Optional adjustment of the left foot:** You can lift the left heel inwards slightly prior to turning the right toes inwards.

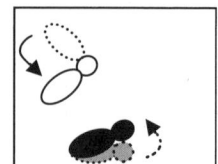

- **Posture:** Keep the body upright as you sit back and turn.

- **The 'arcing' of the hands/arms** is minimal. The fingertips don't need to lift much above the head. Compare the circling of the left arm as you move into the final posture of Single Whip; the movement is almost identical.

- **The open arm position:** Beginners find it very difficult to get the feel of the position of the open arms. They should be opened to either side slightly forwards of the body, with the wrists at shoulder-height, and most importantly the elbows should be sunk. The fingertips will be lifted, and the little finger edges of the hands will be almost vertical and furthest from the body.

- **The shoulders and elbows** should stay relaxed and sunk.

- **'Opening':** This is an 'open' position.

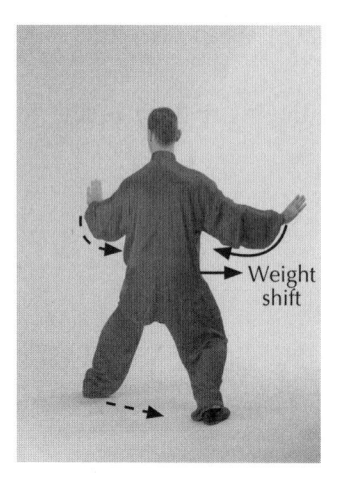

BRIEF 2

Sit back and cross wrists, and left foot draws in.

DETAILS

Move the weight back on to your right foot.

Circle your hands downwards, palms crossed at the wrists at waist height in front of you (see the following page for more details on the crossing of the wrists).

As your hands cross at the wrists, draw your left foot into your right ankle so that it arrives at the same moment as the crossing of the hands.

The eyes look either to the left or to 7.30.

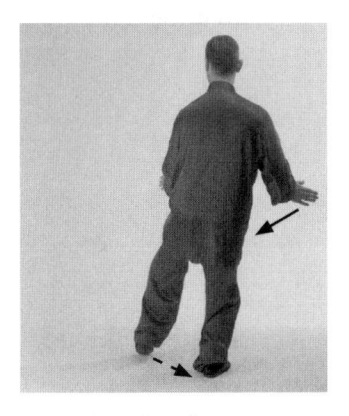

NOTES

- **Method of lowering the arms:** Sink the elbows first, gradually rotating them inwards. Continue to rotate them inwards as you sink the wrists, and then lead the fingertips inwards to cross at the wrists. The energy should be in the forearms.

- **The crossing of the hands** causes beginners a few problems. When crossing them in the lower position, hold the left palm in front of your abdomen, and then place the right wrist against the thumb side (radial side) of your left wrist (the right hand will therefore appear to be on top of, or inside the left hand). The palms are not facing the body, nor are they facing the ceiling, they are somewhere in between.

  Do not hold the hands too close to the body; they should be about 8 inches (20 cm) ahead of the waist.

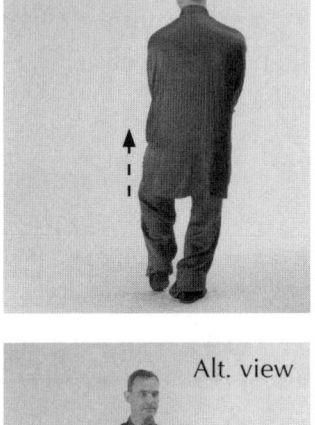

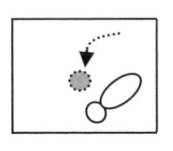

- **The crossed arms:** Keep a space under the armpits – in other words, don't drop the elbows too much – the elbows shouldn't be against the sides of the chest.

- **The right leg** should be bent.

- **The left foot:** Beginners can rest the toes on the floor alongside the right foot.

- **Posture:** Keep the body upright; avoid leaning forwards.

- **The head:** The eyes should be level; avoid dropping the head and looking down – because the hands are dropping, beginners often drop the head at this point.

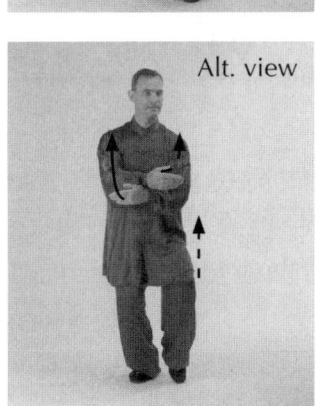

- **The pelvis** should be relaxed and sunk; gently pull in the lower abdominal muscles, allowing the coccyx/tailbone to tuck under.

- **'Closing':** This is a 'closed' position. Coordinate the upper and the lower: Notice how the elbows and knees work together, in particular the left elbow and left knee.

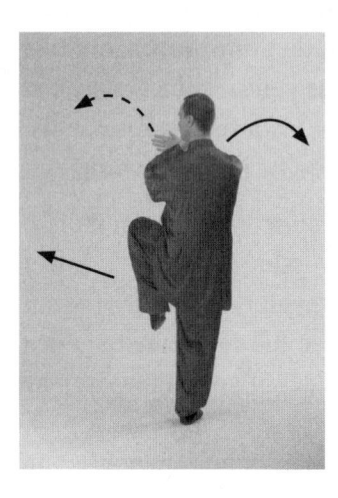

BRIEF 3
Stand up; lift hands and knee.

DETAILS
As you straighten the right leg, raise the left knee.

Lift the crossed hands upwards to in front of your throat. The hands rise up your centreline so that the wrists reach the same height as your shoulders with the left hand on the outside (furthest away from you); the palms should be facing you.

The eyes look between the hands.

NOTES

- **Lifting the hands:** The lifting of the arms and left knee is a little like a puppeteer lifting a puppet's limb – feel as though the elbows are lifting the knee. Keep the hands approximately 4–8 inches (10–20 cm) away from the body as you lift. The knee opens out to point at 4.30/5.00 as it rises.

  Lift the hands leading with the fingertips.

- **Pull in the lower abdominal muscles** as you lift the knee; apart from anything else, it helps the raising of the knee by tucking the buttocks under.

- **Variation:** Some practitioners don't lift the knee all the way up at this stage; they make the final lift of the knee as they separate the hands in the next movement.

  Comments: This is not a variation that I personally use as I feel that it breaks the connection between the upper and the lower body – the elbows and knees no longer working together in unison.

BRIEF 4A
Start to separate hands; turn palms; lift the left toes.

DETAILS
Push the fingertips upwards to begin the separation of the hands. As the hands separate, gradually start to turn your palms to face outwards.
    Raise your left knee higher (without extending the leg yet) and lift the toes. The eyes start to look towards your left.

NOTES

- **Lifting the knee** as high as possible before the kick makes a surprising difference to the height of the kick.

- **The shoulders** should be sunk.

- **Align the left elbow and left knee.**

- **Sink/relax your pelvis** and continue to pull in the lower abdominal muscles as you lift the knee.

- **'Opening':** The body is starting to 'open'.

- **Separation of the arms:** The opening of the arms has the same feel to the movement of the left arm and hand when moving into the final posture of Single Whip (see also 'Opening the arms' note on the following page).

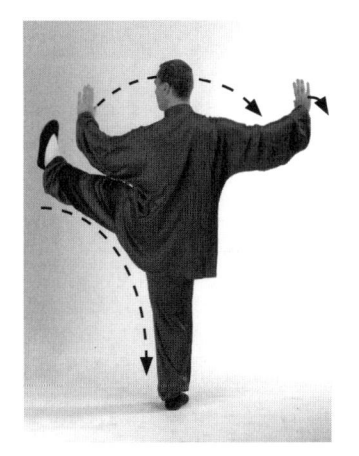

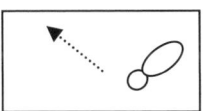

BRIEF 4B
Open arms and kick.

DETAILS
Continue to separate the arms, arcing them upwards and then outwards, and then downwards so that the wrists arrive at shoulder height.
    The left calf extends and kicks with the heel to 4.30/5.00.
    The hands arrive in position on either side of you as the kick is completed.
    The eyes look in the direction of the kick.

NOTES

- **Dēngjiǎo 蹬脚 (heel kick):** Standing in relaxed fashion on the supporting leg which is slightly bent, raise the other leg bent at the knee, hooking the foot back. With the heel as the power point, slowly press the leg out, extending it naturally with the foot above waist height.

- **The shoulders:** Keep them relaxed – most beginners lift the shoulders when kicking (see also note on 'Balance' on the following page).

- **Opening the arms:** The 'arcing' of the hands/arms shouldn't be too exaggerated. There is a feeling of pushing the fingertips upwards as you separate them; the fingertips shouldn't lift much above the head. As you open the arms gradually rotate the palms so that, by the time that the arms are open, the palms have turned outwards.

    Compare the circling of the left arm as you move into the final posture of Single Whip; this arm movement is identical in feel but with only a 'single' arm.

    The open arm position: Beginners find it very difficult to get the feel of the arm position.

    The arms should be slightly forwards of the body with the wrists turned outwards at shoulder-height, and most importantly the elbows should be sunk. The fingertips will be lifted, the hand as vertical as possible (therefore the thumb side of the wrist flexed inwards), and the little finger edge of the hand will be furthest from the body.

    Body/arms relationship: There should be symmetry between the two arms; the centreline of the body should not point more towards the left arm than the right arm. This is a mistake that beginners often make.

- **The left arm** should be on the same line as the left leg.

- **The supporting leg** (on which you are standing) should be straight, neither bent forwards at the knee, nor locked backwards at the knee. Just relax it by relaxing the pelvis and right hip.

- **Timing of kick and arms:** The kick should be timed with the completion of the opening of the arms.

- **The kick** doesn't have to be high. Beginners, and even some experienced practitioners, seem to feel that it is necessary to kick as high as they can at the expense of every other muscle in the body, so they end up leaning backwards and usually losing their balance.

From a martial point of view, it is much more effective to kick low, for example to an opponent's knee, than higher where the foot can easily be caught.

If you do want to practise kicking higher, lift the knee as high as you can before extending the calf.

- **The kick and the left hip:** When kicking, the left hip should be relaxed; many practitioners lift it because they are trying to lift the leg with the wrong muscles. Sink the left buttock and gently pull in the lower abdominal muscles; use the pelvic tilt (under-turn of the pelvis) to create the kick. Doing this connects the legs together, enabling the power of one to be supported by the other. Lifting the left hip breaks both the muscular and energetic connection between the legs, as though you are trying to lift one away from the other and use it independently.

- **Balance** can be a problem. This is usually caused by two things, either 1) the locking of the pelvis which destabilizes the core of the body, or 2) the lifting of the shoulders as the kick is made, i.e. the qì is lifted.

  It is therefore essential (not only for the balance to be maintained but also for the kick to be effective) that both the upper and lower body are relaxed, the elbows sunk, and that you concentrate on sinking into the foot on which you are standing.

  A good 'trick' that works well is to press the supporting foot downwards as you simultaneously kick outwards.

SECTION 6

(2 MOVEMENTS)

These movements have different directions of performance.

16. **Push Down and Stand on One Leg (Left Style) (Snake Creeps Down) (Golden Cockerel/Rooster on One Leg)**
    左下势独立 (Zuǒ Xiàshì Dúlì)

17. **Push Down and Stand on One Leg (Right Style) (Snake Creeps Down) (Golden Cockerel/Rooster on One Leg)**
    右下势独立 (Yòu Xiàshì Dúlì)

FORM 16: PUSH DOWN AND STAND ON ONE LEG (LEFT STYLE) (SNAKE CREEPS DOWN) (GOLDEN COCKEREL/ROOSTER ON ONE LEG)

左下势独立 (Zuǒ Xiàshì Dúlì)

This movement and the one that follows should really be thought of as a single movement, but for descriptive purposes it is easier to break it into two.

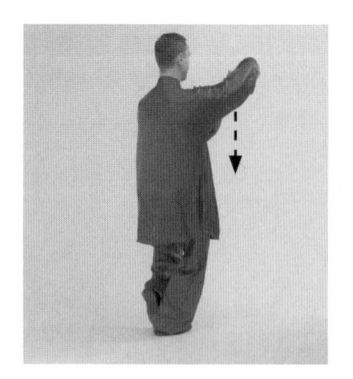

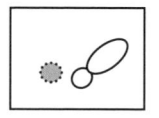

BRIEF 1A
Relax the left calf; start to bend right knee; arc the left hand to the right; bunch and hook the right hand.

DETAILS
Leaving the left knee raised, relax the left calf (and soften the left ankle).

Start to bend the right knee.

Simultaneously, arc the left arm (with palm leading – but see more on 'Closing' on the following page – and with fingers still pointing upwards) to the centreline of the body (the wrist will be opposite the centreline), eventually sinking the elbow so that the arm is moving downwards, the fingers now pointing towards your right elbow crease/upper arm. The forearm will be close to the body.

As this happens, the right hand fingers bunch together, and the hand flexes at the wrist with the fingers therefore hooking downwards into a crane's beak at shoulder-height; the right arm points to 7.00/7.30.

The eyes look to 7.00/7.30.

Notes

- **The right foot** points at 7.00/7.30, the right arm is extended in the same direction, and the eyes also look to 7.00/7.30.

- **The centreline** of the body faces approximately 7.00.

- **The shoulders** should be relaxed to help retain your balance – in particular your right shoulder.

- **Start to bend the right knee** – this is the start of the 'closing' of the body (see below).

- **'Closing':** The body is starting to 'close' at this stage.

  - There is an inwards rotation of both elbows – feel as though the left *elbow* is moving the arc of the left arm, and at the same time, the right elbow is rotating downwards.

  - Simultaneously the centre is starting to pull inwards – the body is drawing into itself and sinking into the right foot.

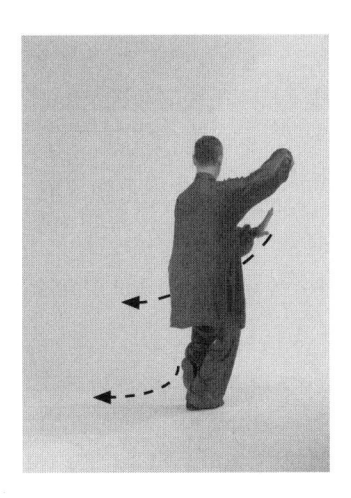

BRIEF 1B
Find the right heel with the left toes; left hand starts to push down to your waist.

DETAILS
Without looking downwards, lower your left toes so that they find the back of your right heel.

As you do so, start to push the left hand down your centreline with the palm facing the floor.

Leave your right hand out to 7.00/7.30 still in the crane's beak position.

The eyes continue to look to 7.00/7.30.

THE YANG TÀIJÍ 24-STEP SHORT FORM

NOTES

- **'Finding the right heel with the left toes'** is not essential, but helps to get the correct alignment of the feet in the move that follows. It is also possible to lower the left foot slightly and then step out towards 3.00 without the foot going so close to the floor.

- **The lowering of the left arm** is done by sinking the elbow, rather than by pushing the hand downwards. The hand does not have to be in front of your centreline, it may be on the right side of the body.

- **Direction of the body:** The body is still turned slightly towards 7.00, but is in the process of turning to the left.

- **The right shoulder** should be relaxed.

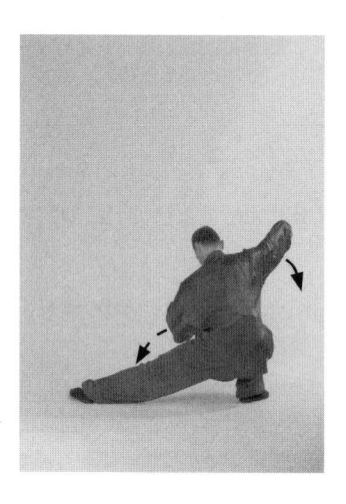

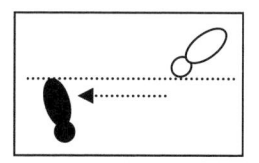

BRIEF 2
Slide left foot to 3.00; left hand arrives at waist.

DETAILS
Slide or step your left foot towards 3.00 leading with the side of the foot – see diagram above (also see Notes below), so that in the final position the *toes* of the left foot and the *heel* of the right foot both touch the 3.00/9.00 axis at the end of the movement.

As the left foot slides out, the left hand continues to push palm down towards your waist.

Leave your right hand out to 7.00/7.30 still in the bunch and hook position. The eyes still look to 7.00/7.30.

NOTES

- **Angle of the right foot:** It is this movement that makes it clear why the right toes should start off by pointing to 7.30 (i.e. in the previous movement – the second kick – they are turned out in this direction). If they don't, and they are pointing to (for example) 6.00, you will need to adjust them to point to 7.30 for this movement to be possible.

- **The left foot:** Slide with the *side* of the foot to 3.00; the toes can be turned to 5.00, but not much more. Beginners often turn the body too early and lead the step or slide-out with the toes pointing to 3.00 or 4.00.

- **The weight:**

  - Keep the weight on the right foot; don't move the weight on to the left foot at all.

  - The main mistake that beginners (and even intermediate practitioners) make is to slide the left foot out *whilst* shifting the weight on to the left foot, so that they finish the movement with the weight somewhere in between both feet.

    As a result, the stance becomes far wider than is necessary, and it therefore becomes much harder to move out of it at the end of the movement.

    The more you are able to keep the centreline of your body over the right heel, therefore, the easier the move.

- **Posture:** Beginners tend to lean forwards too much here, sticking their backsides out. The body can lean forwards slightly, but it should if possible be minimal.

  - Sink your hips, releasing the small of the back. Feel as though you are dropping the tip of your spine into your right heel.

  - Allow the Kuà 胯 of the right hip to close up, and the Kuà of the left hip to open.

- **Height of posture:** It is not essential to go into a very low Crouch Stance. It is far better to have a high Crouch Stance with all the parameters correct, than a flashy low one with several postural errors – mainly because you are more likely to damage your knees! You only have to look at the internet to see several practitioners running the risk of damaging the medial ligaments of their right knees (in this and the next movement) because their 'turn out' is not good enough, and the right knee is no longer supported correctly by the right foot.

- **The right shoulder** should be sunk and relaxed.

- **Variation:** Some practitioners slide the leg out at the same time as pushing the hand down the leg (see Notes at the end of Brief 3, p.226).

THE YANG TÀIJÍ 24-STEP SHORT FORM

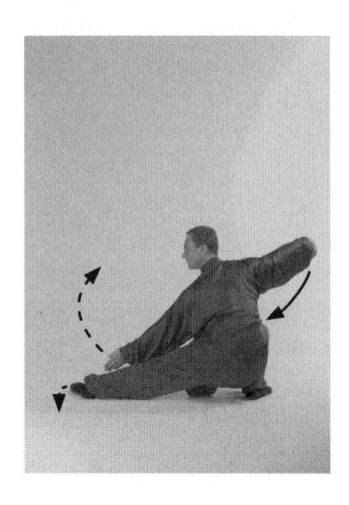

Brief 3

Snake Creeps Down (Push Down). Turn the hips and waist; thread the left fingers to the knee.

Details

Sink further, and turn your hips and waist to your left (to 5.00) – see Notes below for further detail about this.

The left hand (which is by your waist with the palm down and the fingers pointing to your right) now rotates so that the thumb starts to turn upwards. The left elbow moves in close against the left side of the body, and the back of the left hand moves towards your left inner thigh. With the tips of the fingers leading, and the thumb uppermost, the left hand then slides down the length of the inside of the left thigh to the knee or beyond it.

The right hand still stays in a crane's beak facing 7.00/7.30.

The eyes look slightly downwards towards 3.00/4.00.

Notes

- **The body turns to 5.00** as you thread the left hand down the left leg.
- **The 'threading' of the left hand:**
  1. The left hand (which, at the end of Brief 2, is by your waist with the palm down and the fingers pointing to your right) now rotates so that the thumb starts to turn upwards.
  2. Flex the wrist backwards so that there is almost a feeling of trying to touch the middle fingernail against the back of the forearm.
  3. The left elbow moves close to the left hip (this connection is a pivot point for the left arm) and the back of the left hand moves towards your left inner thigh.

     (Note that the movement of the left hand to the left knee comes with the gradual turn of the hips to the left.)
  4. With the tips of the fingers leading, and the thumb uppermost, the left hand then slides down the length of the inside of the left thigh to the knee or beyond it (depending upon how deeply you sink into the stance).

- **The right arm** is starting to lower at this stage, the right elbow leading the sinking of the arm.

- **The weight** should remain on the right foot; don't move the weight on to the left foot at all.

- **Posture:** The body will lean forwards slightly towards 4.30/5.00.

  - Sink your hips, releasing the small of the back. Feel as though you are dropping the tip of your spine into your right heel so that your backside doesn't stick out.

  - Allow the Kuà 胯 of the right hip to open up, and the Kuà of the left hip to begin to close.

  Height of posture: See note on 'Height of posture' in Brief 2 (p.225).

- **Avoid collapsing the right knee:** It is here in particular that the right knee is liable to collapse inwards, running the risk of damaging the medial ligaments (see 'Height of posture' on p.225).

  Keep the lines of the right thigh and right toes pointing in the same direction.

VARIATION TO BRIEFS 1A, 1B AND 2
Some practitioners time the coordination of the limbs slightly differently:

VARIATION DETAILS 1A
Perform the movement identically to the description above with the addition of a little more bend in the right leg, the body starting to sink immediately.

VARIATION DETAILS 1B
The only difference here from the description above is that the left hand has already reached the waist; this is timed with a further sinking of the body (see Notes immediately below).

VARIATION NOTES

- **The 'closing' of the body:** Briefs 1a and 1b should be thought of as the completion of the body 'closing':

  - The right knee is bent.

- The body is sinking, the centre of the body folding and compressing into the right foot.

- The upper body is also compressing towards the dāntián, the elbows moving together, and the left elbow (initially) and then the left hand dropping.

Variation details 2

As the left foot slides out, the fingers of the left hand coordinate with the foot so that both move outwards together.

The left hand 'threads' down the inner left thigh to the inner calf/knee (depending on flexibility).

Turn your hips to your left (to 5.00) (see 'Advantages' notes below for further detail about this).

Your right hand (still in a crane's beak) remains out in the 7.00/7.30 direction, but at this stage the hand is beginning to lower.

The eyes follow the direction of the left arm.

Variation notes

- **Coordinate** the movements of the left ankle and left wrist as they expand outwards together.

- **Advantages/Disadvantages:**

  - **Advantages:** The 'open' and 'close' is much clearer; the lower and upper body 'open' together. In the other method, the left leg opens first followed by the upper body; in other words the 'opening' is not coordinated.

    The direction of flow of energy is clearer in this method. Your aim, after the kick, is to drop the body and immediately move forwards and attack to 3.00, the body drawing a large 'U' bend up into Golden Cockerel.

    The pelvis is making a continuous turn from right to left, and therefore needs to turn to 5.00.

    In the basic method (described at the start of Form 16), there is a tendency to drop first, then to turn with the weight still on the back (right) foot, and then finally to move forwards.

  - **Disadvantage:** There is more strain on the right knee.

Both this movement (Brief 4a) and the next (Brief 4b) finish simultaneously. But when teaching it, I have found it easier to separate them into two moves.

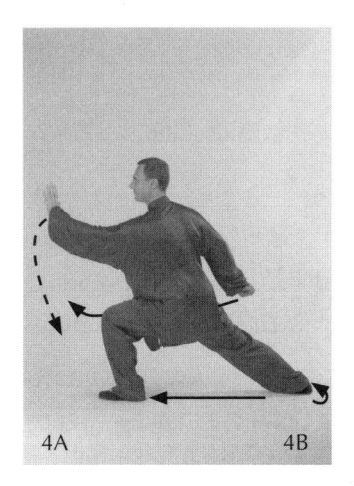

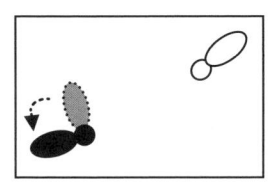

BRIEF 4A
Weight forwards; turn the left toes.

DETAILS
Without standing up, push the weight from the right foot to the left foot. Before the weight fully arrives on the left foot, turn the toes of your left foot to 2.00/2.30 – see the diagram above (also see Notes below).

As the weight transfers to the left foot, raise your left hand (the palm still facing 6.00) directly up the centreline of your body to a height where the index finger is ahead of the tip of your nose. Keep the arm well extended with the hand beyond your left knee.

The right arm drops still further.

The eyes look to 3.00.

N.B. The left foot turns first, and then the right foot on the next movement.

NOTES

- **The turning out of the left toes:**

  - The correct placement of the left foot prepares the footwork for the posture that is about to happen (Brief 5). A large percentage of people find it very difficult to turn the foot out to 2.00/2.30, and although this may sound like a very small detail, the foot being at the wrong angle creates a difficulty in standing on one foot in the move that follows (Push Down and Stand on One Leg) – the posture becomes less stable.

  - First of all the turn of the foot is controlled largely by the hips; you cannot really turn the foot until you start to turn the hips to the left, so do not expect to be able to turn them until towards the end of the movement when there is already some weight on the left heel. Beginners usually try to turn the foot much too early.

- If this still doesn't help, see 'Alternative method for the turning of the left toes' on the following page.

- **The left arm and hand:**
  - Keep the left elbow sunk as you raise the hand.
  - Lift the hand directly up the body between your centreline and 3.00.
  - The left hand should be extended well away from the body at the end of the movement; beginners tend to arrive with the left elbow too bent.
  - Flex the left wrist at the end of the movement so that the hypothenar eminence is extended rather than the fingertips (which should be pointing upwards).

- **Snake Creeps Down:** It is this part of the movement that gives Snake Creeps Down its name. When the posture is done very low, there is a feeling of slithering along the ground as you move forwards and out of it.

BRIEF 4B
Adjust the right toes; hook moves to hip.

DETAILS
The right hand (still in a crane's beak) lowers to beside your right thigh, with the 'beak' pointing behind you.

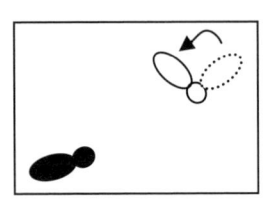

The left hand arrives in position with the index finger ahead of the tip of your nose.

As the weight arrives on the left foot, lift the *toes* of the rear foot and turn them inwards to 4.30 (see the diagram to the left).

The eyes continue to look to 3.00.

NOTES

- **The right hand:** A common fault is to place the back of the right hand against the right buttock. It should finish by the *side* of the right thigh, not behind it.
- **The right foot:** Beginners usually try to slip the rear heel instead of turning the toes. Strictly speaking this isn't correct because it increases the length of the stance; this makes moving out of the stance much harder. So although you will not notice any difference if you are not doing a low Crouch Stance,

as your flexibility gradually improves and you start to sink lower, a habit of slipping the right heel will begin to cause problems.

- **Problems associated with turning the rear toes:** The most common fault is to stick the backside out during the turn of the back foot. This is due to either:

  1. the feet being too far apart in the first place (see Brief 3)

  2. the inflexibility of the front of the right hip, making it impossible to sink and relax the hip, or

  3. the right Achilles tendon being too tight, making it impossible to lift the toes.

Additionally, the back foot is difficult to adjust correctly if the weight isn't completely over the left foot.

ALTERNATIVE METHOD FOR THE TURNING OF THE LEFT TOES

Not everyone is able to turn the left toes out to 2.00/2.30. If it is too difficult, then initially point them to 3.00 (see Alt. method 1). Then, just before the movement that follows (i.e. Brief 5) which requires that you stand, either: 1) turn the toes outwards just before standing, or 2) turn the *heel* inwards just before standing (see Alt. method 2).

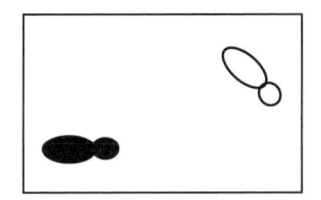

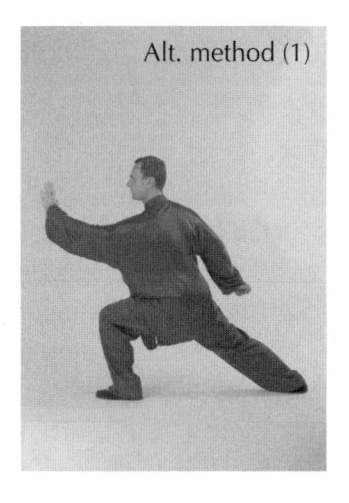

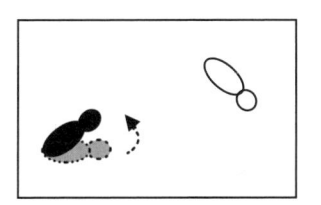

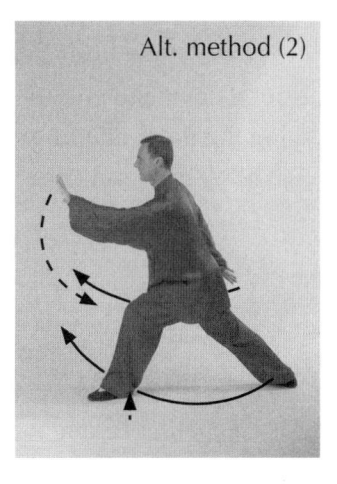

THE YANG TÀIJÍ 24-STEP SHORT FORM

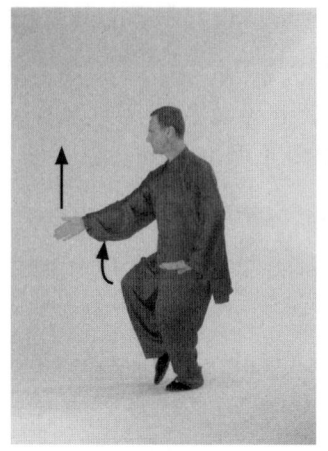

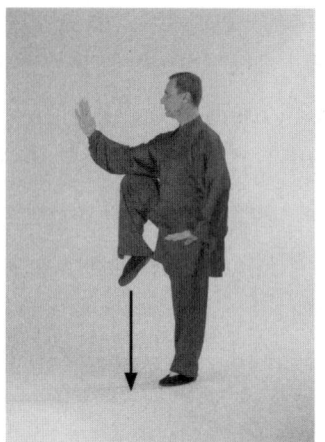

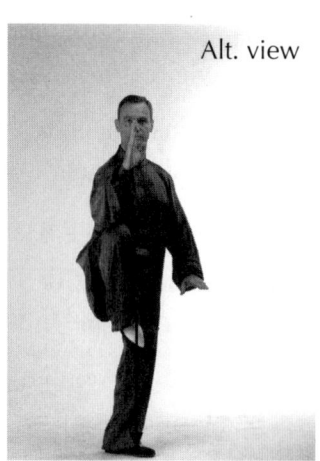

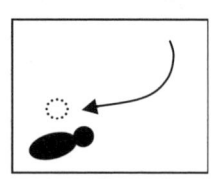

Alt. view

Brief 5

Golden Cockerel (Left Side) (Stand on Left Leg). Push the left hand down; raise the right hand and right knee.

Details

As you move the weight fully on to your left foot, push your left palm downwards with the fingers pointing to your right (4.30).

As you start to straighten your left leg, the right hand moves from your right thigh, the fingers opening, and simultaneously the right leg moves forwards.

The right hand and knee move towards 3.00, and both lift; the right hand moves up the centreline of the body with the arm well extended – the palm facing left (12.00), the fingers vertical, to arrive with the hand ahead of the mouth (the index finger level with the tip of the nose) and directly between your centreline and 3.00.

The right knee lifts so that it touches your right elbow (or as near as possible).

As the right hand and leg move into position, the left hand has finished pushing down the midline of the body and has moved to your left side with palm facing the floor, and fingers pointing to 3.00.

The eyes continue to look to 3.00.

Notes

- **Connections:**
  - There should be a feeling of the right elbow and right knee working together throughout the lift.

- Feel the 'opposites' working together, i.e. right and left wrists; left knee straightening and right knee bending; left wrist pushing down, right wrist lifting up, etc.

- **Lifting the right knee:**
  - When raising the right knee, keep the body upright. To get the feel, have a partner push down on your knee as you lift it.
  - The lifting of the knee is partly achieved by a pelvic tilt; therefore gently pull in the lower abdominal muscles as you lift the knee.
  - The right knee should rise to, and touch, your right elbow. Lift the *knee* to the elbow, rather than lower the *elbow* to the knee. If trying to touch the knee with the elbow means that you have to bend the body at the waist to get it there, then only lift it as high as you are able.
  - The right ankle is relaxed.

- **The left leg** finishes straight but not locked.

- **Lifting the right hand:**
  - Extend the arm towards 3.00 as you lift, allowing the body to turn slightly further to your left.
  - When lifting the right hand, there should be a feeling of initially lifting the heel of the thumb, followed by a feeling of lifting the fingers and pushing the little finger edge of the palm away from you towards 3.00.
  - The hand should finish with the hand *beyond* the knee, i.e. further towards 3.00 than the knee.

- **The left hand:**
  - Sink the left elbow and forearm to lower the left hand, and push down with the *heel* of the hand.
  - This movement can also be called Push Down and Stand on One Leg. The pushing down is therefore very important, particularly as you arrive in the final posture of the movement. Feel the simultaneous pushing down of the left hand and the lifting of the right hand.
  - When pushing down with the left hand, there should be a sense of Péng in the upper arm.

- **Application:** Visualize the left hand as blocking down, and the rising right hand as striking upwards to the groin.

THE YANG TÀIJÍ 24-STEP SHORT FORM

- **Balance:**

    - Relax the hips and the buttocks allowing the small of the back to relax. Balance becomes much harder if this area is locked.

    - For purposes of balance, the left foot needs to be turned outwards very slightly (see note 'The turning out of the left toes' on p.229 and 'Alternative method for the turning of the left toes' on p.231). It is noticeable that if the foot is pointing directly to 3.00, the balance is far more precarious; this is to do with the lie of the iliofemoral joint in the hip, i.e. the hip/thigh joint.

- **'Closed':** The body is 'closed' in this posture.

FORM 17: PUSH DOWN AND STAND ON ONE LEG (RIGHT STYLE) (SNAKE CREEPS DOWN) (GOLDEN COCKEREL/ROOSTER ON ONE LEG)

右下势独立 (Yòu Xiàshì Dúlì)

This movement and the two that follow should really be thought of as one 'closing' movement, but for descriptive purposes it is easier to break it into three. Please see 'General notes on combined Briefs 1a, 1b and 1c' on p.237 for the combined feeling of the movements.

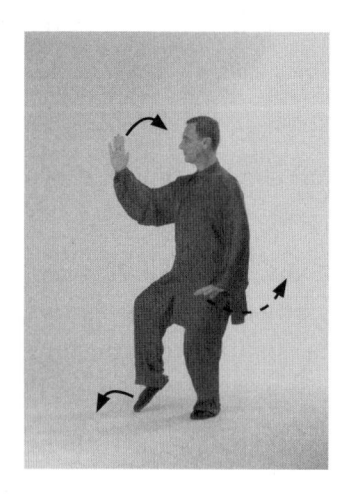

BRIEF 1A
Sink; place right toes ahead.

DETAILS
Bend your left knee.
  Lower and place your right toes to 9.00, one foot's length ahead of you.
  The eyes continue to look to 3.00.

NOTES

- **The feet:** You will need approximately 8 inches (20 cm) between the feet.

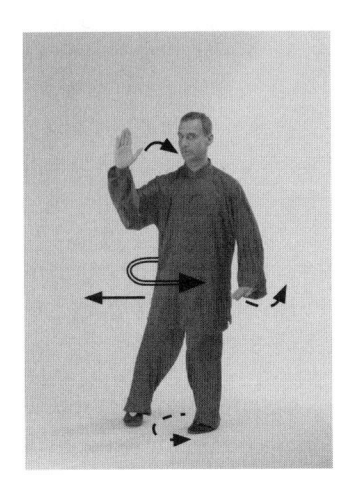

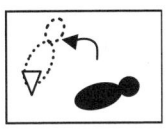

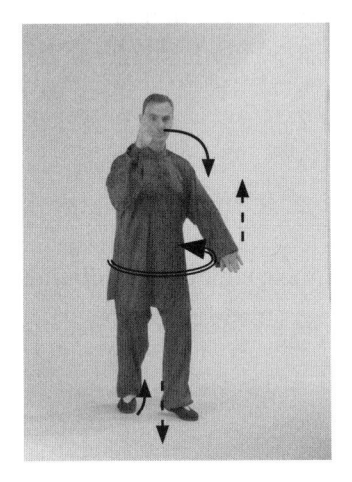

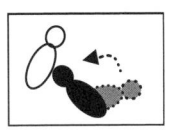

BRIEF 1B

Turn body left; adjust right foot; *fractional* shift weight; adjust left foot.

DETAILS

As you start to turn the hips to the left, pivot the right foot on the ball of the foot, so that the foot points to 1.00/1.30.

Very briefly move your weight on to the right foot (see Notes below); your feet will be approximately parallel to each other.

As the weight shifts fractionally over the right foot, turn your centre still further to the left, lift the left heel *slightly* and pivot the heel inwards (see Notes below), so that the left foot now points to 10.30/11.00. Your feet will now be approximately perpendicular to one other.

The arms move around with the turn of the body, the left arm remaining by your side.

The right arm arcs towards the midline of the body (with palm leading and with fingers temporarily still pointing upwards). The right elbow then sinks so that the arm is moving downwards, the fingers pointing towards your left elbow crease/upper arm. The forearm will be close to the body.

The eyes follow the right hand.

NOTES

- **Weight shift and foot-changes:** With this foot movement you are, in effect, pivoting the body on the spot.

The weight shift on to the right foot is very slight so that anyone watching you would be unaware that you have shifted any weight; it should be just enough to enable the left foot to alter angle before the weight moves back over it.

- **Turning the right foot:** Use the turn of the body (centre) to turn the right heel outwards.

- **Pivoting the left heel inwards:**
  - Use the centre to turn the left heel inwards (as you place the weight briefly on the right foot).
  - Some practitioners turn the left *toes* outwards instead. As the movement has the feeling of pivoting on the spot, I prefer to pivot on the *ball* of the foot.

- **The right hand** appears to have moved to your left side, although it is really the turn of the body that gives this illusion and, *relative to the body*, the arm has made virtually no lateral movement at all.

- **The right arm:** This is a 'closing' of the right arm, so feel as though the elbow and forearm are pushing to the left.

- **The left arm:** There is a slight push downwards with the palm, and the left elbow starts to rotate inwards slightly; in other words, the left side of the body is also 'closing'.

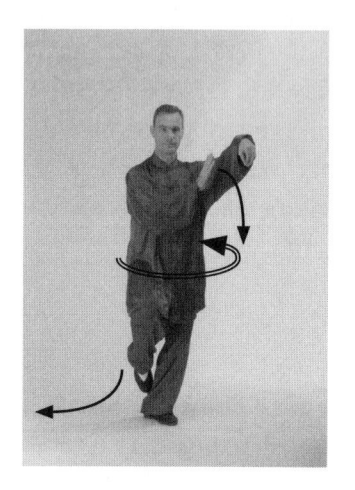

BRIEF 1C

Weight back on to the left foot; sink the right hand; Form the crane's beak as you raise the left arm; start to bend the left knee.

DETAILS

Move the weight back on to the left foot and lift the right heel.

As you do so, start to bend the left knee and sink into the left foot.

The right hand pushes down the front of your body to your waist with the palm facing downwards.

The left hand simultaneously rises from your left side, and forms into a crane's beak as it lifts. The wrist is pulled strongly downwards with the beak pointing down. The left arm is parallel to the ground and points to 10.30/11.00.

The eyes look in the direction of the left arm.

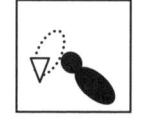

Notes

- **The right arm:**
  - From Briefs 1b to 1c, the beginner's version of the right hand/arm movement is just to leave the arm where it is (relative to the body) and only turn the body. The arm will therefore seem to move from 9.00 to 10.30/11.00, whereas, in relation to the centreline, it is only the centreline that has moved and the arm itself has merely stayed in the centre of the body.
  - A slightly smoother (and more circular) method is to lift the fingertips of the right hand as you turn the centreline to your left. This gives the *appearance* of forming an arc – an arc which continues in the movements that follow.

See also below...

- **'Closing':** The body is 'closing'. There is an inwards rotation of both elbows – feel as though the right elbow is leading the sinking of the right arm, and at the same time, the left elbow is rotating downwards as the left arm lifts.

  Simultaneously the centre is starting to pull inwards – the body is drawing into itself.

- **The arms:** Feel the arms moving in opposite directions – the left hand rising, the right hand sinking.

- **Left side alignments:**
  - The left foot is turned towards 10.30/11.00.
  - The left arm is extended towards 10.30/11.00.
  - The eyes look towards 10.30/11.00.

- **The left leg** is bent; the centre/abdomen has folded.

- **The centreline** of the body faces approximately 12.00.

- **The shoulders** should be relaxed to help retain the balance; beginners tend to lift the left shoulder.

General notes on combined Briefs 1a, 1b and 1c

- **The overview of all three movements** should be one of 'closing'. Therefore, from the end of the first Golden Cockerel, you should feel the gradual

THE YANG TÀIJÍ 24-STEP SHORT FORM

'compressing' of the elbows (as they rotate inwards) and of the body whilst simultaneously feeling the body sinking.

Notice the connections of elbows working with the knees.

- **The transition:** Beginners find this small transition quite difficult.

    It is important not to make it too ponderous – although I've described it as three movements, it is really only one, and is also only a 'link' movement between the two Golden Cockerels, and should happen fairly rapidly.

    When pivoting on the ball of the left foot (Brief 1c), try to put as little weight as possible on to the right foot. Because you are attempting to pivot 'on the spot' (in effect), the weight shifts should be minimal and not exaggerated.

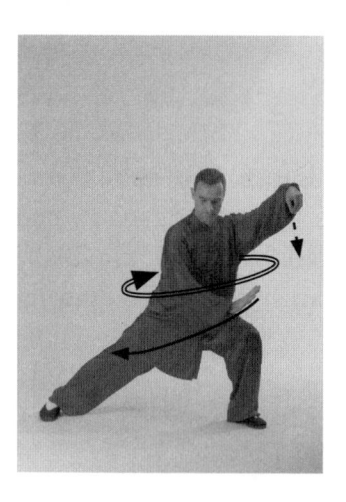

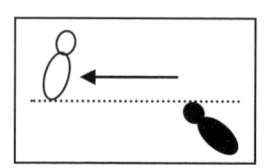

BRIEF 2
Slide right foot to 3.00; right hand arrives at waist.

DETAILS
Slide or step your right foot towards 3.00 leading with the side of the foot – see diagram above (and Notes below), so that in the final position the *toes* of the right foot and the *heel* of the left foot both touch the 3.00/9.00 axis at the end of the movement.

As the right foot slides out, the right hand continues to push palm down towards your waist. Leave your left hand out to 10.30/11.00 still in the crane's beak position. The eyes still look to 10.30.

NOTES

- **Angle of the left foot:** It is this movement that makes it clear why the left toes should start off by pointing to 10.30. If they don't, and they are pointing to (for example) 12.00, you will need to adjust them to point to 10.30 for this movement to be possible.

- **The right foot:** Slide with the *side* of the foot to 3.00; the toes can be turned to 1.00, but not much more. Beginners often turn the body too early and lead the step or slide-out with the toes pointing to 2.00 or 3.00.

- **The weight:**

  - Keep the weight on the left foot; don't move the weight on to the right foot at all.

  - The main mistake that beginners (and even intermediate practitioners) make is to slide the right foot out *whilst* shifting the weight on to it, so that they finish the movement with the weight somewhere in between both feet.

    As a result, the stance becomes far wider than is necessary, and it therefore becomes much harder to move out of it at the end of the movement.

    The more you are able to keep the centreline of your body over the left heel, therefore, the easier the move.

- **Posture:** Beginners tend to lean forwards too much here, sticking their backsides out. The body can lean forwards slightly, but it should if possible be minimal.

  - Sink your hips, releasing the small of the back. Feel as though you are dropping the tip of your spine into your left heel.

  - Allow the Kuà 胯 of the left hip to close up, and the Kuà of the right hip to open.

  Height of posture: It is not essential to go into a very low Crouch Stance. It is far better to have a high Crouch Stance with all the parameters correct, than a flashy low one with several postural errors – mainly because you are more likely to damage your knees! You only have to look at the internet to see several practitioners running the risk of damaging the medial ligaments of their left knees (in this and the previous movement) because their 'turn out' is not good enough, and the left knee is no longer supported correctly by the left foot.

- **The left shoulder** should be sunk and relaxed.

- **Variation:** Some practitioners slide the leg out at the same time as pushing the hand down the leg (see Notes at the end of Brief 3, p.240).

THE YANG TÀIJÍ 24-STEP SHORT FORM

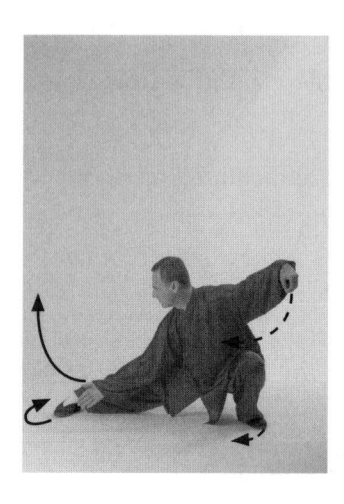

Brief 3

Snake Creeps Down (Push Down). Turn the hips and waist; thread the right fingers to the knee.

Details

Sink further, and turn your hips and waist to your right (to 1.00) (see Notes below for further detail about this).

The right hand (which is by your waist with the palm down and the fingers pointing to your left) now rotates so that the thumb starts to turn upwards. The right elbow moves in close against the right side of the body, and the back of the right hand moves towards your right inner thigh. With the tips of the fingers leading, and the thumb uppermost, the right hand then slides down the length of the inside of the right thigh to the knee or beyond it.

The left hand still stays in a crane's beak facing 10.30/11.00.

The eyes look slightly downwards towards 2.00/3.00.

Notes

- **The body turns to 1.00** as you thread the right hand down the right leg.
- **The 'threading' of the right hand:**

  1. The right hand (which, at the end of Brief 2), is by your waist with the palm down and the fingers pointing to your left) now rotates so that the thumb starts to turn upwards.

  2. Flex the wrist backwards so that there is almost a feeling of trying to touch the middle fingernail against the back of the forearm.

  3. The right elbow moves close to the right hip (this connection is a pivot point for the right arm) and the back of the right hand moves towards your right inner thigh.

     Note that the movement of the right hand to the right knee comes with the gradual turn of the hips to the right.

  4. With the tips of the fingers leading, and the thumb uppermost, the right hand then slides down the length of the inside of the right thigh to the knee or beyond it (depending upon how deeply you sink into the stance).

- **The left arm** is starting to lower at this stage, the left elbow leading the sinking of the arm.

- **The weight** should remain on the left foot; don't move the weight on to the right foot at all.

- **Posture:** The body will lean forwards slightly towards 1.00/1.30.

  - Sink your hips, releasing the small of the back. Feel as though you are dropping the tip of your spine into your left heel so that your backside doesn't stick out.

  - Allow the Kuà 胯 of the left hip to open up, and the Kuà of the right hip to begin to close.

  Height of posture: See note in Brief 2 (p.239).

- **Avoid collapsing the right knee:** It is here in particular that the left knee is liable to collapse inwards, running the risk of damaging the medial ligaments (see 'Height of posture' note on p.239).

  Keep the lines of the left thigh and left toes pointing in the same direction.

VARIATION TO BRIEFS 1A, 1B AND 2

Some practitioners time the coordination of the limbs slightly differently:

VARIATION DETAILS 1A

Perform the movement identically to the description above with the addition of a little more bend in the left leg, the body starting to sink immediately.

VARIATION DETAILS 1B

The only difference here from the description above is that the right hand has already reached the waist; this is timed with a further sinking of the body (see Notes immediately below).

VARIATION NOTES

- **The 'closing' of the body:** Briefs 1a and 1b should be thought of as the completion of the body 'closing':

  - The left knee is bent.

- The body is sinking, the centre of the body folding and compressing into the left foot.

- The upper body is also compressing towards the dāntián, the elbows moving together, and the right elbow (initially) and then the right hand dropping.

VARIATION DETAILS 2

As the right foot slides out, the fingers of the right hand coordinate with the foot so that both move outwards together.

The right hand 'threads' down the inner right thigh to the inner calf/knee (depending on flexibility) (see Notes below).

Turn your hips to your right (to 1.00) (see Notes below for further detail about this).

Your left hand (still in a crane's beak) remains out in the 10.30/11.00 direction, but at this stage the hand is beginning to lower.

The eyes follow the direction of the right arm.

VARIATION NOTES

- **Coordinate** the movements of the right ankle and right wrist as they expand outwards together.

- **Advantages/Disadvantages:**

  - **Advantages:** The 'open' and 'close' is much clearer; the lower and upper body 'open' together. In the other method, the right leg opens first followed by the upper body; in other words the 'opening' is not coordinated.

    The direction of flow of energy is clearer in this method. Your aim, after the kick, is to drop the body and immediately move forwards and attack to 3.00, the body drawing a large 'U' bend up into Golden Cockerel.

    In the basic method (described at the start of Form 17), there is a tendency to drop first, then to turn with the weight still on the back (left) foot, and then finally to move forwards.

  - **Disadvantage:** There is more strain on the left knee.

DESCRIPTION OF THE YANG TÀIJÍ 24-STEP SHORT FORM

Both this movement (Brief 4a) and the next (Brief 4b) finish simultaneously. But when teaching it, I have found it easier to separate them into two moves.

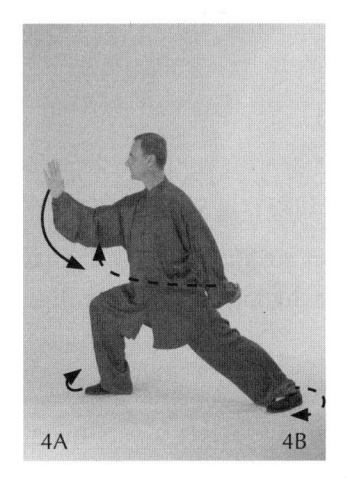

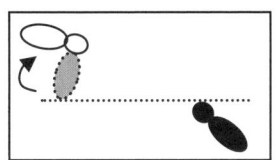

BRIEF 4A
Weight forwards; turn the right toes.

DETAILS
Without standing up, push the weight from the left foot to the right foot. Before the weight fully arrives on the right foot, turn the toes of your right foot to 3.30/4.00 – see diagram above (also see Notes below).

As the weight transfers to the right foot, raise your right hand (the palm still facing 12.00) directly up the centreline of your body to a height where the index finger is ahead of the tip of your nose. Keep the arm well extended with the hand beyond your right knee.

The left arm drops still further.

The eyes look to 3.00.

N.B. The right foot turns first, and then the left foot in the next movement.

NOTES

- **The turning out of the right toes:**

  - The correct placement of the right foot prepares the footwork for the posture that is about to happen (Brief 5).

  - A large percentage of people find it very difficult to turn the foot out to 3.30/4.00, and although this may sound like a very small detail, the foot being at the wrong angle creates a difficulty in standing on one foot in the move that follows (Golden Cockerel on One Leg) – the posture becomes less stable.

  - First of all the turn of the foot is controlled largely by the hips; you cannot really turn the foot until you start to turn the hips to the right, so do not expect to be able to turn them until towards the end of the movement when there is already some weight on the right heel. Beginners usually try to turn the foot much too early.

- If this still doesn't help, see 'Alternative method for the turning of the right toes' on the following page.

- **The right arm and hand:**
  - Keep the right elbow sunk as you raise the hand.
  - Lift the hand directly up the body between your centreline and 3.00.
  - The right hand should be extended well away from the body at the end of the movement; beginners tend to arrive with the right elbow too bent.
  - Flex the right wrist at the end of the movement so that the hypothenar eminence is extended rather than the fingertips (which should be pointing upwards).

- **Snake Creeps Down:** It is this part of the movement that gives Snake Creeps Down its name. When the posture is done very low, there is a feeling of slithering along the ground as you move forwards and out of it.

BRIEF 4B
Adjust the left toes; crane's beak moves to hip.

DETAILS
The left hand (still in a crane's beak) lowers to beside your left thigh, with the 'beak' pointing behind you.

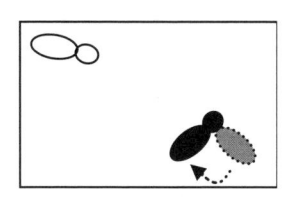

The right hand arrives in position with the index finger ahead of the tip of your nose.

As the weight arrives on the right foot, lift the *toes* of the rear foot and turn them inwards to 1.30 (see the diagram to the left).

The eyes continue to look to 3.00.

NOTES

- **The left hand:** A common fault is to place the back of the left hand against the left buttock. It should finish by the *side* of the left thigh, not behind it.

- **The left foot:** Beginners usually try to slip the rear heel instead of turning the toes. Strictly speaking this isn't correct because it increases the length of the stance; this makes moving out of the stance much harder. So although you will not notice any difference if you are not doing a low Crouch Stance, as your flexibility gradually improves and you start to sink lower, a habit of slipping the left heel will begin to cause problems.

- **Problems associated with turning the rear toes:** The most common fault is to stick the backside out during the turn of the back foot. This is due to either:

  1. the feet being too far apart in the first place (see Brief 3)

  2. the inflexibility of the front of the left hip, making it impossible to sink and relax the hip, or

  3. the left Achilles tendon being too tight, making it impossible to lift the toes.

Additionally, the back foot is difficult to adjust correctly if the weight isn't completely over the right foot.

ALTERNATIVE METHOD FOR THE TURNING OF THE RIGHT TOES

Not everyone is able to turn the left toes out to 3.30/4.00. If it is too difficult, then initially point them to 3.00 (see Alt. method 1). Then, just before the movement that follows (i.e. Brief 5) which requires that you stand, either: 1) turn the toes outwards just before standing, or 2) turn the *heel* inwards just before standing (see Alt. method 2).

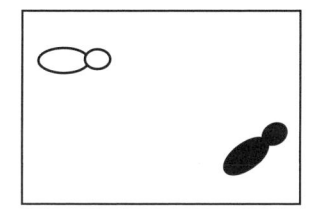

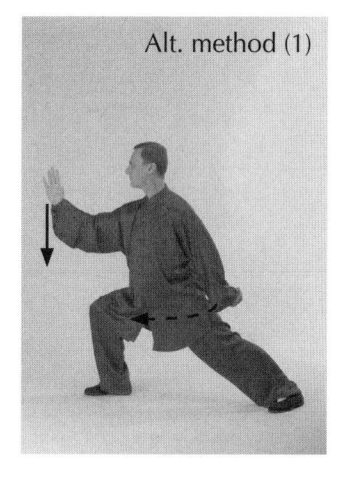

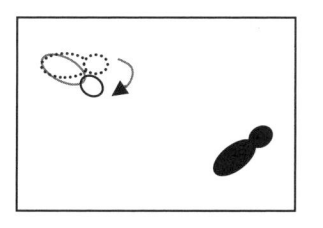

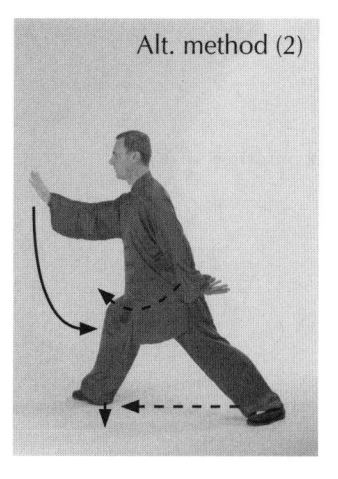

THE YANG TÀIJÍ 24-STEP SHORT FORM

Brief 4

Golden Cockerel (Right Side) (Stand on Right Leg). Push the right hand down; raise the left hand and left knee.

Details

As you move the weight fully on to your right foot, push your right palm downwards with the fingers pointing to your right (1.30).

As you start to straighten your right leg, the left hand moves from your left thigh, the fingers opening, and simultaneously the left leg moves forwards.

The left hand and knee move towards 3.00, and both lift; the left hand moves up the centreline of the body with the arm well extended – the palm facing right (6.00), the fingers vertical, to arrive with the hand ahead of the mouth (the index finger level with the tip of the nose) and directly between your centreline and 3.00.

The left knee lifts so that it touches your left elbow (or as near as possible).

As the left hand and leg move into position, the right hand has finished pushing down the midline of the body and has moved to your right side with palm facing the floor, and fingers pointing to 3.00.

The eyes continue to look to 3.00.

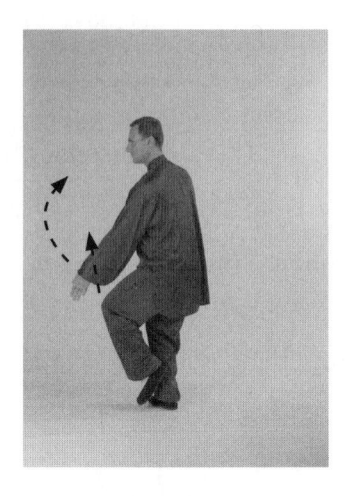

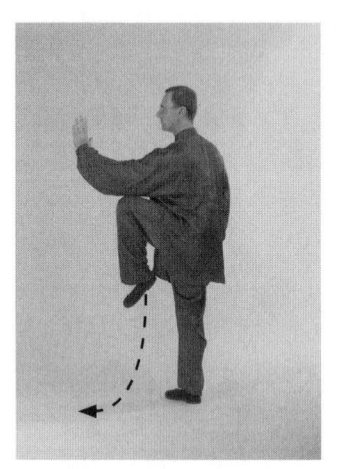

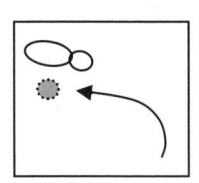

Notes

- **Connections:**

    - There should be a feeling of the left elbow and left knee working together throughout the lift.

    - Feel the 'opposites' working together, i.e. left and right wrists; right knee straightening and left knee bending; right wrist pushing down, left wrist lifting up, etc.

- **Lifting the left knee:**
  - When raising the left knee, keep the body upright. To get the feel, have a partner push down on your knee as you lift it.
  - The lifting of the knee is partly achieved by a pelvic tilt; therefore gently pull in the lower abdominal muscles as you lift the knee.
  - The left knee should rise to, and touch, your left elbow. Lift the *knee* to the elbow, rather than lower the *elbow* to the knee. If trying to touch the knee with the elbow means that you have to bend the body at the waist to get it there, then only lift it as high as you are able.
  - The left ankle is relaxed.
- **The right leg** finishes straight but not locked.
- **Lifting the left hand:**
  - Extend the arm towards 3.00 as you lift, allowing the body to turn slightly further to your right.
  - When lifting the left hand, there should be a feeling of initially lifting the heel of the thumb, followed by a feeling of lifting the fingers and pushing the little finger edge of the palm away from you towards 3.00.
  - The hand should finish with the hand *beyond* the knee, i.e. further towards 3.00 than the knee.
- **The right hand:**
  - Sink the right elbow and forearm to lower the right hand, and push down with the *heel* of the hand.
  - This movement can also be called Push Down and Stand on One Leg. The pushing down is therefore very important, particularly as you arrive in the final posture of the movement. Feel the simultaneous pushing down of the right hand and the lifting of the left hand.
  - When pushing down with the right hand, there should be a sense of Péng in the upper arm.
- **Application:** Visualize the right hand as blocking down, and the rising left hand as striking upwards to the groin.

- **Balance:**
    - Relax the hips and the buttocks allowing the small of the back to relax. Balance becomes much harder if this area is locked.
    - For purposes of balance, the right foot needs to be turned outwards very slightly (see notes 'The turning out of the right toes' on p.243 and 'Alternative method for the turning of the right toes' on p.245). It is noticeable that if the foot is pointing directly to 3.00, the balance is far more precarious; this is to do with the lie of the iliofemoral joint in the hip, i.e. the hip/thigh joint.
- **'Closed':** The body is 'closed' in this posture.

SECTION 7

(3 MOVEMENTS)

18. **Jade Lady Weaves Shuttles (Fair Lady Weaves her Shuttle Left and Right) (Shuttle Back and Forth) (Move the Shuttle Left and Right) (Work at Shuttles on Both Sides)**
左右穿梭 (Zuǒyòu Chuānsuō)

19. **Needle at Sea Bottom (Needle at the Bottom of the Sea)**
海底针 (Hǎidǐzhēn)

20. **Flash Arms (Fan Through Back) (Send a Flash Through the Arms)**
闪通臂 (Shǎntōngbì)

FORM 18: JADE LADY WEAVES SHUTTLES (FAIR LADY WEAVES HER SHUTTLE LEFT AND RIGHT) (SHUTTLE BACK AND FORTH) (MOVE THE SHUTTLE LEFT AND RIGHT) (WORK AT SHUTTLES ON BOTH SIDES)

左右穿梭 (Zuǒyòu Chuānsuō)

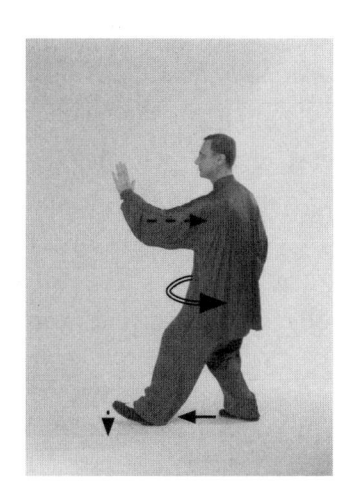

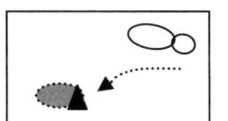

BRIEF 1
Sink and step ahead placing the left heel.

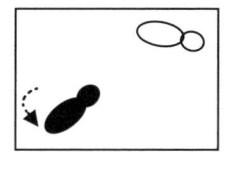

DETAILS
Bend the right knee and place the left heel to approximately 2.00.

The hands begin to change position into a 'holding the ball' gesture.

The eyes follow the left hand.

THE YANG TÀIJÍ 24-STEP SHORT FORM

NOTES

- **Stepping:** Sink into the right foot in order to place the left heel. As you move the foot forwards, widen the stance slightly by stepping towards 1.30/2.00.

- **The arms:** In the movement that follows you will be 'holding the ball', so at this stage the arms begin to alter.

  - **The left arm:** The left elbow starts to lift (and left fingertips to lower). Because the body is turning to the left, the left arm will begin to 'fold' at the elbow (with the turn of the centre) so that, by the end of the move that follows, the forearm will be in front of the body (the folded arm therefore moving nearer to your chest).

  - **The right arm:** As you sink into the right foot (see note above), relax the right wrist so that the fingers start to point downwards, and make a screwdriver turn with the hand so that the palm turns upwards. Start to lead the right fingertips forwards to in front of the body.

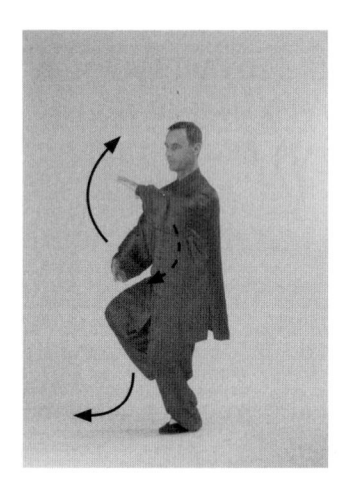

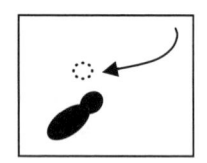

BRIEF 2
Weight forwards turning the toes out (1.30/2.00); hold the ball; bring right foot in.

DETAILS
As you move the weight on to the left foot, turn the toes of the left foot outwards to approximately 1.30/2.00; the body turns to the left diagonal (1.30).

Bring the right foot into the left.

The left hand completes changing angle, the forearm now approximately parallel to the ground (open up under the left armpit as well) at upper chest height.

The right hand, with the turn of the hips to the left, moves below the left hand in a relaxed 'holding the ball' gesture at waist height.

The eyes look over and beyond the left hand.

Notes

- **The centre** turns left towards 1.30.

- **Turning the left toes:** As the weight moves forwards, use the left turn of the hips to turn the left toes outwards.

- **The right hand:** As you place the left foot and move the weight completely over it, the right fingertips lead upwards (the hand with palm upwards) to Form the lower hand of the ball.

- **Position of hands:**
  - The left hand will be palm down at approximately upper chest height.
  - The right hand will be palm up at approximately waist height.

- **Connections:**
  - Keep a feeling of connection between the right elbow and right hip, and the right wrist and right ankle, as you move forwards.
  - As you move forwards, feel as though you are bringing the right shoulder towards the left hip.

- **Coordinate** the turn of the right palm upwards (rotating like a screw-driver) with the turn of the hips to the left.

- **'Holding the ball' gesture:** This is the only place in the Form where the hands actually 'hold the ball'.

  As pointed out previously, many teachers teach the 'holding the ball' gesture as an actual 'posture' in a variety of places throughout the Yang Tàijí 24-Step Short Form, but in all cases – apart from this one – there is no 'ball' gesture as such, as the arms are merely in the process of 'closing'.

  However, here the 'ball' *is* formed, and the shape is used in the movement that follows.

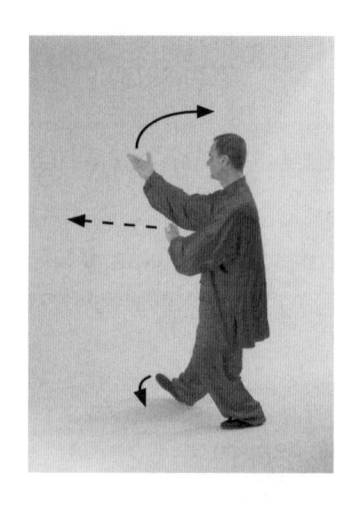

Brief 3

Rotate ball; extend right foot to 4.30; left hand below sternum.

Details

The right hand continues its circle upwards, initially towards 1.30, but soon turning to the right (because of the turn of the body) towards 4.00/4.30 at approximately heart height (see 'The hands rotate the ball' on the following page).

The left elbow sinks, the arm rotating downwards with palm facing away to just below the sternum/breastbone (see 'The hands rotate the ball' on the following page).

Your weight remains on the left foot, but place your right heel to 4.00/4.30.

As your right hand starts to move into your peripheral vision, your eyes look beyond your *right* hand to the 4.00/4.30 corner.

Notes

- **Angle of body:** At this stage the centreline will face 3.00/4.00.

- **The left hand** is close to the body.

- **The right shoulder** should be relaxed and sunk.

    The right heel (width of stance): When placing the right heel, the movement requires a wide stance (12 inches (30 cm) between the feet on the diagonal axis); therefore you need to step *wide* to 4.30. In effect this means almost stepping *sideways* with the toes pointing to 4.30.

    Alternative method: However, there is some flexibility in the posture and it can also be done to 4.00. Oddly enough, this makes a considerable difference to the way in which it is performed. It means that you can step directly to the 4.30 corner ahead of the left heel, but that, as you place your right toes, you turn them slightly inwards to face 4.00. This has the effect of widening your stance.

- **The waist:** Sink further into the left foot and turn the waist initially a little further to the *left* and then to the right.

- **The hands rotate the ball:** There is a feeling of rotating the hands around a ball in this movement – the left hand rotates down to lower chest height (the elbow dropping and the palm altering angle so that it faces 4.30), and the right hand rotates upwards to throat height (the elbow lifting and the palm altering angle so that it initially faces you, and then eventually turns to face downwards).

The main point is that the arms should rotate as though there were a ball between the hands; in order to get the feel of this, hold a football (or something slightly larger) between the palms and then rotate it.

The rotation is slightly more complicated that this in that it is not exactly a *vertical* rotation. In the previous two movements the right hand direction of movement has formed a pathway from right to left on an upwards diagonal. Because of this the line/angle of movement needs to be continued, so the right hand actually continues to the left as it rotates the ball, and then back to the right as it completes the rotation. This means that the shape of the ball rotation resembles the double helix of a strand of DNA or, to put it another way, it looks like the line connecting the two 'fish' in the Yin/Yang symbol.

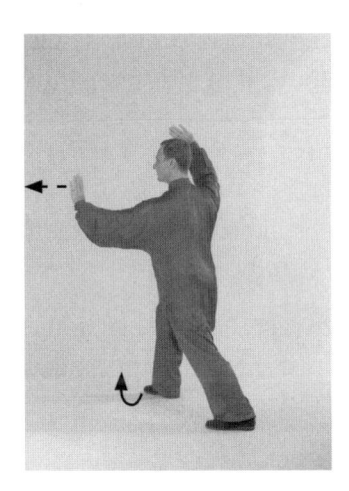

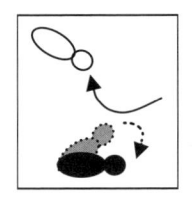

BRIEF 4
Weight forwards; left hand push; right arm rotates upwards; slip the rear heel.

DETAILS
Transfer your weight to the right foot into a right Bow Stance.

Your left hand pushes ahead of you (index finger level with the tip of your nose).

Your right hand continues to arc upwards to the height of the top of your head, or slightly above the head.

As you complete the move, use the turn of the hips to slip your rear heel.
The eyes look to 4.30.

Notes

- **Angle of body:** Your centreline will be turned slightly towards your right knee, i.e. the body is turned to approximately 5.00.

- **Width of stance:** See note in previous movement (p.252).

- **The left hand:** The index finger of the left hand will be directly ahead of the tip of your nose.

- **The right arm:** Beginners tend to try to pull the upper arm backwards.

  The upper hand is higher than your head, with the palm turned upwards, but the hand is still in front of your face, not level with the side of your head.

  To get the feeling of the hand, salute with the nails against the upper right corner of your forehead, then lift the hand just above the head, and push it slightly forwards.

  From the end of Brief 2 (palm up low) to the end of Brief 4 (palm up high) the right hand has made almost a 360° rotation.

  The right shoulder should be relaxed and sunk.

  Movement of energy in the rising right arm: The spiralling energy travels from fingertips to shoulder as you lift the arm between Briefs 3 and 4. By the end of Brief 3 it has reached the elbow (or slightly above it in the upper arm) and by Brief 4 it has reached the shoulder.

- **The hands (relative to each other):**

  - At the end of the move, your right hand is nearer the body than the left hand.

  - The most common fault amongst beginners is to have both hands at the same distance from the body as though pushing forwards with both hands.

  - There is a feeling of pushing *up* with the right hand and *away* with the left hand.

- **Similarities to Brush Knee and Twist Step:** Note the similarities and differences between this posture and Brush Knee and Twist Step.

  The only differences are 1) the angle – one is angled to the diagonal, and one is square to the cardinal points; and 2) the hand not pushing directly ahead – one has a hand raised above head height, and the other has the hand by the side of the leg.

- **'Opening':** Overall this is an 'open' movement.

Jade Lady Weaves Shuttles (Second Side)

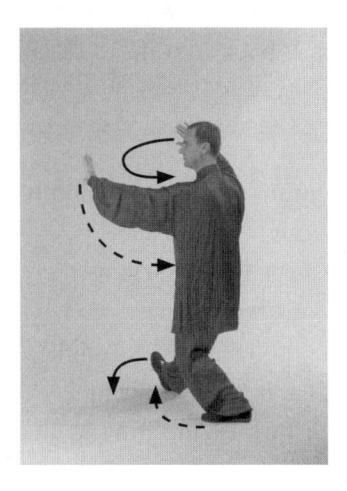

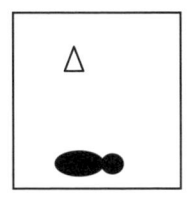

BRIEF 1
Sit back (see Notes below); turn to 3.00; start to lower the arms.

DETAILS
Sit back briefly on to the left foot (see Notes below), turning the body slightly towards 3.00.
 Simultaneously start to lower your arms.
 The eyes continue to look to 4.30.

NOTES

- **Sitting back:** It is optional as to whether you sit back or not. Options are that you can either 1) not sit back at all, and shift the weight immediately further *forwards* on to the right foot, 2) you can sit back on to the left foot fractionally as you turn the body to the left. If you do the latter, it is only a very small shift, and you should move straight back to the right foot in the movement that follows.

  Or 3) you can lift the right toes or not if you sit back. Personally I think that there is nothing to be gained by sitting back.

- **The hands** are going to be 'holding the ball' in the next movement, so the arms are in the process of lowering and circling to reach this position.

  - **The right hand** extends out towards 4.30 as you turn the body towards 3.00.

  - **The left arm** moves to the left with the turn of the body.

- **Sinking the arms:** As you shift the weight forwards, there is a feeling of sinking the arms to sink the qì in the upper body.

- **Direction of body turn:** Turn the body towards 3.00.

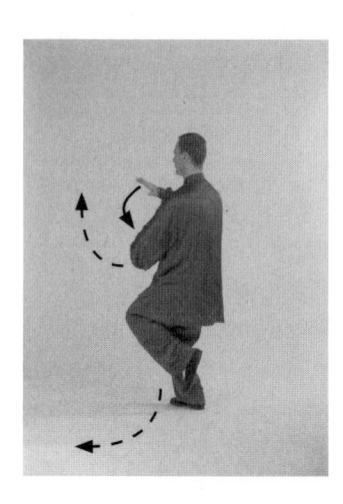

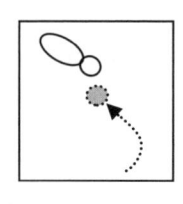

BRIEF 2

Weight forwards (if shifted back); hold the ball; back foot in.

DETAILS

As the weight arrives on your right foot, the body turns back to the right diagonal (4.30).

Bring the left foot forwards into the right.

The right hand finishes lowering, the forearm now approximately parallel to the ground (open up slightly under the left armpit as well) at upper chest height.

The left hand, with the turn of the hips to the right, moves below the right hand in a relaxed 'holding the ball' gesture at waist height.

The eyes look over and beyond the right hand.

NOTES

- **The centre** turns left towards 4.30.

- **The left hand:** As you re-place the right foot (if you have lifted the toes) and move the weight completely over it, the left fingertips lead inwards (the hand with palm upwards) to form the lower hand of the ball.

- **The right hand:** As you turn back to the 4.30 corner, the right arm makes a small anti-clockwise circle to end up folding in front of your upper chest.

- **Position of hands:**
  - The right hand will be palm down at approximately upper chest height.
  - The left hand will be palm up at approximately waist height.

- **Connections:**
  - Keep a feeling of connection between the left elbow and left hip, and the left wrist and left ankle, as you move forwards.
  - As you move forwards, feel as though you are bringing the left shoulder towards the right hip.

- **Coordinate** the turn of the left palm upwards (rotating like a screw-driver) with the turn of the hips to the right.

- **'Holding the ball' gesture:** This is the only other place in the Form where the hands actually 'hold the ball' – the first place was in the previous 'Jade Lady' movement.

   As pointed out previously, many teachers teach the 'holding the ball' gesture as an actual 'posture' in a variety of places throughout the Yang Tàijí 24-Step Short Form, but in all cases – apart from this one – there is no 'ball' gesture as such, as the arms are merely in the process of 'closing'.

   However, here the 'ball' *is* formed, and the shape is used in the movement that follows.

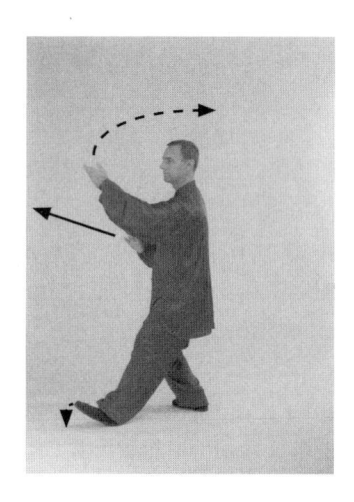

BRIEF 3

Rotate ball; extend left foot to 1.30; right hand below sternum.

DETAILS

The left hand continues its circle upwards, initially towards 4.30, but soon turning to the left (because of the turn of the body) towards 1.30/2.00 at approximately heart height (see 'The hands rotate the ball' on the following page).

The right elbow sinks, the arm rotating downwards with palm facing away to just below the sternum/breastbone (see 'The hands rotate the ball' on the following page).

Your weight remains on the right foot, but place your right heel to 1.30/2.00.

As your left hand starts to move into your peripheral vision, your eyes look beyond your *left* hand to the 1.30/2.00 corner.

NOTES

- **Angle of body:** At this stage the centreline will face 2.00/3.00.

- **The right hand** is close to the body.

- **The left shoulder** should be relaxed and sunk.

- **The left heel (width of stance):** When placing the left heel, the movement requires a wide stance; therefore you need to step *wide* to 1.30 (12 inches (30 cm) between the feet on the diagonal axis). In effect this means almost stepping *sideways* with the toes pointing to 1.30.

- **Alternative method:** However there is some flexibility in the posture and it can also be done to 2.00. Oddly enough, this makes a considerable difference to the way in which it is performed. It means that you can step directly to the 1.30 corner ahead of the right heel, but that, as you place your left toes, you turn them slightly inwards to face 2.00. This has the effect of widening your stance.

- **The waist:** Sink further into the right foot and turn the waist initially a little further to the *right* and then to the left.

- **The hands rotate the ball:** There is a feeling of rotating the hands around a ball in this movement – the right hand rotates down to lower chest height (the elbow dropping and the palm altering angle so that it faces 1.30), and the left hand rotates upwards to throat height (the elbow lifting and the palm altering angle so that it initially faces you, and then eventually turns to face downwards).

  The main point is that the arms should rotate as though there were a ball between the hands; in order to get the feel of this, hold a football (or something slightly larger) between the palms and then rotate it.

  The rotation is slightly more complicated than this in that it is not exactly a *vertical* rotation. In the previous two movements, the left hand direction of movement has formed a pathway from left to right on an upwards diagonal. Because of this, the line/angle of movement needs to be continued, so the left hand actually continues to the right as it rotates the ball, and then back to the left as it completes the rotation. This means that the shape of the ball rotation resembles the double helix of a strand of DNA or, to put it another way, it looks like the line connecting the two 'fish' in the Yin/Yang symbol.

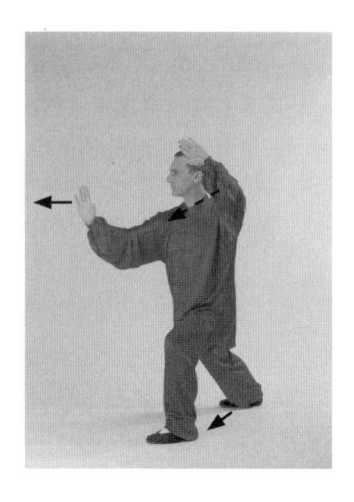

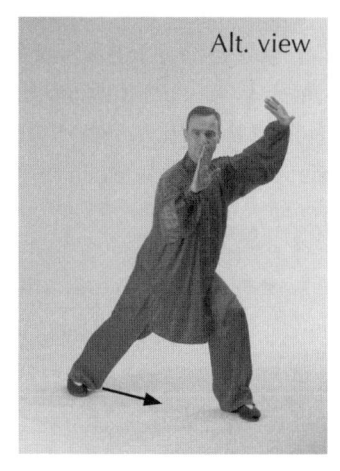

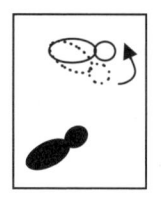

DESCRIPTION OF THE YANG TÀIJÍ 24-STEP SHORT FORM

BRIEF 4
Weight forwards; right hand push; left hand rotates upwards; slip the rear heel.

DETAILS

Transfer your weight to the left foot into a left Bow Stance.

Your right hand pushes ahead of you (index finger level with the tip of your nose).

Your left hand continues to arc upwards to the height of the top of your head, or slightly above the head.

As you complete the move, use the turn of the hips to slip your rear heel.

The eyes look to 1.30.

NOTES

- **Angle of body:** Your centreline will be turned slightly towards your left knee, i.e. the body is turned to approximately 1.00.

- **Width of stance:** See note in previous movement (p.258).

- **The right hand:** The index finger of the right hand will be directly ahead of the tip of your nose.

- **The left arm:** Beginners tend to try to pull the upper arm backwards.

    The upper hand is higher than your head, with the palm turned upwards, but the hand is still in front of your face, not level with the side of your head.

    To get the feeling of the hand, salute with the nails against the upper left corner of your forehead, then lift the hand just above the head, and push it slightly forwards.

    From the end of Brief 2 (palm up low) to the end of Brief 4 (palm up high) the left hand has made almost a 360° rotation.

    The left shoulder should be relaxed and sunk.

Movement of energy in the rising left arm: The spiralling energy travels from fingertips to shoulder as you lift the arm between Briefs 3 and 4. By the end of Brief 3 it has reached the elbow (or slightly above it in the upper arm) and by Brief 4 it has reached the shoulder.

- **The hands (relative to each other):**

  - At the end of the move, your left hand is nearer the body than the right hand.

  - The most common fault amongst beginners is to have both hands at the same distance from the body as though pushing forwards with both hands.

  - There is a feeling of pushing *up* with the left hand and *away* with the right hand.

- **Similarities with Brush Knee and Twist Step:** Note the similarities and differences between this posture and Brush Knee and Twist Step.

  The only differences are 1) the angle – one is angled to the diagonal, and one is square to the cardinal points; and 2) the hand not pushing directly ahead – one has a hand raised above head height, and the other has the hand by the side of the leg.

- **'Opening':** Overall this is an 'open' movement.

FORM 19: NEEDLE AT SEA BOTTOM (NEEDLE AT THE BOTTOM OF THE SEA)

海底针 (Hǎidǐzhēn)

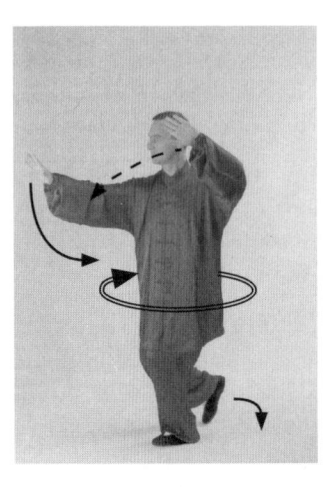

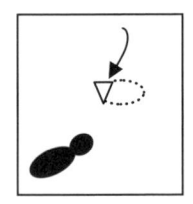

BRIEF 1
Back foot forwards.

DETAILS
Put the weight fully on to your left foot, and bring your right toes forwards towards 3.00.

The eyes look beyond the right hand.

DESCRIPTION OF THE YANG TÀIJÍ 24-STEP SHORT FORM

Notes

- **Coordinate** the movement of bringing in the rear foot with pushing slightly further forwards with the right hand, and upwards with the left hand. In other words, continue both hands' direction of energy from the previous movement.

- **The right hand**, having pushed forwards, immediately relaxes as the weight finishes moving forwards on to the left foot.

  The right elbow sinks (starts to rotate inwards) as the wrist releases – starting the process of 'closing'.

- **The left elbow** begins to 'close' inwards.

- **The right foot** step is similar to a Sun style step.

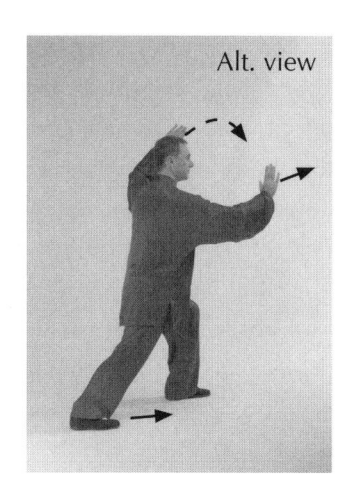

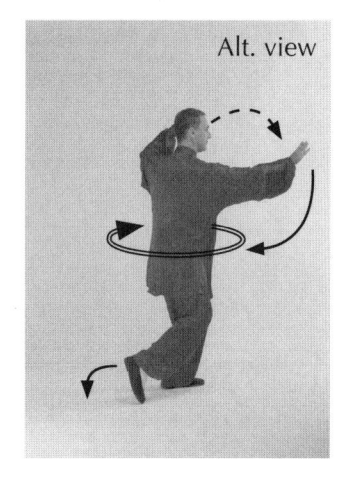

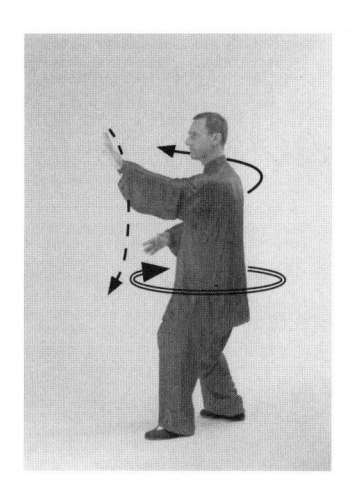

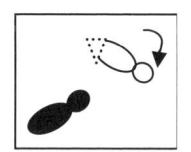

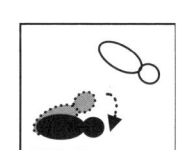

Alt. view

Alt. view

BRIEF 2
Sit back; left hand lowering to the right; right hand rotating palm up to right side of the waist.

DETAILS
Sit back on to the right foot, turning the right toes to 4.30, and turn the centreline towards 4.30.

261

As you do so, the left arm sinks further from above head height in the previous movement, to throat/chest height (it will therefore lie between the body and 3.00/4.00), the forearm pushing downwards and to the right side (see 'The left arm' below).

Simultaneously, the right hand lowers with the turn of the body, and as the palm rotates upwards, it draws back to the right side of the waist.

The eyes follow the left forearm.

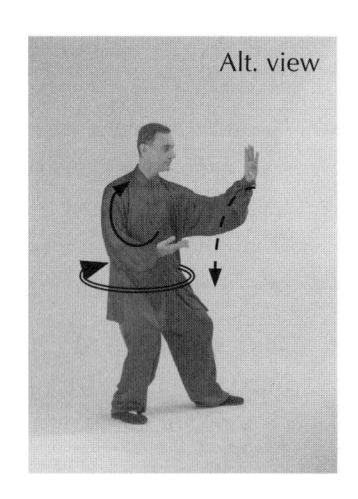

Alt. view

NOTES

- **Connections:** The whole movement should be coordinated with the turn of the waist and hips to the right. Make a connection between the hips and the elbows as you turn the body.

- **The left arm** is in the process of moving from the left corner (1.30) to the right, and there should be a sense of sinking the forearm as though to block something downwards and slightly rightwards.

  The left elbow should lead the sinking of the forearm ('closing').

- **The right elbow** rotates inwards, the right palm spiralling/rotating upwards as the arm draws back as though breaking out of a wrist grip.

- **The left foot:** As you turn the body to the right (3.00/4.00), free the left heel so that the foot pivots on the left toes to point to 3.00. This is less strain on the medial aspect of the left knee.

- **This is a 'closed' movement:** Feel the elbows and hips working together in the closing. This is easily felt if you have a partner take hold of your right wrist and gently pull away from you as you sit back on to the right foot.

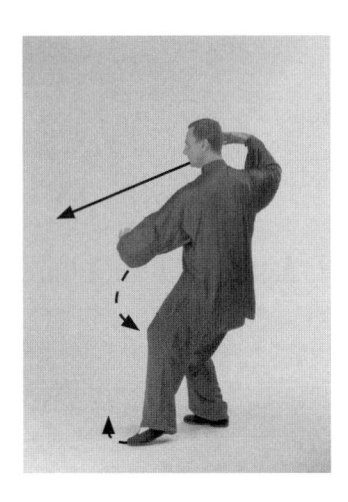

DESCRIPTION OF THE YANG TÀIJÍ 24-STEP SHORT FORM

Brief 3
Change the hands.

Details
The weight stays on the right foot.

As the body turns further to the right the right hand rises from the waist to head height, the tips of the fingers as high as the ear with the fingers pointing upwards at approximately 45°. The right palm faces the body.

The left hand pushes (palm down) down the centreline of the body to the waist.

The centreline turns further to the right.
The eyes are looking back to 3.00.

Notes

- **The right hand** rises upwards in a *circular* anti-clockwise vertical lift, i.e. the right forearm and hand will continuously point towards 3.00. (Beginners tend to circle the hand/arm out sideways to the right so that the fingers point towards 6.00, as though they were performing the circling of the arm between Lù and Jí in Forms 7 and 8.)

  Direction of circle: This is very much a circular movement of the right arm (not unlike the side rods on an old fashioned steam train). With the right elbow doing very little other than moving with the turn of the body (i.e. the elbow neither lifts nor lowers), the right hand circles from your waist, backwards (but only because the body is turning further to the right), then rises and starts to move forwards (because the body is now starting to turn back to the left), to the height of your right shoulder/ear.

  The right palm faces the body continuously as it rises.

  The right elbow *does* lift slightly towards the end of the movement, but the majority of the movement is in the forearm.

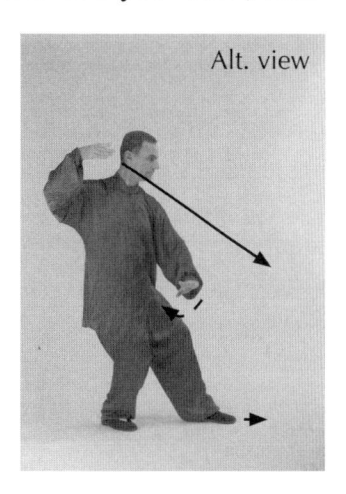

Alt. view

N.B. The movement of the right elbow should coordinate with the movement of the right hip.

The right shoulder should remain relaxed as you raise the right hand.

- **Connections:** The right elbow and right hip have already been mentioned, but also be aware of the left elbow and left hip.

- **The knees and hips:** The left knee has a tendency to collapse inwards if not watched, and the right knee should open during this part of the movement. There is therefore an 'opening' of the Kuà here.

- **Posture:** Keep the body upright in this movement; beginners tend to lean the body forwards in anticipation of the final movement.

- **The arms:** Note the 'opening' of the arms here – one hand up and one hand down in preparation for the 'close' in the movement that follows.

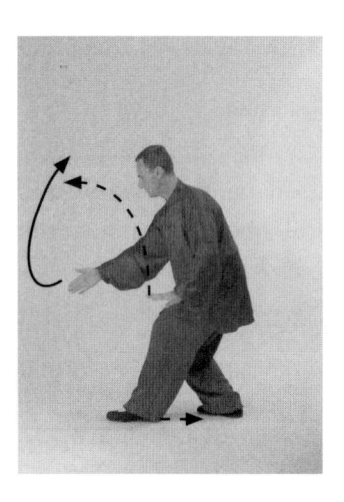

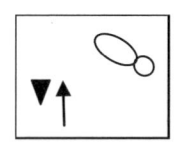

BRIEF 4

Left hand sweeps knee; right hand fingers 'dive' downwards; adjust left toes.

DETAILS

With the weight on the right foot, turn the centreline back to face 3.00.

The left hand sweeps across the front of the body at waist height to the left side of the left knee with the turn of the body (palm down; the fingers pointing to 3.00).

The right hand 'dives' from the right ear to directly ahead of the body at pelvis height (palm facing left, arm and fingers angled at 45° downwards).

The body is angled no further forwards than 45° (and can be less than that if required).

As the hands arrive in their final position, adjust the left toes into an empty step ahead of you.

Notes

- **The right hand:** There are a number of ways of moving the right hand and fingers as they move from the ear. My preference is to slightly tilt the little finger downwards (the palm still facing 12.00), so that the wrist flexes slightly, and then to thrust downwards with the tips of the fingers leading.

    You do see this move done a number of different ways however, the most popular being the pushing down of the right hand leading with the entire little finger *edge* as though 'chopping' downwards. (As one of the applications for this movement is a sword-like thrust with the fingertips, I don't personally agree with this interpretation.)

- **The left hand**, in sweeping across the front of the body, pushes *down* at the same time.

- **Bending forwards:**

    - Lead the movement by drawing in the lower abdominal muscles and relaxing the small of the back.

    - **Angle of the body:** This is a fairly demanding posture if you bend forwards too much, and can be quite stressful on the right knee. Bend forwards to an angle between vertical and 45°.

- **The spine:**

    - The bend forwards should come from the hips and not from the lower thoracic vertebrae.

    - When leaning forwards, the spine should be fairly straight; avoiding excessive bowing or rounding of the back.

    - **The head and neck** should remain aligned with the spine.

- **The eyes:** In this posture you *are* looking downwards, but don't look at your left foot; the eyes in the final posture look approximately a metre ahead of

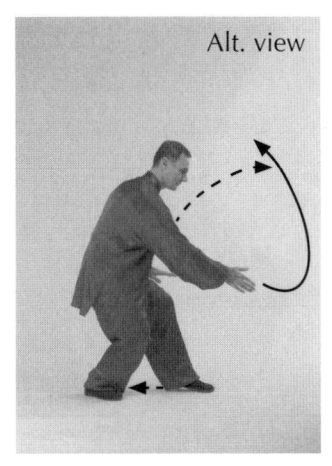

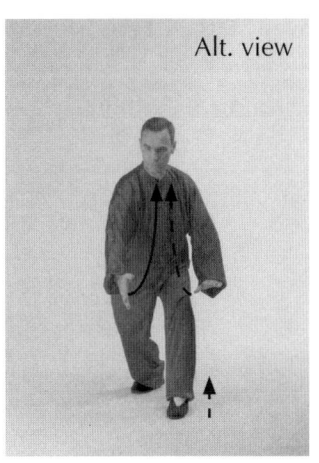

THE YANG TÀIJÍ 24-STEP SHORT FORM

the point at which the right hand is pointing; this avoids the neck bending downwards too much.

- **'Closing'**: This is a 'closed' movement.

- **General note for all 4 movements**: Throughout, use the centre to create the rotation of the right arm as described above. There is a circling in the dāntián that moves: left (Brief 1), right (Brief 2), right, up and left (Brief 3), before moving down (Brief 4).

FORM 20: FLASH ARMS (FAN THROUGH BACK) (SEND A FLASH THROUGH THE ARMS)

闪通臂 (Shǎntōngbì)

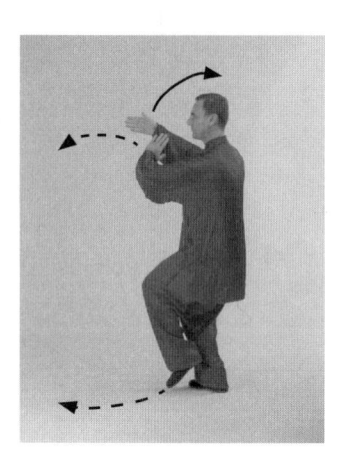

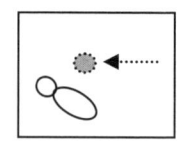

BRIEF 1
Extend right arm; straighten the body; start to lift the hands; left foot empty.

DETAILS
Keeping the right knee bent, turn your waist to the left (2.00), extending the right arm ahead of you.

As you start to straighten the body, the extended right arm rises ahead of you (still pointing to 3.00) and with the weight still on the right foot, turn your centreline towards 4.30.

The left hand also rises with the straightening body directly ahead of the centreline (approximately to the height of the sternum).

The palms face inwards, the right palm facing 12.00, the left palm facing 6.00.

Partially draw the left foot into the right foot (but see Notes on the following page).

The eyes look to 3.00.

NOTES

- **The upper body** turns to the left slightly, not the hips. This continues the line of energy in the right hand from the previous Form (Needle at Sea Bottom).

- **The left foot** can come back as far as the right ankle (the toes do not touch the floor) or you can simply only lift the left foot. (See Variation photo to the right.)

    From a martial point of view, the weight should not shift too much on to the right foot, i.e. there shouldn't be a feeling of the body retreating; the aim of the movement from the previous Form is to advance further to 3.00. Excessive sitting back would therefore give an opponent, who is pushing you from 3.00, an added advantage. The 'energy' of these movements is therefore not backwards – you should be thinking forwards (unless to avoid an attack to the foot itself).

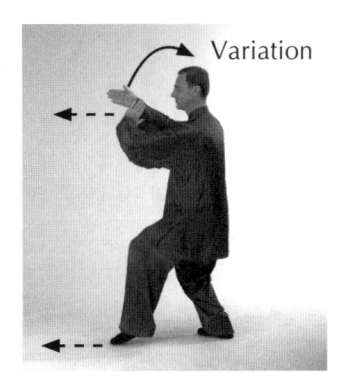

    Having said that – this is a tàijí form, and not everyone is doing it with martial intention in mind! In which case, observation of weight-control and balance play a role.

- **'Closing'**: The body is 'closing'.

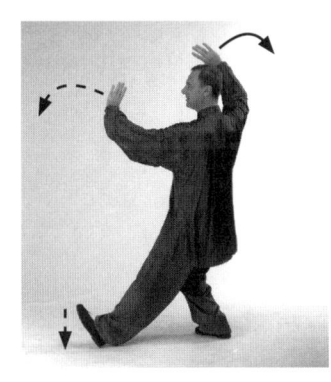

BRIEF 2
Hands continue to rise; re-step to 3.00.

DETAILS
Place the left heel to 3.00.

The right hand continues to rise, the palm beginning to rotate downwards.

The left hand rises to meet the right wrist at approximately shoulder/throat height.

The eyes continue to look to 3.00.

Notes

- **The right hand** is in the process of rising above your head with palm facing upwards. The arm therefore makes a gradual screwdriver turn, and at this stage of the turn the palm is turning to face downwards. There is no flexing of the wrist involved.

    The energy is in the forearm, i.e. feel as though you are lifting the right *forearm*, not the hand.

- **The left hand** rises and the fingers touch the medial aspect of the right wrist (or are held very close to it). This comes from the Traditional Long Form (108) where the left hand is used to lock an opponent's fingers to your right wrist if he were to grip your right hand.

- **Left hand alternative version:** Some practitioners don't place the left fingers on the right wrist. Both hands rise upwards at the same speed, and by the time that the left hand is ahead of the upper chest/right shoulder, the right hand will therefore be at face height. The hands therefore never meet.

    Which version you use is unimportant; the applications are slightly different, but the feeling is the same.

- **Sink the shoulders** when lifting the hands.

- **'Closing':** The body 'closing'.

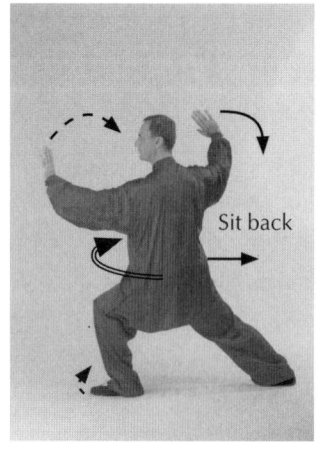

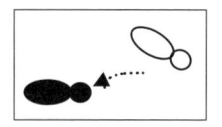

BRIEF 3
Weight forwards; lift right hand; push left hand.

Details

Move forwards into a left Bow Stance.

As you move forwards, the hands start to separate: The right arm rises higher, rotating to face first away from the body, and then turning upwards to finish with hand just higher than the head – the palm facing outwards (diagonally upwards).

The left hand, from being in front of the right shoulder, pushes ahead to 3.00 to finish directly ahead of your body with the index finger at the height of the tip of your nose.

The eyes look towards 3.00.

Notes

- **Width of stance:** There should be about the width of one fist (4 inches; 10 cm) between your heels on the 3.00/9.00 axis.

- **Angle of body:** The centreline is turned about 30°–45° to your right.

- **The right arm:** There is a feeling of the right arm lifting and pulling slightly backwards, but don't pull it too far behind the head.

  The right shoulder should be relaxed.

- **The left hand:** If not using the 'alternative version' outlined in Brief 2 on p.268, the aim of the left hand throughout Briefs 1 to 3 is to rise from the side of the left knee and push out ahead to 3.00. It doesn't need to move too closely into the body therefore.

  The best way to get the feel of it is to have a partner stand in front of you whilst you are in the final position of Needle at Sea Bottom, and then as quickly as possible to lift the left hand whilst straightening the body and push your partner away with your hand on his chest.

- **'Opening':** This is an 'open' movement.

- **Shǎn** is often translated as 'flash' meaning 'quick as lightning'. **Tōng** means 'through', and **Bì** means 'back'.

  (As a point of interest, Tōng Bèi (also spelt as Tōngbì) is the name of a Northern China martial art (Tōngbèiquán) that uses movements involving the turning of the torso in coordination with whirling of the arms.)

SECTION 8

(4 MOVEMENTS)

21. **Turn, Deflect Downwards, Parry and Punch (Turn the Body, Deflect, Block and Punch)**
    转身搬拦捶 (Zhuǎnshēn Bānlánchuí)

22. **Apparent Close-Up (Appearing to Seal and Close) (Pull Back then Push, as if to Close)**
    如封似闭 (Rúfēng Sìbì)

23. **Cross Hands**
    十字手 (Shízìshǒu)

24. **Closing Form**
    收势 (Shōushì)

FORM 21: TURN, DEFLECT DOWNWARDS, PARRY AND PUNCH (TURN THE BODY, DEFLECT, BLOCK AND PUNCH)

转身搬拦捶 (Zhuǎnshēn Bānlánchuí)

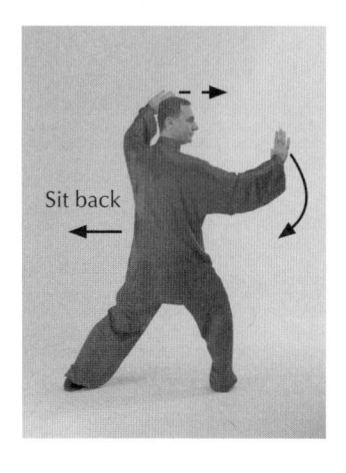

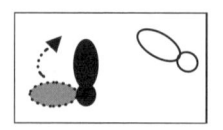

BRIEF 1
Sit back; turn the body; arc the arms.

DETAILS
As you sit back, shifting the weight on to the right foot, lift the left toes slightly and turn the centre/hips to 6.00, pivoting the left foot on the heel to face 6.00.

Simultaneously, arc the arms from the left side of the body, upwards in front of the face, and down to the right side of the body; the palms face away from you throughout.

The eyes look beyond the right hand at the end.

NOTES

- **The left hand:** Continue the feeling of pushing to 3.00 to convert the change of energy-direction in the arm.

- **Sitting back:** Bend the back knee to sit back, and sink the tip of the tailbone into the rear heel. Sit back only enough to free the left foot so that it can turn on the heel.

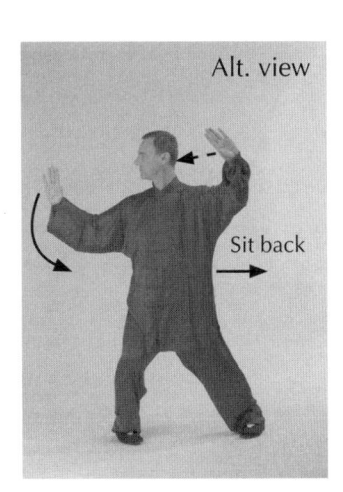

- **The weight** is on the right foot (beginners often take the weight back on to the left foot at this stage).

- **The 'arcing of the arms'** often causes a problem; try moving the arms as though drawing a rainbow with *both* palms (beginners often arc only the right arm).

- **The shoulders** should remain relaxed (beginners often lift the left shoulder).

- **Posture:**
    - **The right hip** should relax as you sit back.
    - **The right hip** should sink as you turn, the waist and lower back being allowed to open.
    - **The body should be upright** throughout (beginners sometimes lean the torso to the right).
    - **The coccyx/tailbone** should be tucked under.

- **Connections:** Feel the turn of the hips, and keep a feeling of connection between the hips and elbows, or alternatively the elbows and the knees.

- **The final position of the hands** (at this stage of the movement) is almost a mirror of the starting hand position. The left hand will be slightly above your head, and the right hand will be out to your right side with the wrist at approximately shoulder-height; both hands will have palms facing outwards.

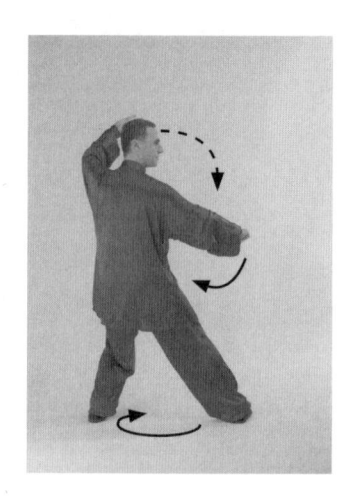

BRIEF 2

Shift weight; right hand into a fist palm down.

DETAILS

Move the weight back on to the left foot.

Simultaneously, the right hand continues its circle from shoulder-height downwards (the palm now downwards) and inwards to in front of the waist, where the open palm becomes a fist. The eye of the fist faces the dāntián (the palm of the fist therefore facing downwards).

The left hand (still with palm facing away) moves slightly further around to the right and starts to lower to arrive between the throat and 6.00.

At the end of the move, the body faces 7.00.

The eyes look towards 7.30.

NOTES

- **The weight** has shifted back on to the left foot.

- **The right elbow** should be sunk – there is a feeling of connecting it to the right knee.

- **The left shoulder** should be relaxed.

- **The left knee** 'opens' outwards slightly – avoid letting it collapse inwards.

- **'Closing'**: The body is starting to 'close' at this stage; the elbows are beginning to move together.

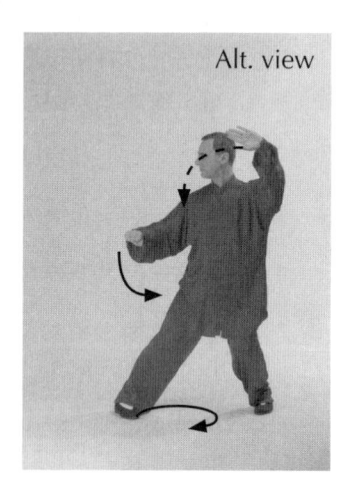

The following two movements should be thought of as one movement, but for the purposes of description and learning, it is easier to break them into two.

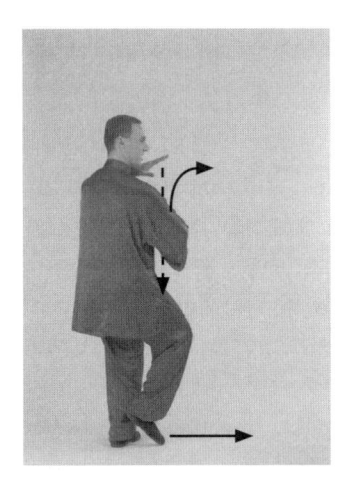

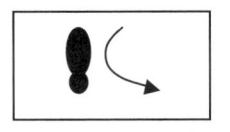

Brief 3a
Deflect Downwards (Bān). Left hand palm down the centreline; right foot lifts to step.

Details
The left hand starts to push palm down the centreline towards the waist.

The right fist starts to rise up the centreline between the left hand and the body.

The right foot briefly circles towards the left foot (but see Notes below).

Notes

- **Hand positions:**

  - The *palm* of the left hand pushes down; the *back* of the right fist rises.

  - Note that the rising fist is closer to the body than the sinking left hand.

- **The right foot** does not have to move into the left foot before re-stepping; some practitioners bring it alongside the left foot, some bring it in slightly, and some not at all. The reason for this is that the energetic direction of Bān is to 9.00. Some practitioners feel that the bringing in of the right foot has a tendency to reverse the sense of energetic direction (i.e. to 3.00). It does not matter if you do bring the foot back, but if you bear the energetic-direction concept in mind, it will alter the way in which you practise the movement. (See also 'General remarks on Briefs 1 to 3b' on p.275.)

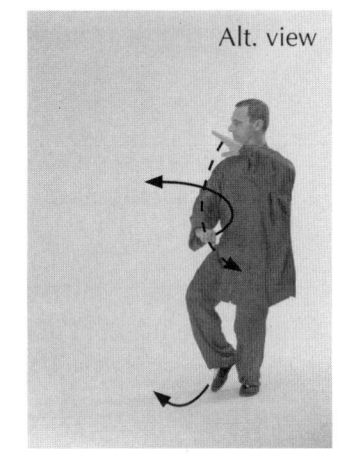

- **Connections:** Feel a connection between the hips and elbows; they should feel as though they are working together.

THE YANG TÀIJÍ 24-STEP SHORT FORM

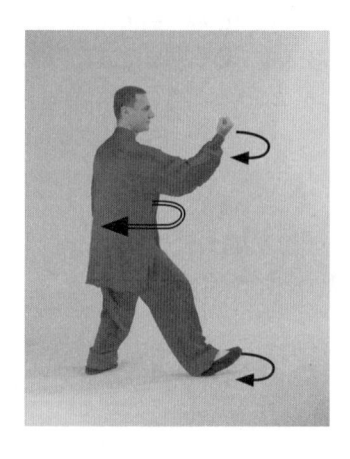

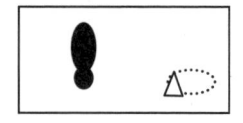

BRIEF 3B

Left palm continues to push downwards; right fist up and over; place right heel.

DETAILS

The right fist rises up the centreline of the body (nearer the body than the left arm) with the knuckles leading. It arcs upwards and then away to 9.00 in a vertical circle to arrive with the right forearm at 45° – the palm of the fist facing towards you but diagonally upwards.

The left hand continues to push downwards, the palm moving close to, or just below, the right elbow.

Although the body is in the process of turning towards 9.00, the centreline is still facing to 8.00 approximately; move the right foot around to 9.00.

The eyes look to 9.00.

NOTES:

- **Movements in Briefs 3a and 3b are simultaneous:** As the left hand pushes down the centreline, the right fist starts to rise up the centreline to strike outwards with the back of the fist.

- **The weight** remains on the left foot; the right foot does not even have to be placed on the floor at this stage. Beginners often try to move it on to the right foot.

- **The rotation of the right arm** is a rotation from the *elbow*, not from the shoulder.

The right fist: The vertically arcing fist rises to approximately the height of your mouth. In its final position, your right forearm is at an angle, with the elbow sunk and the fist directly ahead of you. Avoid pulling the elbow into the centreline of the body excessively, once again it is a feeling of elbow and right hip working together; if you are able to feel this, you will not over-contract the right arm.

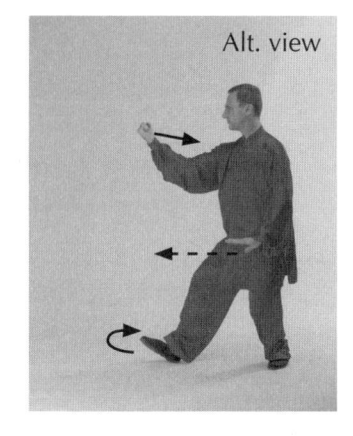

Alt. view

- **'Deflect Downwards' (Bān):** This movement is a simultaneous deflection and strike.

- **'Closed':** This is a 'closed' movement.

- **General remarks on Briefs 1 to 3b:** These movements should be thought of as a defence/attack to the 9.00 direction, and should be performed as one energetic movement in that direction. Although they have been divided up for the purpose of teaching them, from the point of view of the 'direction of energy' the intention (yǐ 意) throughout is very much to the 9.00 direction, and it should be felt and performed in this way. So, although the weight shifts back to the left foot in Brief 3, the feeling is *not* of moving back to 3.00.

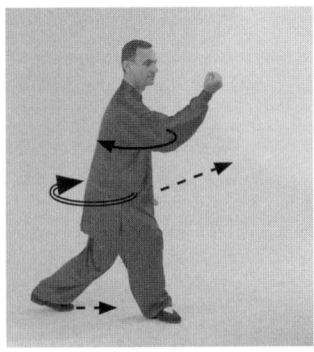

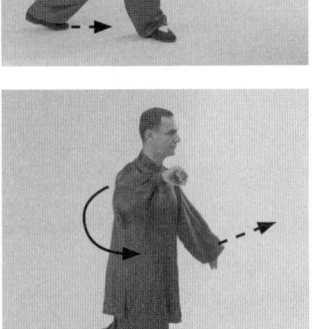

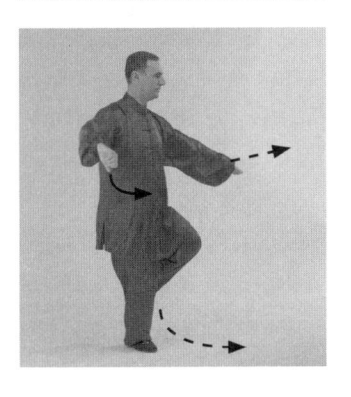

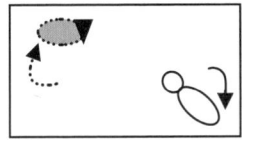

BRIEF 4

Parry (Lán). Weight forwards; turn right toes out; separate arms; rear heel off the ground.

DETAILS

Place and move the weight on to the right foot simultaneously turning the toes outwards to 45°. Lift your left heel off the ground.

Your right fist swings sideways to your right side lowering further to approximately waist height with the palm of the fist gradually rotating downwards.

At the same time your left palm continues the line of its push downwards before swinging out to your left side at approximately waist height with the palm of the hand downwards.

There should be a feeling of 'balancing' the arms (almost a horizontal windmilling of the arms around the body) – one hand in a fist, and the other with open palm, but both (whether open or in a fist) are palm down.

The eyes continue to look to 9.00.

Notes

- **Rotation of the hips:** The hips are in the process of turning to the right in both this and the next movement.

- **Connections:**
  - Use the turn of the hips to turn the right foot outwards.
  - Feel the relationship between the movement of the elbows and the turning of the hips.
  - Note the connections of hips turning the shoulders.

- **Turning the right foot:** Beginners often underestimate the importance of turning out the right foot. If the foot isn't turned out, the hips are unable to rotate to the right in the movement that follows.

- **The left foot** is in the process of stepping forwards. If the toes remain on the ground, it should therefore have no weight on it; some practitioners start to bring it towards the right foot at this stage.

- **The elbows and shoulders** should stay relaxed and sunk throughout.

- **Vertical and horizontal circles:** Briefs 1 to 3b form vertical circles with the arms; Briefs 4a and 4b form a horizontal circle.

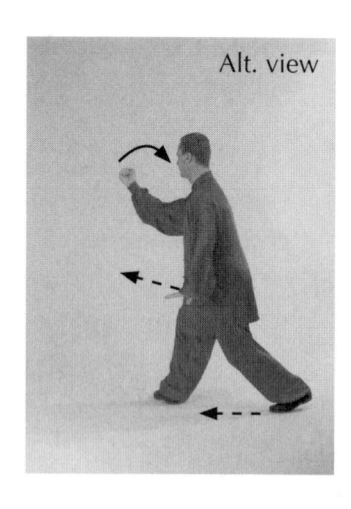

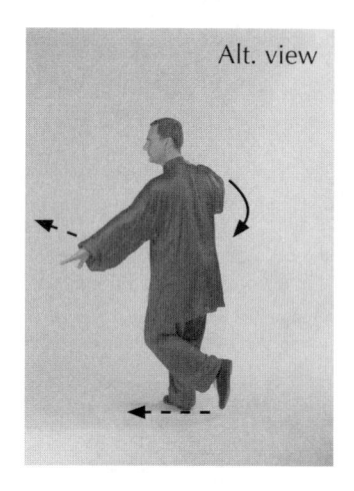

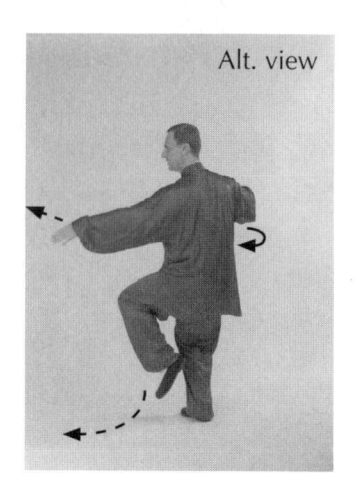

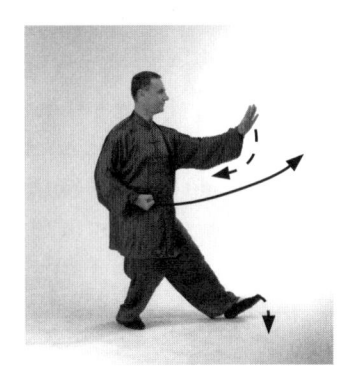

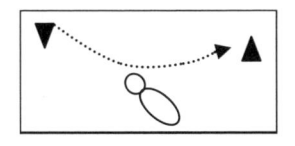

Brief 5

Bring left foot through to 9.00; left hand 'parry'; right hand into waist.

Details

Turn your centreline to your right (10.30).

The left foot moves past the right ankle and beyond it towards 9.00; keep it relaxed and 'empty' as you step through.

As you do so, the left palm (rising diagonally upwards from low left to centre) sweeps around to 9.00 at chest height, the palm of the hand rotating so that the thumb is uppermost, and the palm therefore pushing towards the right (12.00). The hand finishes with the arm pointing towards 9.00 (the palm still facing 12.00) and the fingers slightly raised.

The right fist circles into the side of your waist, with the palm of the fist facing upwards.

The eyes look to 9.00.

Notes

- **'Parry' (Lán):** The movements in Briefs 4 and 5 are both Lán.

- **Connection:** It is important to feel that the turn of the hips to 10.30 is controlling the movement of the elbows, and therefore the arms.

- **The left leg** should be very relaxed; if you are going to place the heel, place it lightly.

  Width of stance: The stance should be between 4–8 inches (10–20 cm) wide.

- **The right foot:** If the right foot wasn't turned out at 45° in the previous movement, it is not possible to execute this movement correctly as it will be impossible to turn the hips to the right.

- **Angle of body:** The body is still turned to 10.00/10.30.

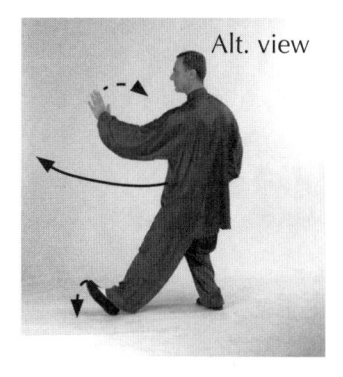

- **The coccyx/tailbone** should be tucked under, the lower abdominal muscles should be gently pulled in, and the right hip should be relaxed and sunk.

- **The rotation of the right fist in 4 and 5:** From the end of Bān (Brief 3b) the right fist (initially palm upwards) moves out to the right side and, as it does so, the palm rotates to face downwards. By the time that it has circled back into the waist again, the palm is upwards again.

  The reason for this twisting and turning of the arm/palm is that the arms are 'opening' and 'closing': They are 'closed' in Bān, but then if you observe the rotation of the elbows as the arms circle out sideways, you will see that they 'open', and by the time that you reach Lán (Brief 5), they have 'closed' again.

  There is therefore a feeling in the upper body of 'close', 'open', 'close'.

- **'Closing':** As you arrive in this position, sink the left elbow still further, pushing it gently towards 12.00, and complete the twisting upwards of the right fist.

  The pushing to 12.00 of the left elbow will cause the left palm to turn away slightly, and the turning upwards of the right palm closes the right elbow. The elbows should feel as though they are working together. Feel the body beginning to 'close' as you sink into the right foot.

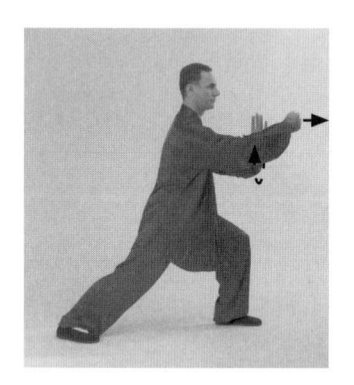

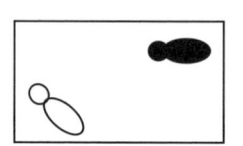

BRIEF 6

Punch (Chuí). Weight forwards; punch (rotating eye of fist uppermost); left hand to right forearm.

DETAILS

Transfer the weight on to the left foot into a left Bow Stance.

The right fist moves from the waist to 9.00 at solar plexus height, with the eye of the fist rotating upwards.

The left palm draws backwards slightly to face the left arm, with the fingers vertical.

The eyes look to 9.00.

NOTES

- **The width of the stance** is approximately 8 inches (20 cm).

- **The right fist** makes a quarter anti-clockwise rotation as it moves from the right hip to 9.00.

- **The punch:** Extend the punch but avoid over-straightening the right arm.

    The punch is to the height of the heart/solar plexus.

    Sink the right elbow as you punch.

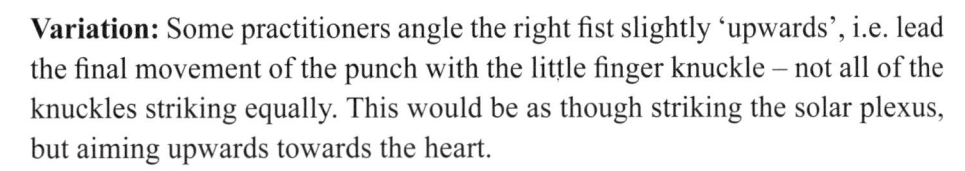

Variation: Some practitioners angle the right fist slightly 'upwards', i.e. lead the final movement of the punch with the little finger knuckle – not all of the knuckles striking equally. This would be as though striking the solar plexus, but aiming upwards towards the heart.

- **The left palm** draws back to either the right wrist, or the right forearm.

- **The elbows** should be relaxed and sunk.

FORM 22: APPARENT CLOSE-UP (APPEARING TO SEAL AND CLOSE) (PULL BACK THEN PUSH, AS IF TO CLOSE)

如封似闭 (Rúfēng Sìbì)

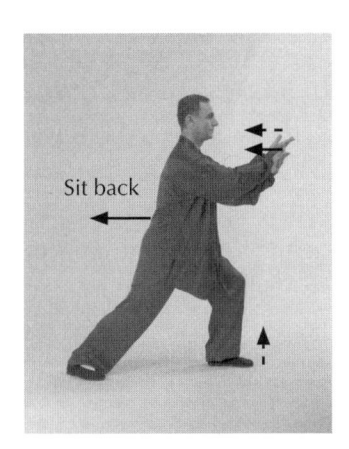

BRIEF 1

Sink into front foot; left hand under arm; separate hands.

DETAILS

As you start to sink slightly into the left foot, extend the arms slightly further towards 9.00, and, turning the left palm upwards, slide the left fingers and palm under and to the outside of the right wrist, initially keeping the fingertips in contact with the wrist (see 'Further clarification' note on p.280).

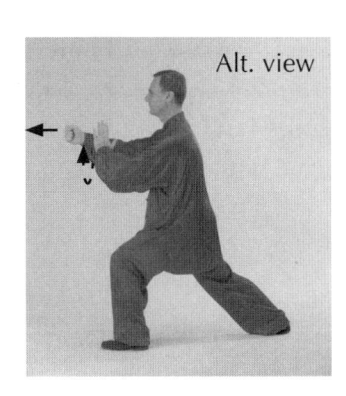

The wrists will now be crossed in front of you, with the right wrist under the left wrist (i.e. the entire left hand will be on the right side of the right hand with the palm facing the ceiling).

As the hand arrives on the other side of the right wrist, open the right fist, and turn the right palm upwards also. As this happens, the upturned palms will start to rise to shoulder-height.

As you finish sinking the weight into the left foot, separate the palms to a shoulder's width apart – the palms still facing upwards.

The eyes continue to look at 9.00.

NOTES

- **Sink into the front foot** slightly as you make this movement.

  Relax the right hip as you do so.

- **Further clarification on the left hand movement:** In order to explain the position that the hands arrive at: if you grasp your right wrist from underneath with your left hand, but then also slip the thumb through to the other side, you will have got the correct position almost!

- **The upturned palms:** Turned up as though holding a large beach ball.

- **Variations:** There are a couple of ways of moving the hand under the wrist.

  The description above is what you might term the 'modern' way.

  The other (perhaps more 'traditional') way is to keep the left fingers vertical with the palm continuously facing your right (12.00) and then to slide the tips of the left fingers under the right wrist. You will therefore end up with the backs of the wrists together, the wrists being crossed. All you do then is to turn the palms upwards.

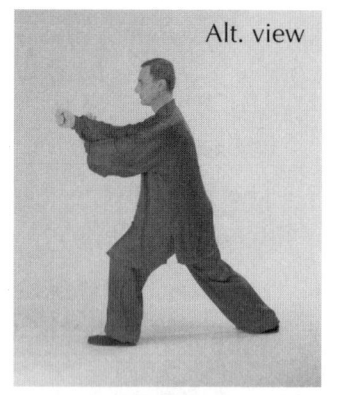

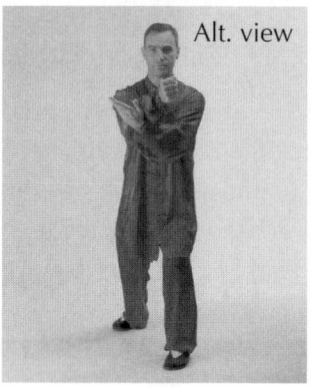

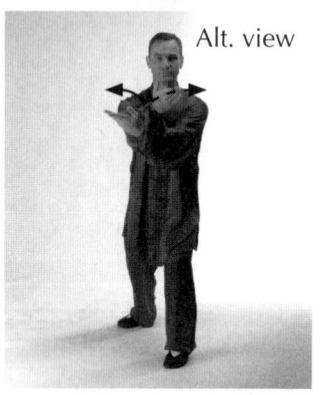

- **The separated hands:** At the end of the description above, when the hands have separated to left and right ahead of your shoulders, if someone were pushing towards you with both hands, your palms would be underneath his elbows.

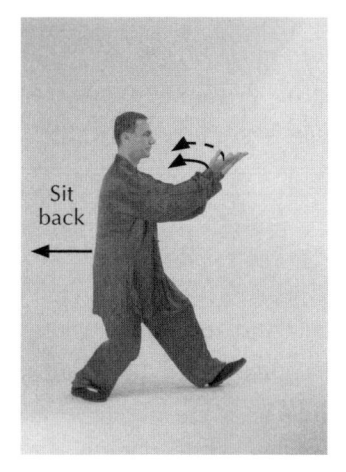

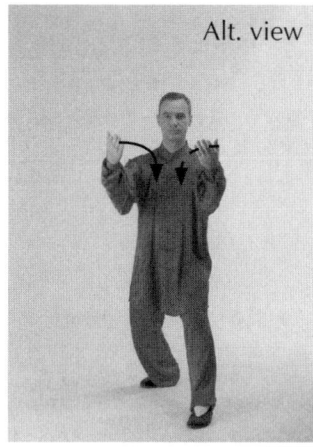

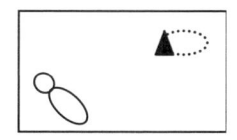

BRIEF 2
Sit back; rotate palms; sink elbows and hands.

DETAILS
Sit back on to the right foot, lifting the left toes.

Start to draw the wrists back towards your chest (fingers no higher than your shoulders) gradually sinking the elbows and rotating the palms so that, by the time your hands have moved approximately 12 inches (30 cm) from the chest, the palms have turned to face palm down.

The eyes continue to look to 9.00.

NOTES

- **'Closing' in the arms:** The elbows will initially be 'open' with a space under the armpits, but start to 'close' (sink) as you sit backwards.

- **The coccyx/tailbone** should be tucked under as you sit back. Gently pull in the lower abdominal muscles, and sink/relax the right hip.

- **Method of visualization:** Your palms, from being underneath your opponent's elbows (see 'The separated hands', p.280) have now rotated around the outside of the elbow joints and are now on the insides of the elbow-creases.

Brief 3

Àn 按. Sink further into the right foot; push palms down to waist.

Details

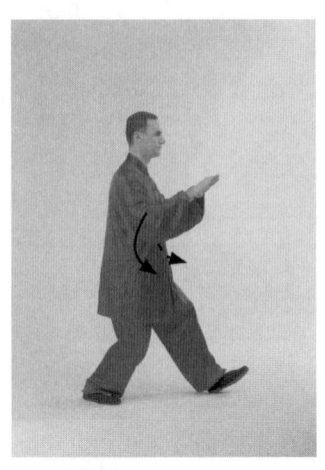

Sink the weight further into the right foot.

Sink the elbows, the palms pushing downwards to waist-height with the fingers slightly lifted.

The eyes continue to look to 9.00.

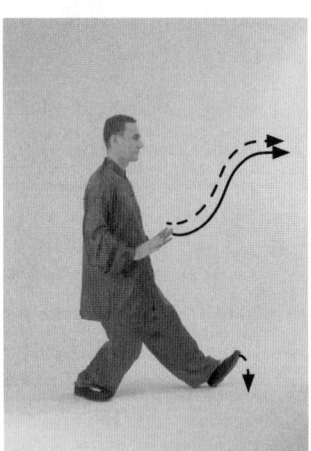

Notes

- **Sink the elbows** but don't compress them against the sides of the body – still maintain a small space in the armpits.

   Beginners tend to pull the elbows behind the back; this should be avoided.

- **The coccyx/tailbone** should be tucked under as you sit back. Gently pull in the lower abdominal muscles, and sink/relax the right hip. Avoid leaning backwards.

- **Variation:** Some practitioners turn the body slightly to the right here. I personally prefer this.

- **'Closing':** Drawing everything into the centre.

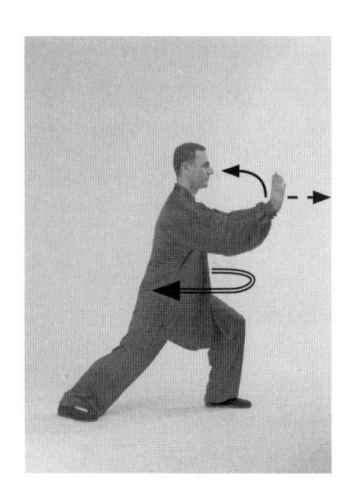

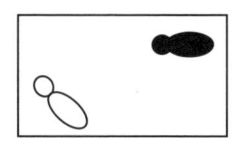

BRIEF 4
Weight forwards; push ahead – hands up to shoulder-height.

DETAILS
Place the left foot flat.
Move the weight forwards into a left Bow Stance.
Push the palms forwards to 9.00 with fingers pointing upwards, the wrists arriving at shoulder height at the end of the push.
The eyes continue to look to 9.00.

NOTES

- **Àn 按**: Although technically Àn is the downwards push prior to the push ahead, usually the push ahead is considered to be part of the Àn movement.

- **The push** is not a direct line from waist to shoulder-height (i.e. on a diagonal). Initially push more upwards towards shoulder-height, and then ease the gradient off by pushing away with a less steep ascent – more on the horizontal.

- **Variation:** Some teachers teach a discontinuous circle for Briefs 3 and 4; they drop the hands to the waist at the end of Brief 3 and then lift the hands up along the same path on which they've just travelled downwards before pushing away.
  I cannot personally agree with this as it breaks the thread of energy in the movement; I agree that this might apply to a Fā jìn application, but not to the textbook version of the Yang 24-Step Form.

- **The elbows when pushing:** As you push, sink the elbows further. The feeling is of slightly 'squeezing' something with the elbows.

- **The palms when pushing** are very slightly rounded as though pushing a very large beach-ball.

- **The arms at the end of the movement:** Beginners often try to straighten the arms in the final position; keep the elbows slightly bent at the end of the movement.

- **Final hand position:** The heels of the hands will finish at shoulder-height.

FORM 23: CROSS HANDS

十字手 (Shízìshǒu)

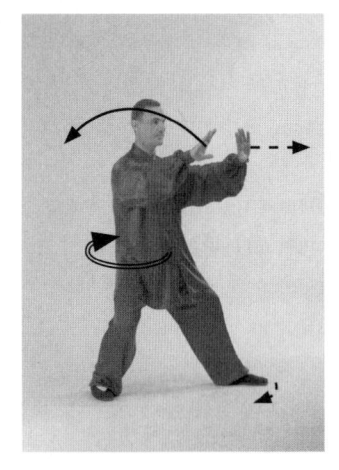

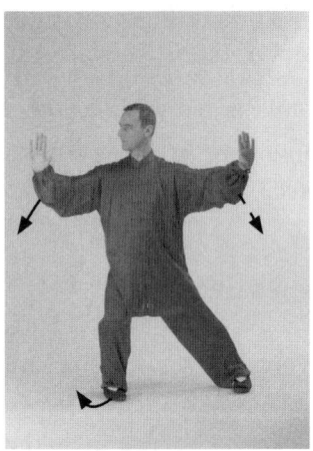

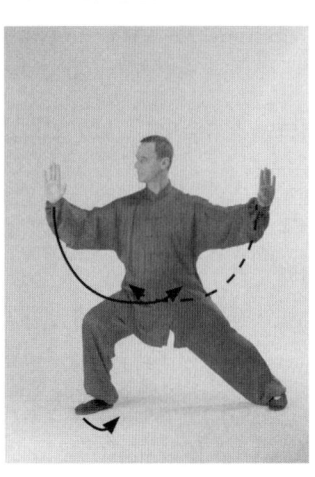

Brief 1
Sit back; turn left toes, turn right toes; open arms.

Details
Start to sit back on to the right foot, and as soon as the weight has moved back enough for you to lift up your left toes, turn the hips and toes towards 12.00, placing the left foot (with the toes facing 12.00). This should be done *before* the weight has fully transferred to the right foot.

Follow this by immediately pivoting the right toes to 1.30.

The body arrives slightly on the diagonal with the weight on the right foot.

As you turn the body, the hands move with the palms continuously facing away from you: the left hand remains parallel to the ground, and although it doesn't move very much (compared to the right arm), it has a feeling of pushing the palm away as it makes a small change of direction to extend to 10.00 (see also Notes on the following page).

The right hand makes a slight arc (upwards and downwards) following the turn of the body to finish with the elbow approximately over the right knee and the arm pushing to 1.30.

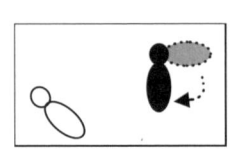

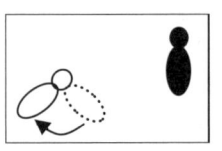

As you arrive in this position, there should be a sensation of sinking into the right foot (see Notes on the following page).

The eyes look to 1.30.

NOTES

- **Sitting back:** Avoid sitting back too much because you will not be able to pivot the right foot. (This isn't obvious on a solid floor, but quickly becomes apparent when you try to perform the move on e.g. grass).

    This is almost a 'double pivot', but the feet don't pivot at the same time. The left foot pivot is *immediately* followed by the right foot pivot with no gap in between. The transfer of the weight from left foot to right foot is therefore a *continuous* movement from one to the other.

    Beginners very often transfer the weight from left to right foot, then return the weight slightly to the left foot so they can turn the right foot, and then move back on to the right foot again.

    When sitting back at the start of the movement, relax the hips, tuck the pelvis/tailbone under, and continue to do so as you turn the body.

- **The left hand:** The previous form (Apparent Close-up) finished with the left hand pushing to 9.00. This move therefore starts with your feeling as though the left hand is continuing the push to 9.00; don't alter the direction abruptly. Continue to maintain this feeling as you turn the body.

    A common fault with beginners is to drop the left hand during the turn.

- **The arms:** As you turn the body the gap between the hands widens; the left hand moving slower than the right hand, because it is retaining the feeling of pushing to 9.00. Both hands finish with the palms facing away from you at shoulder-height, the left palm facing 10.00, and the right palm facing 1.30.

- **'Opening':** This is an 'open' movement (but see also next note).

- **Sinking into the right foot:** As the weight arrives on the right foot and the arms arrive in position, start to sink the elbows and body into the foot. This is the start of the 'closing' movement.

THE YANG TÀIJÍ 24-STEP SHORT FORM

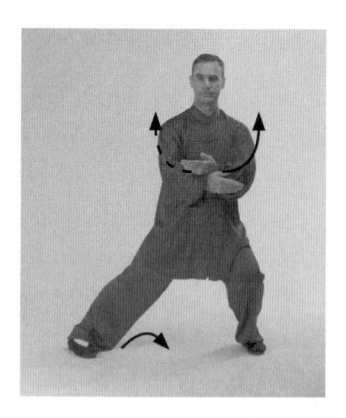

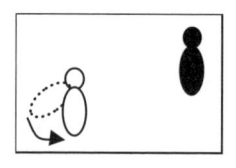

Brief 2
Sit back; lower arms; turn hips; turn right toes.

Details
Begin to sit back on to the left foot.

The arms continue to lower further, the elbows sinking.

As the weight shifts, turn the hips and right toes to approximately 12.00.

The weight is now about 50/50, and the arms are drawing together low at about pelvis height. (The body can be angled forwards slightly.)

The hands continue to circle downwards to cross at the wrists – with the right hand on the outside/underneath (see 'Angle of palms' below).

As the hands move together, the weight moves over the left foot and the right heel starts to lift.

The eyes throughout follow the direction of movement of the right arm (without looking down) so will finish looking to 12.00.

Notes

- **The weight in Briefs 1 and 2:** The weight shifts on to the right foot (via the double pivot on the feet) and then back to the left foot, the arms crossing. The shift of weight should be smooth and continuous.

- **The right toes:** It isn't essential to turn the right toes, but it makes it easier to lift the right foot inwards in the movement that follows.

- **Sinking the arms:** Lower the arms by feeling the weight of the elbows sinking, and then the energy should be in the forearms as the arms draw together.

  There is a feeling of gathering something.

- **Angle of palms when crossing:** The palms are turned so that they don't exactly face your body, but neither do they face the ceiling; they will therefore be somewhere in between – angled slightly inwards towards you.

  The right wrist will be under (or on the outside of) the left wrist at the end of the movement.

  The arms should not be too close against the body – somewhere between 35–45° from the vertical (i.e. if they were hanging by your sides).

- **The coccyx/tailbone** should be tucked under.

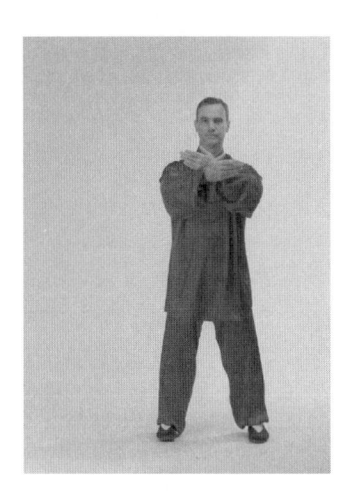

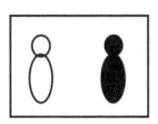

Brief 3
Right foot in; crossed hands rise up centreline.

Details
Gently press your right toes into the ground, thereby moving 100 per cent of weight on to the left foot and, as you straighten your legs, lift your right foot towards your left foot to a shoulder's width apart (see 'Weight distribution' below).

Simultaneously, the hands, which are crossed at waist/pelvis height, continue to rise up your centreline to ahead of your throat. Because you right hand is underneath your left hand, there might be a feeling of the right hand lifting the left hand; at the end of the movement your right hand will therefore be on the outside (furthest away from you).

The eyes look to 12.00.

Notes

- **Weight distribution:** The placement of the weight is usually taught as 50/50 at this point.

  Variation: There is a variation where you leave the weight on the left foot, and the right toes just off the ground at this point.

  There is a reason for this that involves the movement that follows. (See note 'Form 23:3 to 24:2 variation' on p.290.)

- **The wrists** finish at shoulder/top-of-sternum height.

- **The shoulders** should be relaxed.

- **The knees** should remain 'soft'.

- **'Opening and closing' in Briefs 1, 2 and 3:** The body 'opens' in 1, and 'closes' from the end of 1 onwards.

- **The arms:** The forearms, as you look at them, will be angled at about 45°, i.e. there needs to be a space under each armpit.

  The area between the hands and the body should be 'rounded' as though holding a beach ball, i.e. the elbows should not be bent less than 90°.

FORM 24: CLOSING FORM

收势 (Shōushì)

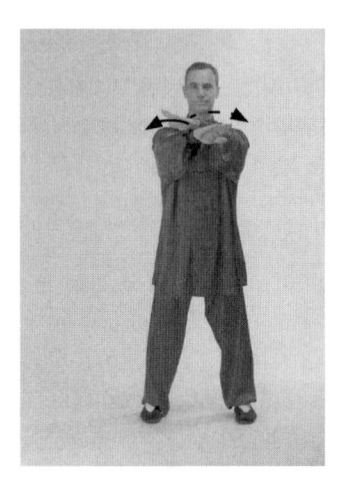

BRIEF 1
Extend arms turning palms down.

DETAILS
Rotate the palms to face downwards (still crossed at the wrists), pushing the wrists directly ahead of you at shoulder-height. As the palms start to move apart, separate the hands to a shoulder's width apart, and begin to sink the elbows.

NOTES

- **The weight** should remain on the heels (approximately 70%); if you are not careful it will automatically shift over the toes because of the additional weight of the arms ahead of you (but see 'Form 23:3 to 24:2 variation' on p.290).
- **The shoulders** should be soft as you extend the arms.
- **The centre:** There is a feeling of the centre moving backwards.
- **'Opening/closing':** This is an 'opening' movement.

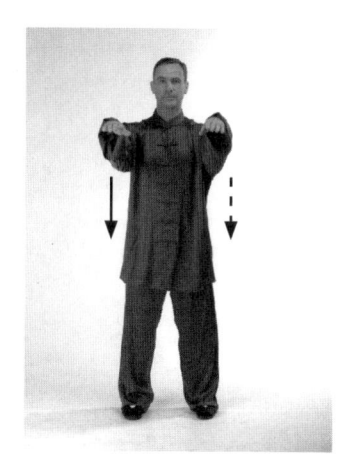

Brief 2
Lower arms to sides.

Details
Slowly lower your hands to your sides with the fingers pointing towards 12.00, the palms still facing downwards.

The eyes continue to look to 12.00.

Notes

- **Lowering the arms:** This is achieved by releasing the *elbows*, i.e. you don't exactly *bend* them, you let the weight of them sink and rotate slightly inwards/downwards.

  Once this movement has been initiated, feel as though you are pushing downwards with your forearms; your yì 意 (intention) moves to the forearms so that the energy moves down the arms.

  You then sink the wrists and palms – feel as though you are pushing down with them.

- **Over-bending the elbows:** Beginners often continue to bend the elbows so that they arrive at the sides of the body before the hands.

- **Sink the qì** by relaxing the chest (hollow the chest slightly), allowing the shoulders to sink into the hips, and by gently relaxing the small of the back (the coccyx/tailbone tucking under slightly).

  As you do so, the lowering of the arms is initiated – the elbows working with the relaxing knees.

- **'Opening/closing':** This is a 'closing' movement.

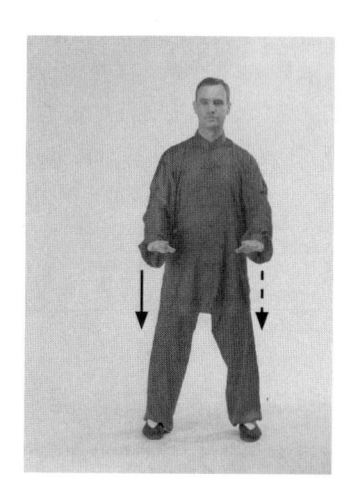

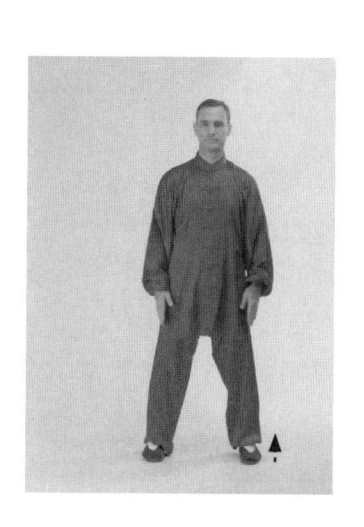

- **Form 23:3–24:2 variation:** When teaching beginners it is easier to teach the weight as being 50/50 from the end of Form 23 to the end of Form 24. It's clear, and there is less to think about.

    However, it had always bothered me that there didn't appear to be any reciprocal movement in the legs for this part of the tàijí Form – the centre was to a certain extent involved, but not in a body-integrated way. Other than the arms, the body seemed to have virtually stagnated at this point.

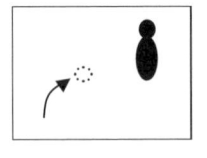

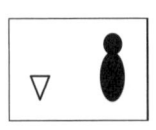

    However, there is a variation that I personally prefer…

    First of all it's necessary to understand that the energy of Form 23 is initially a 'rising' energy (23:1 – the opening arms, etc.) followed by a 'sinking' energy (23:2 – the closing of the centre, and the sinking and crossing of the arms, etc.). After this the energy begins to rise again (23:3 – the hands rising).

    1. To apply this also to the body (and legs) in 23:3, leave the weight on the left foot and the right toes just off the ground; don't move the weight on to the right foot yet.

        In the movements that follow (Form 24), you are going to sink your energy again.

    2. As you push your hands away from you, separating them, place your right toes and begin to move the weight into the *ball* of the foot only. We now have a corresponding centre action (the preliminary sinking into the right foot) to work with the action of the arms.

    3. Then, as you sink the arms, gradually place the entire foot, shifting the weight from the ball of the right foot along the outside 'ridge' of the foot to the heel.

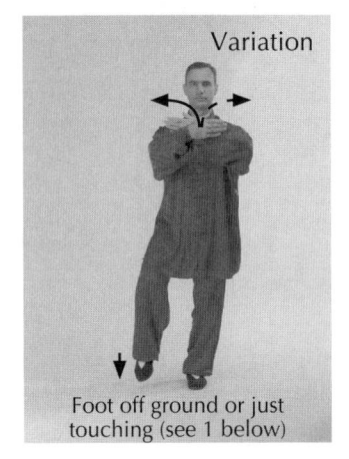

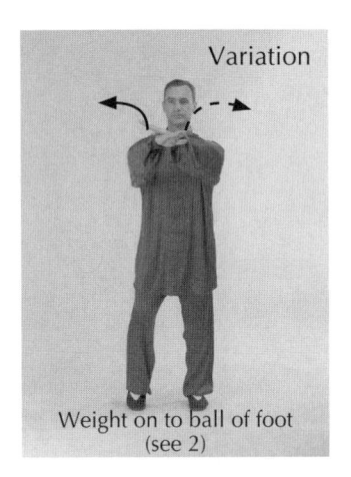

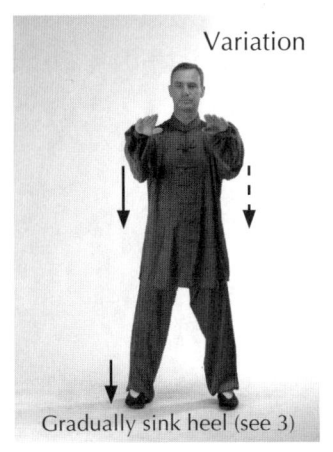

As you do this, sink the shoulders into the hips, the elbows into the knees, and the wrists into the ankles – the knees not exactly bent, but definitely not straight. You have 'sunk the qì' to complete Form 24.

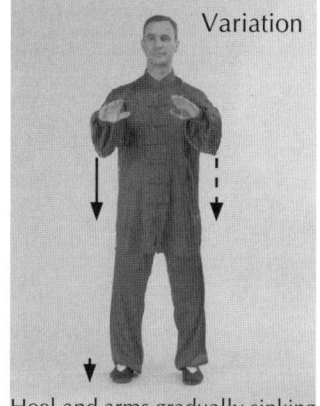

Variation

Heel and arms gradually sinking

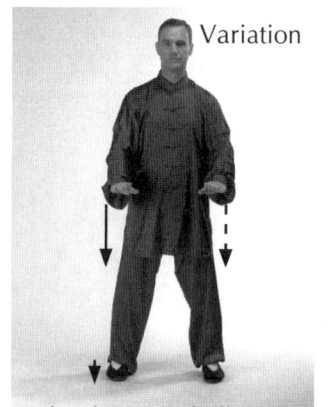

Variation

Heel and arms gradually sinking

Variation

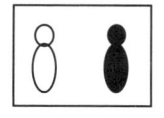

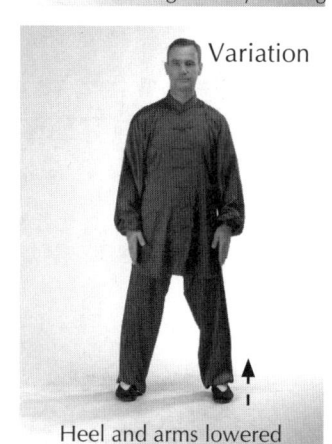

Heel and arms lowered

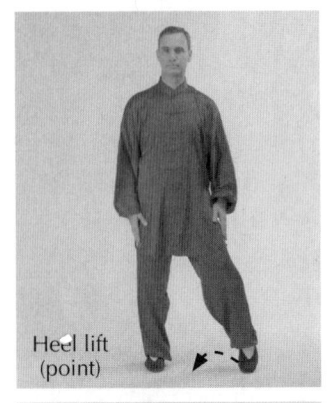

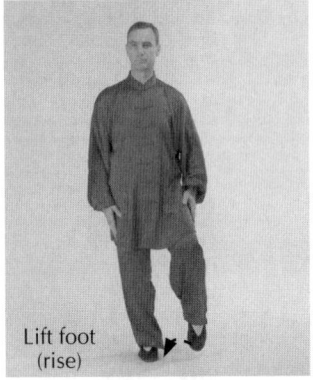

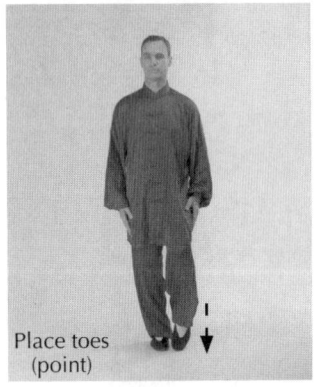

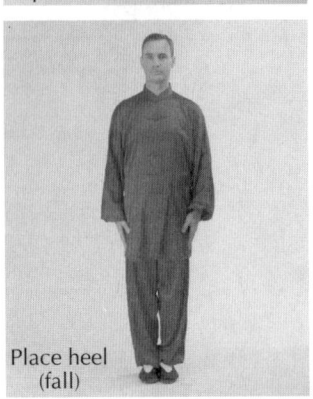

Brief 3
Left foot in.

Details
Allow the back of your neck to release and the crown (Bǎihuì 百會) to rise as you move your weight on to the right foot. As the weight shifts over the right foot, free up the left heel and lift the left foot off the ground.

Place the left toes alongside your right foot and then put the heel down.

Turn the palms to face the thighs.

The eyes continue to look to 12.00.

Notes

- **Point, rise, point, fall:** When lifting the left foot, raise the heel first (pointing the toes), lift the foot (rise), bring the foot into the right foot and touch the toes to the ground (point), and joint by joint sink the heel (fall).

- **The weight:** As you move the weight on to the right foot, make sure that you have approximately 70 per cent of weight on the right *heel*.

  Avoid 'kicking' the weight across on to the right foot. Be aware of the shifting of the weight, and lift the left foot in under control.

- **Posture:** The neck should be released, lengthened, and relaxed; the body upright 'connecting Heaven and Earth'.

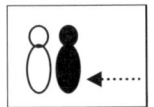

16

Easy Reference

Here I give just the photographs and form headings for easy reference.

READY POSITION

预备势 (Yùbèishì)

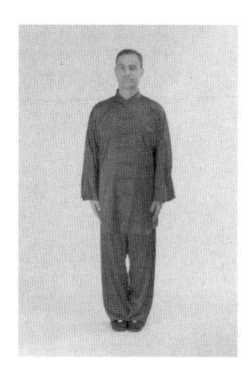

SECTION 1 (3 MOVEMENTS)

1. COMMENCING FORM

起势 (Qǐshì)

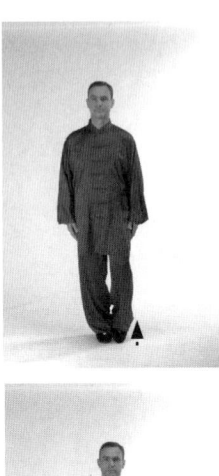

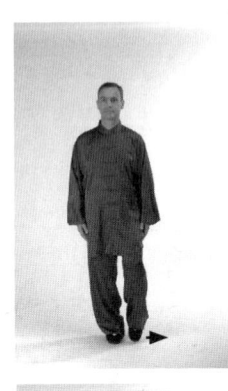

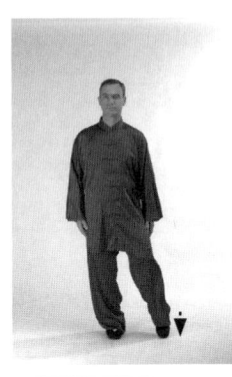

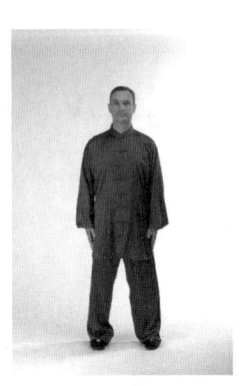

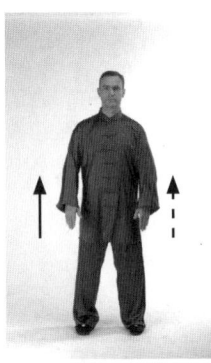

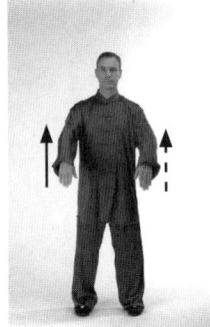

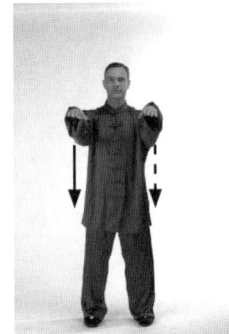

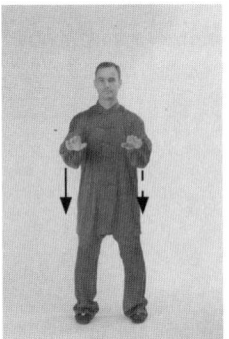

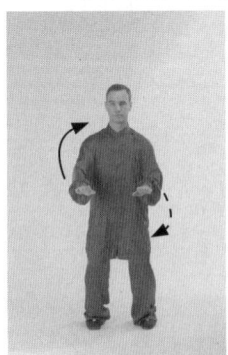

EASY REFERENCE

2. PARTING THE WILD HORSE'S MANE (LEFT AND RIGHT)

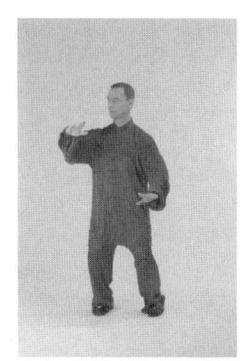

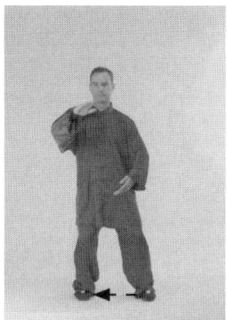

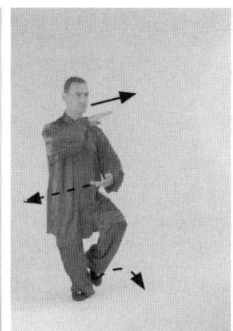

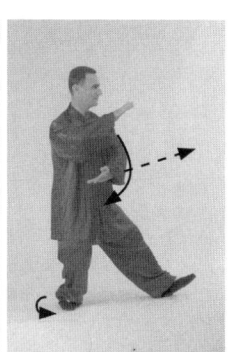

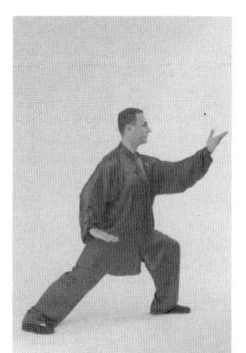

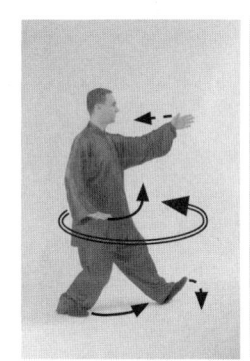

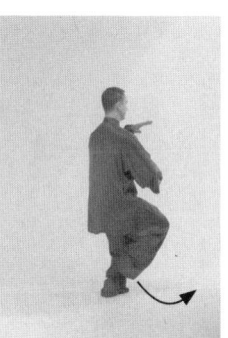

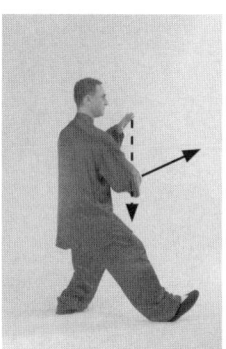

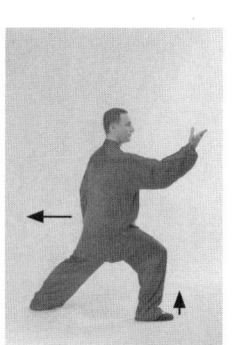

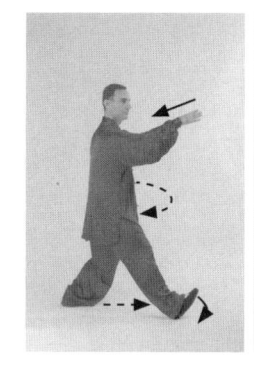

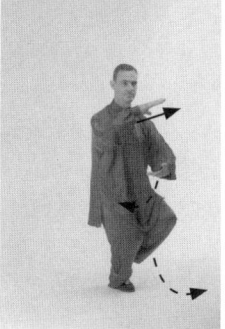

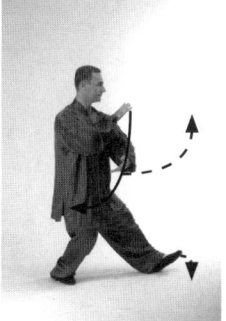

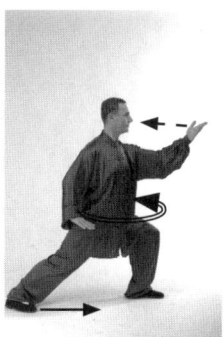

左右野马分鬃 (Zuǒyòu Yěmǎ Fēnzōng)

1)

2)

3)

295

THE YANG TÀIJÍ 24-STEP SHORT FORM

3. STORK SPREADS ITS WINGS

白鶴亮翅 (Baíhè Liàngchì)

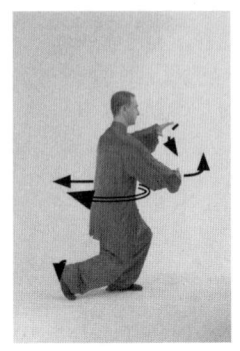

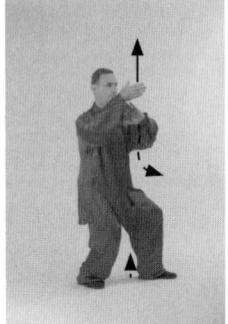

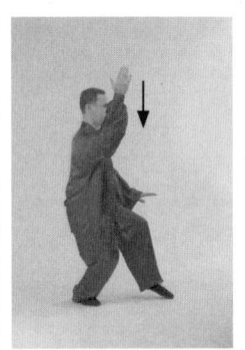

SECTION 2 (3 MOVEMENTS)

4. BRUSH KNEE AND TWIST STEP (LEFT AND RIGHT)

左右摟膝拗步 (Zuǒyòu Lōuxī Àobù)

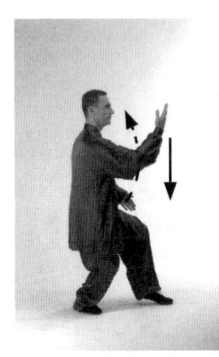

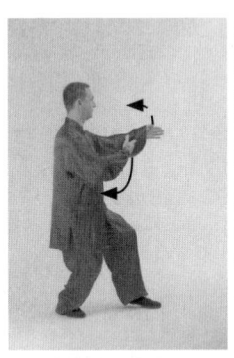

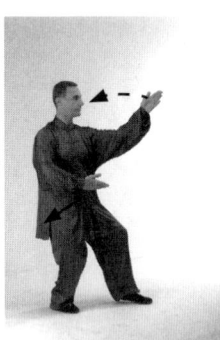

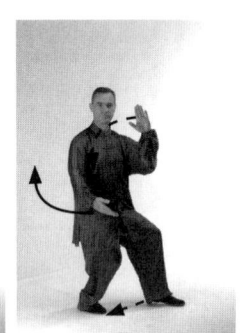

1)

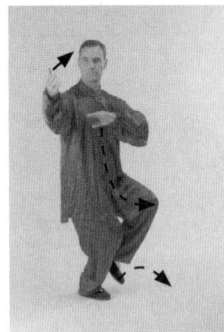

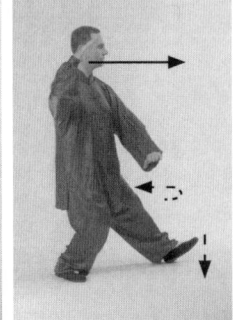

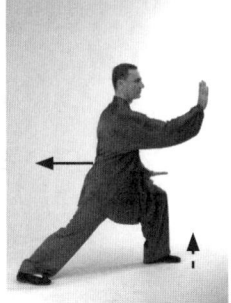

EASY REFERENCE

2)

3)

297

5. PLAY THE PIPA

手挥琵琶 (Shǒuhuī Pípā)

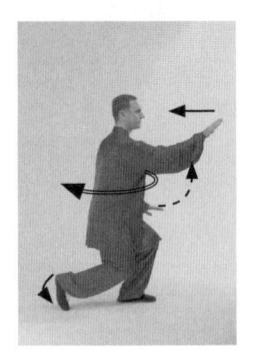

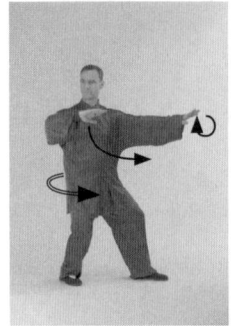

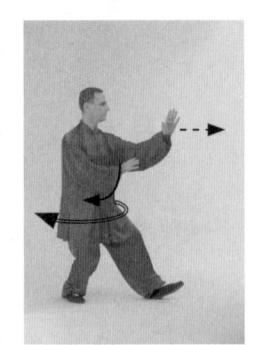

6. CURVE BACK ARMS (LEFT AND RIGHT)

左右倒卷肱 (Zuǒyòu Dàojuǎngōng)

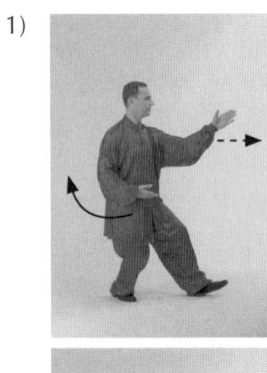

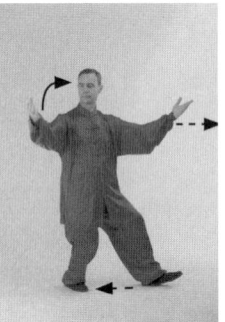

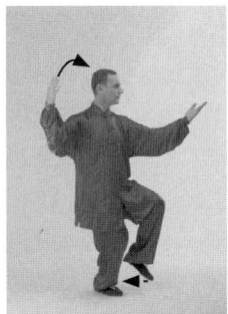

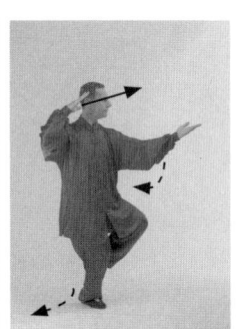

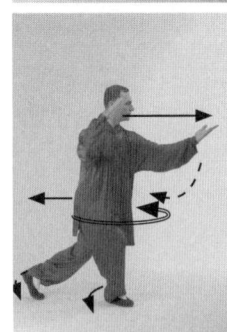

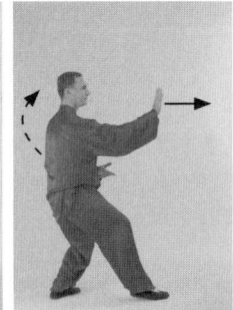

1)

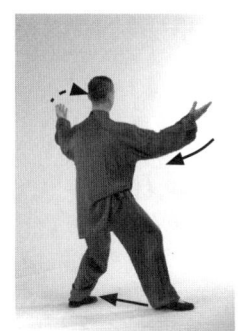

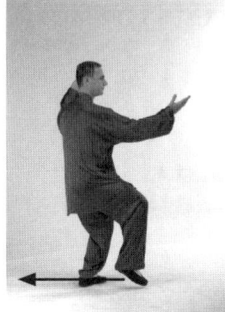

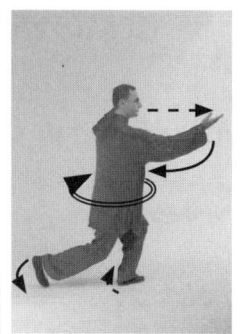

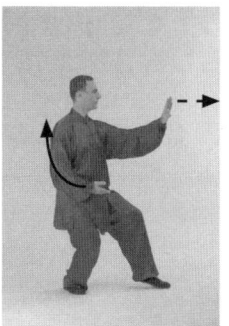

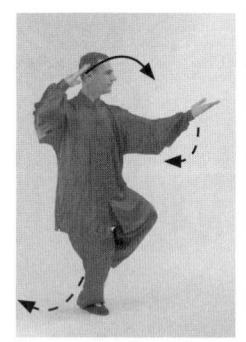

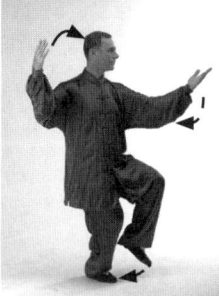

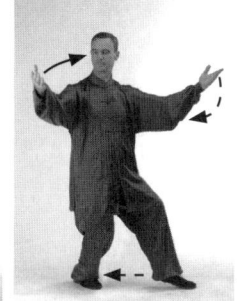

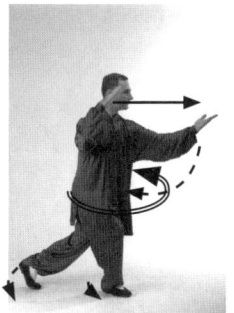

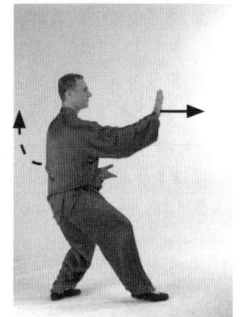

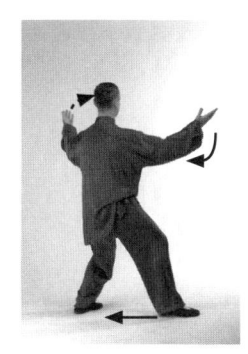

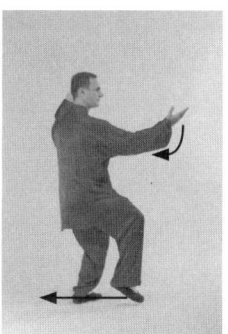

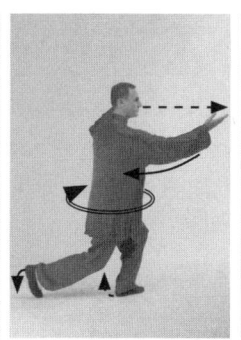

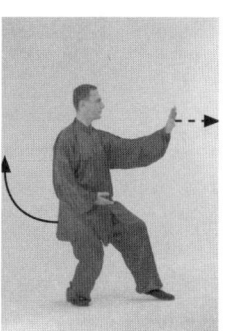

EASY REFERENCE

2)

3)

4)

299

THE YANG TÀIJÍ 24-STEP SHORT FORM

SECTION 3 (2 MOVEMENTS)

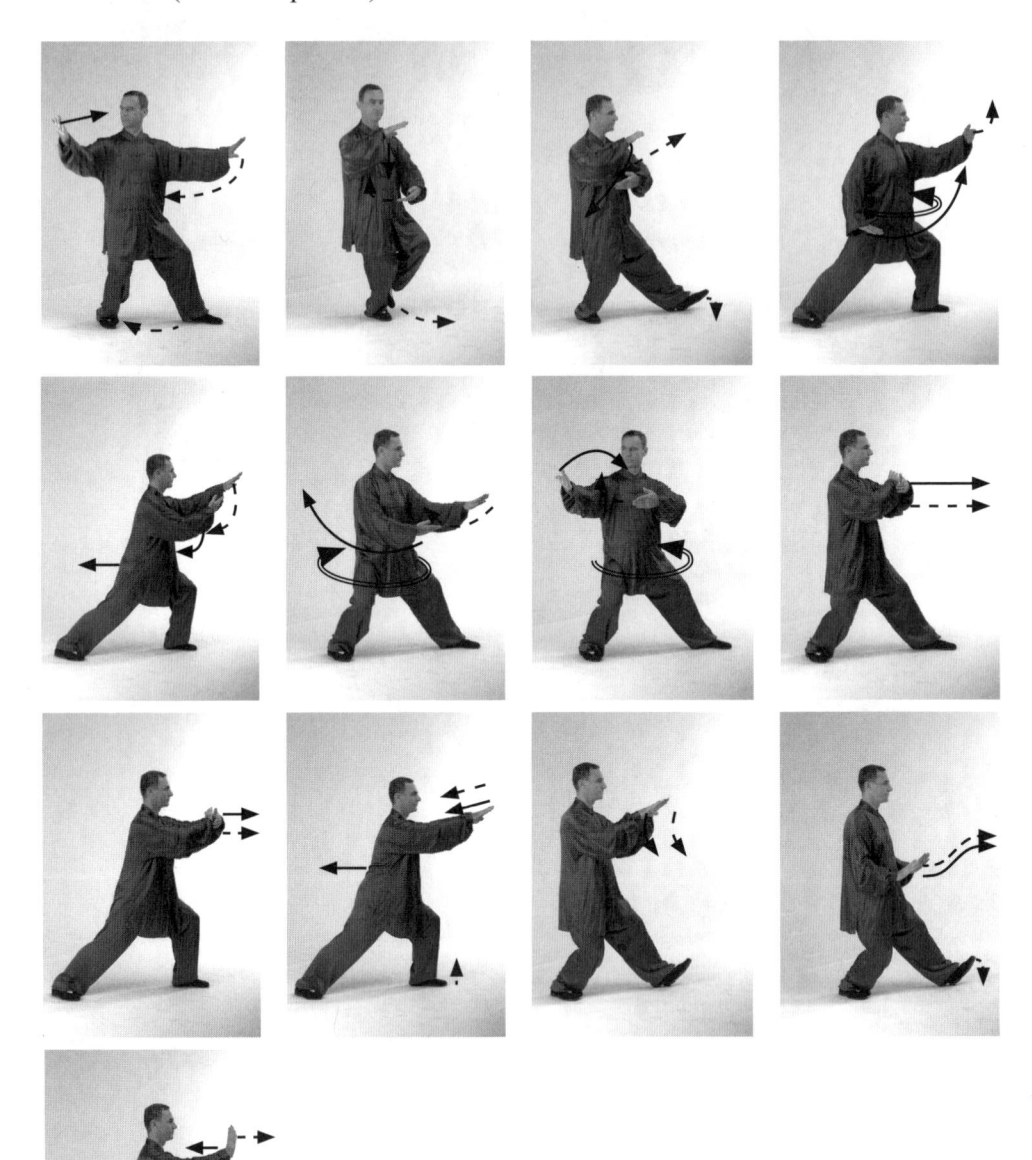

7. GRASP THE BIRD'S TAIL (LEFT STYLE)
左揽雀尾 (Zuǒ Lǎnquèwěi)

8. GRASP THE BIRD'S TAIL (RIGHT STYLE)
右揽雀尾 (Yòu Lǎnquèwěi)

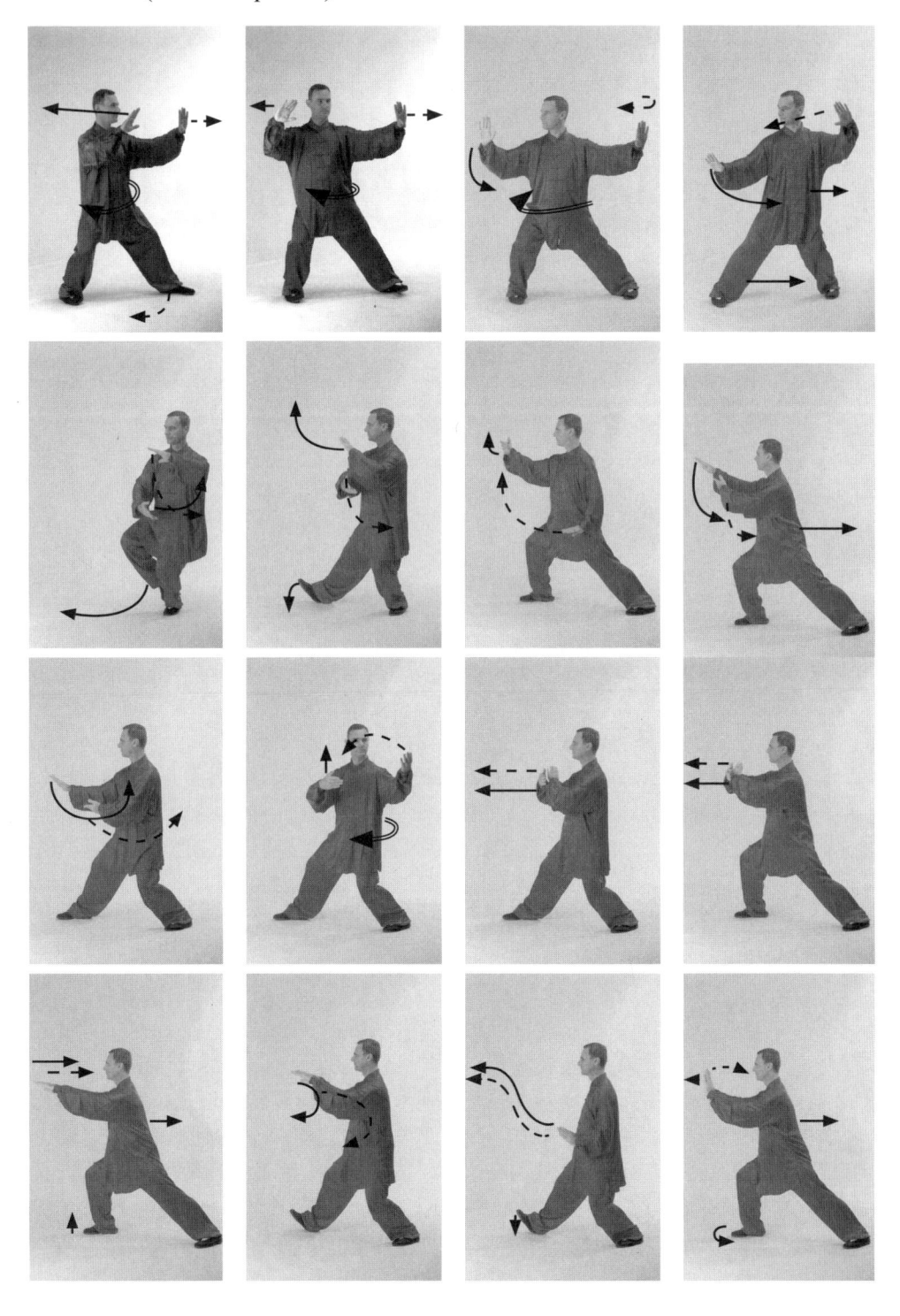

SECTION 4 (3 MOVEMENTS)

9. SINGLE WHIP

单鞭 (Dānbiān)

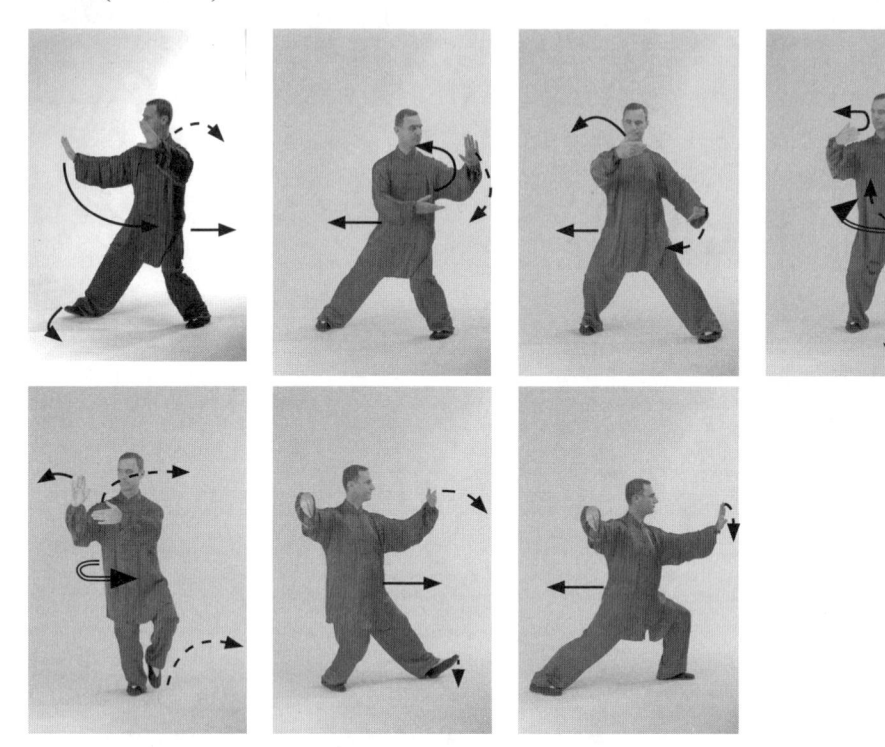

10. CLOUD HANDS

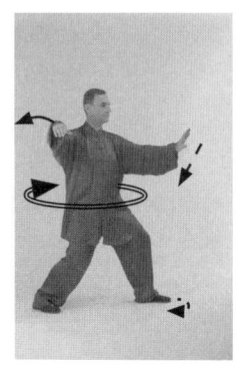

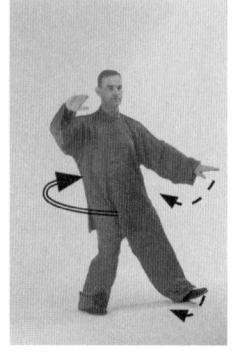

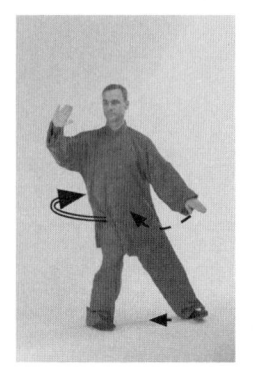

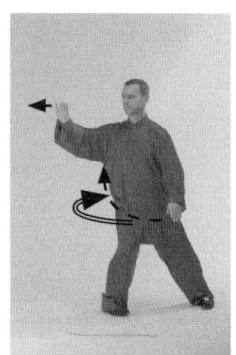

云手 (Yúnshǒu)

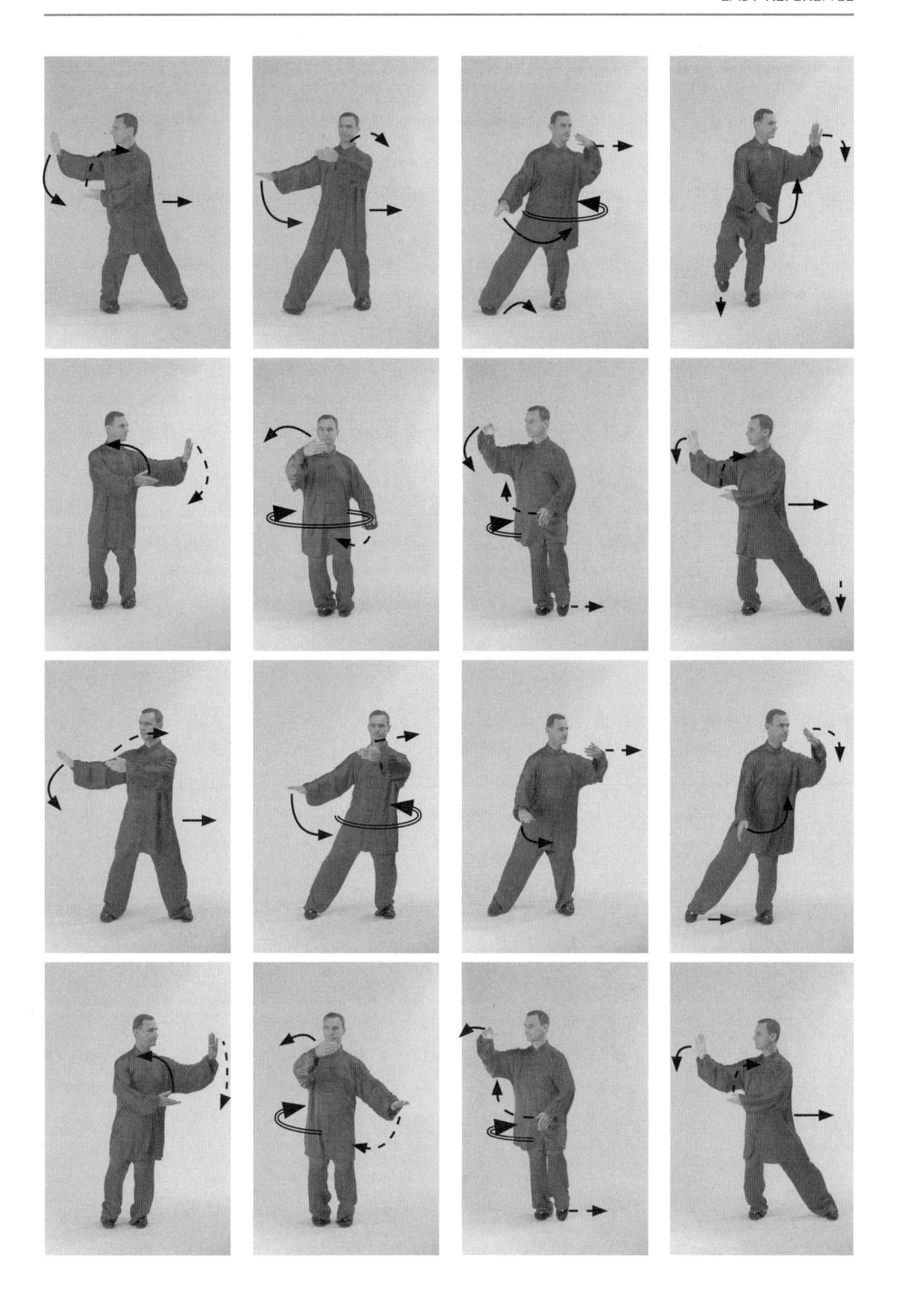

EASY REFERENCE

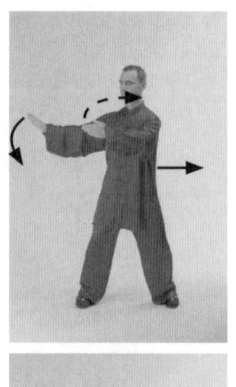

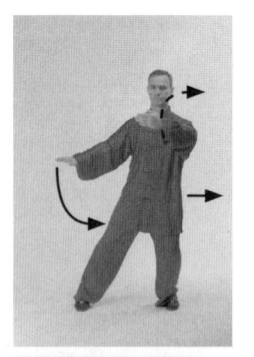

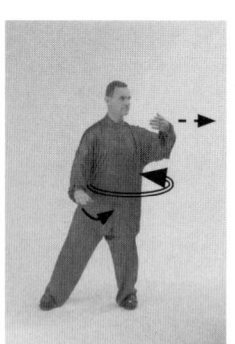

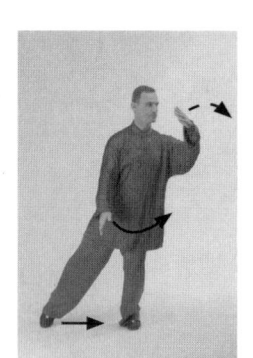

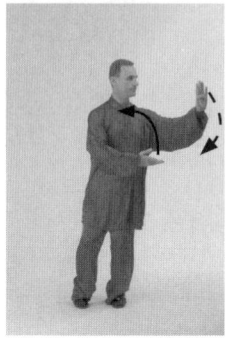

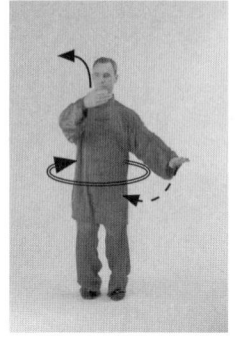

11. SINGLE WHIP

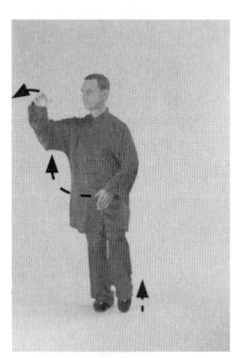

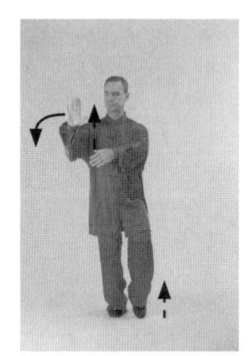

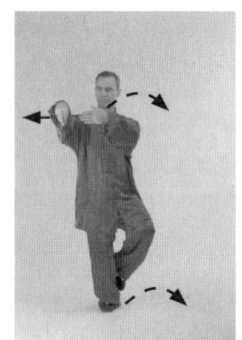

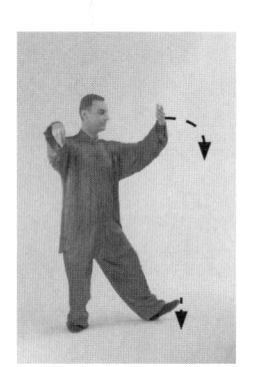

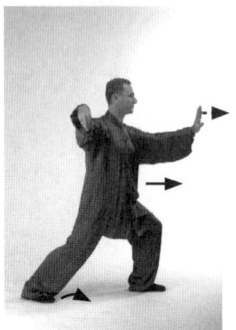

单鞭 (Dānbiān)

SECTION 5 (4 MOVEMENTS)

12. HIGH PAT ON HORSE

高探马 (Gāotànmǎ)

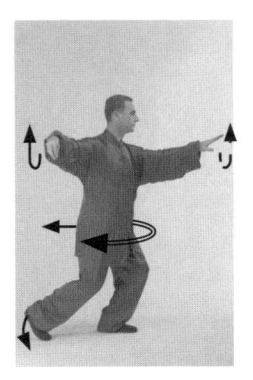

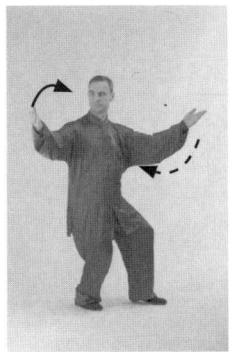

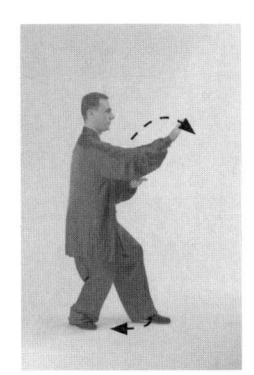

13. KICK WITH RIGHT HEEL

右蹬脚 (Yòu Dēngjiǎo)

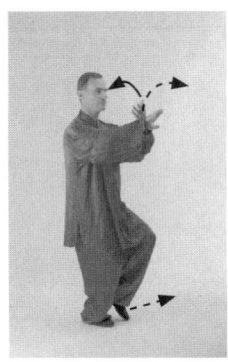

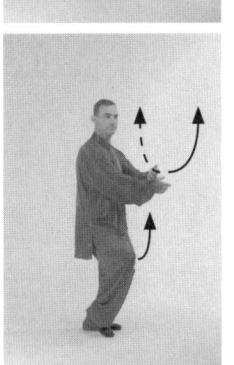

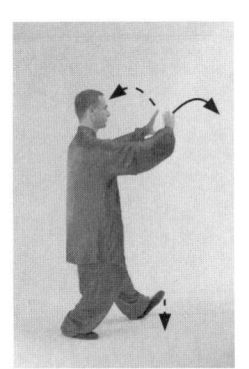

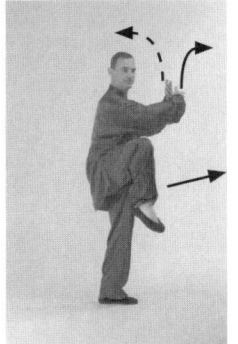

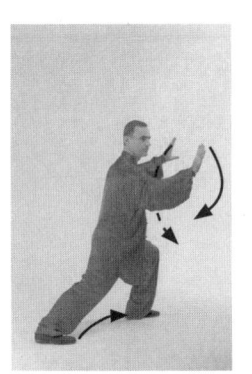

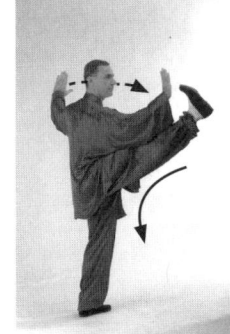

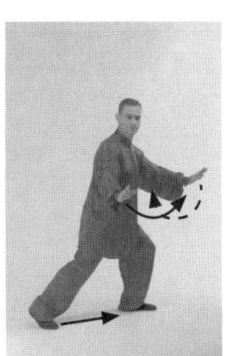

THE YANG TÀIJÍ 24-STEP SHORT FORM

14. STRIKE (OPPONENT'S) EARS WITH BOTH FISTS

双峰贯耳 (Shuāngfēng Guàn'ěr)

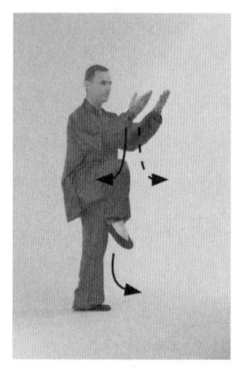

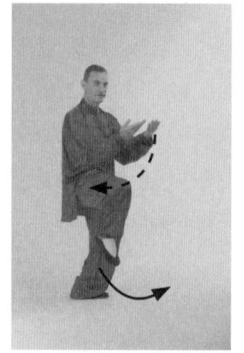

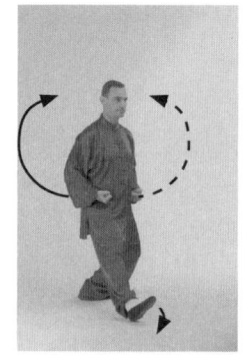

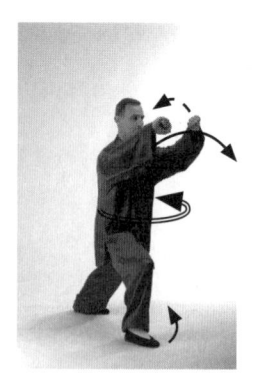

15. TURN AND KICK WITH LEFT HEEL

转身左蹬脚 (Zhuǎnshēn Zuǒ Dēngjiǎo)

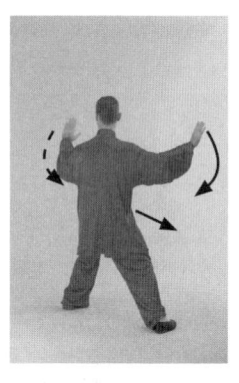

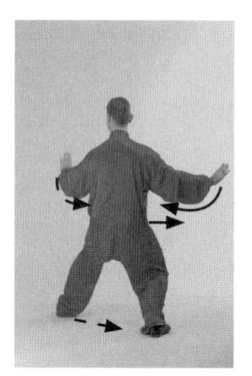

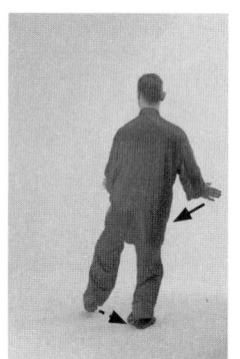

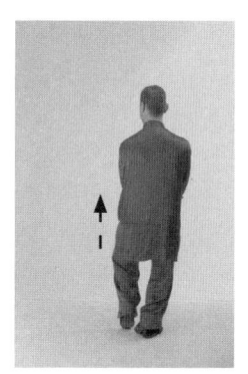

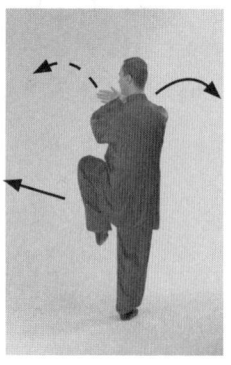

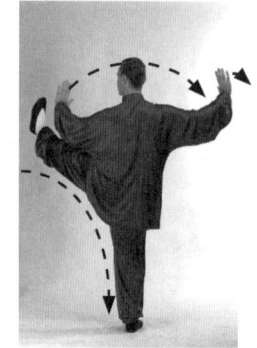

SECTION 6 (2 MOVEMENTS)

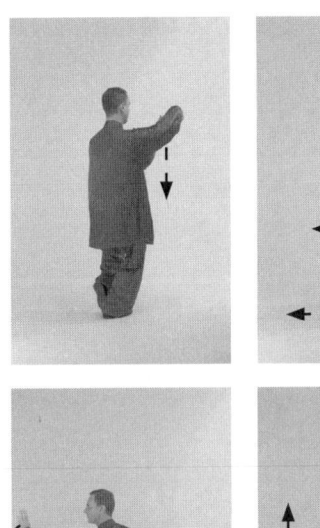

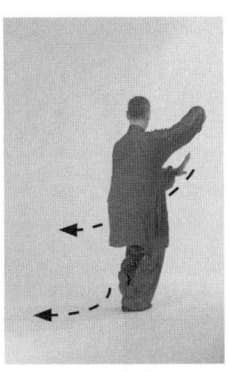

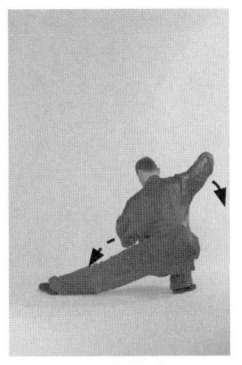

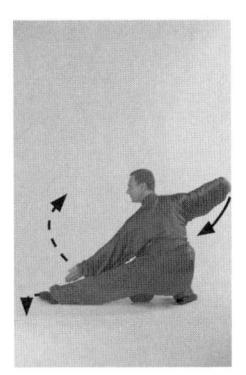

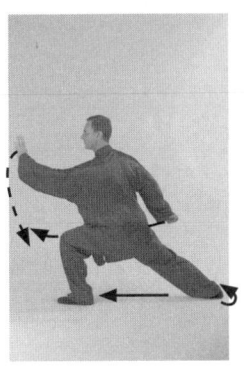

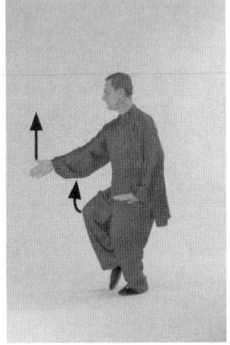

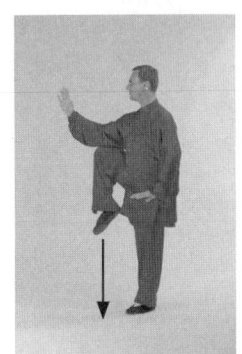

16. PUSH DOWN AND STAND ON ONE LEG (LEFT STYLE)

左下势独立 (Zuǒ Xiàshì Dúlì)

17. PUSH DOWN AND STAND ON ONE LEG (RIGHT STYLE)

右下势独立 (Yòu Xiàshì Dúlì)

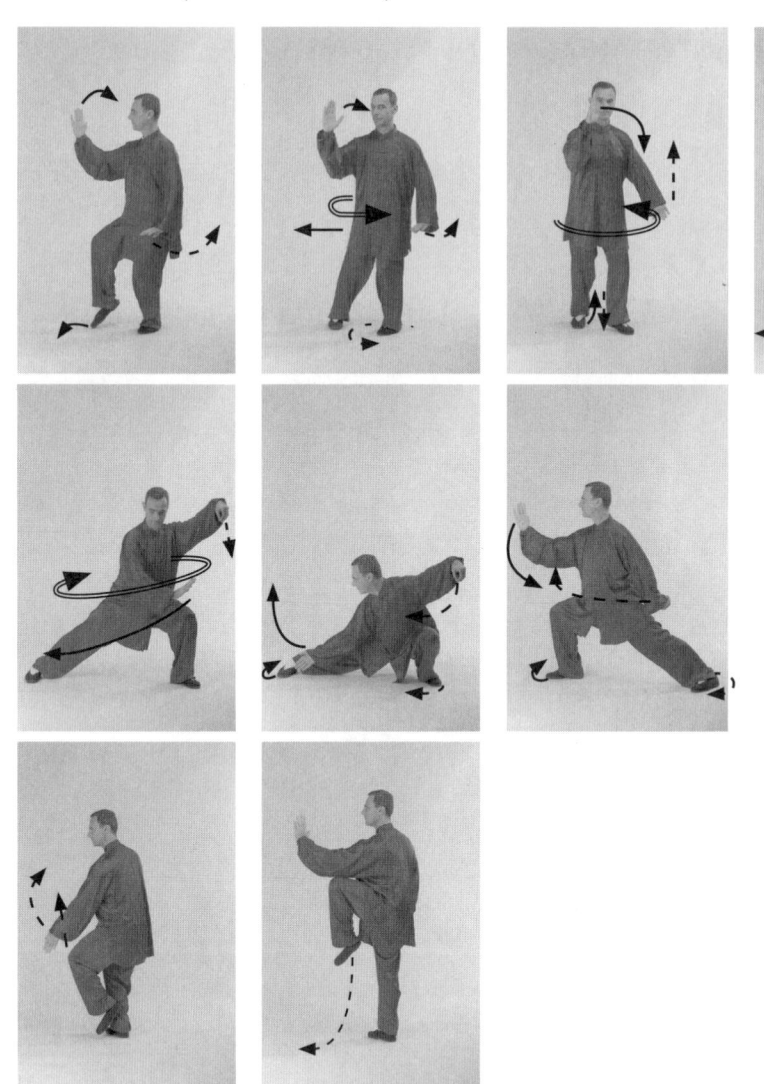

SECTION 7 (3 MOVEMENTS)

18. JADE LADY WEAVES SHUTTLES

左右穿梭 (Zuǒyòu Chuānsuō)

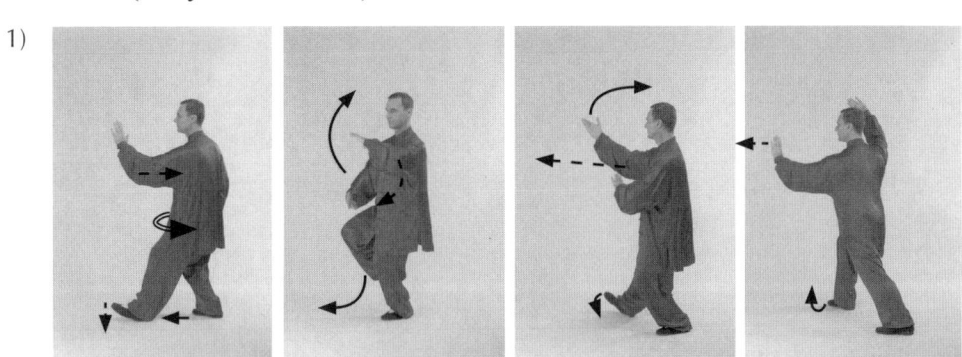

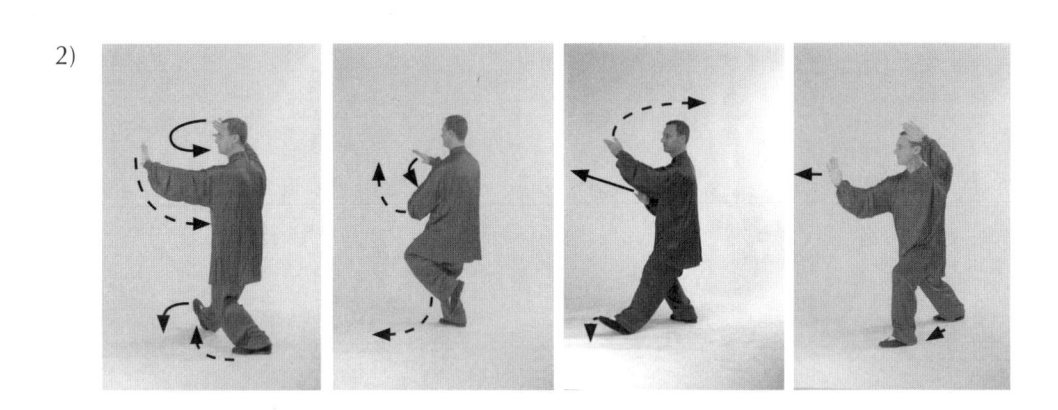

1)

2)

THE YANG TÀIJÍ 24-STEP SHORT FORM

19. NEEDLE AT SEA BOTTOM

海底针 (Hǎidǐzhēn)

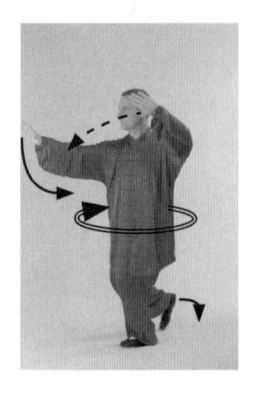

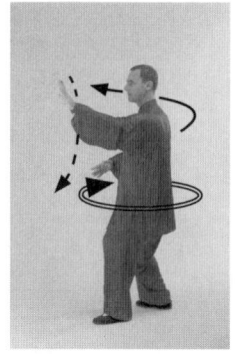

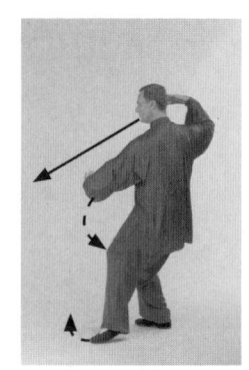

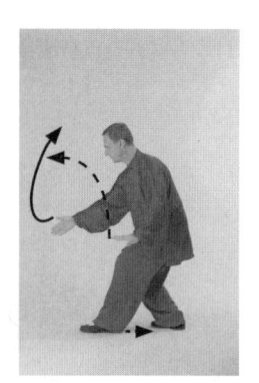

20. FLASH ARMS

闪通臂 (Shǎntōngbì)

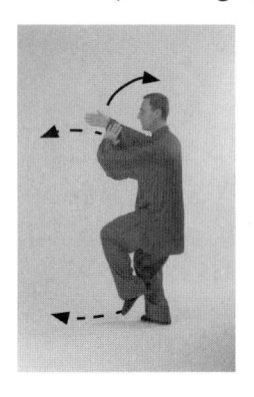

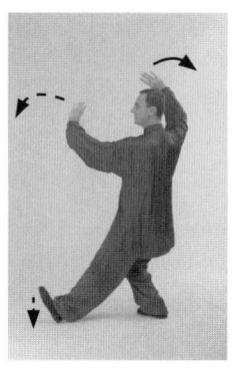

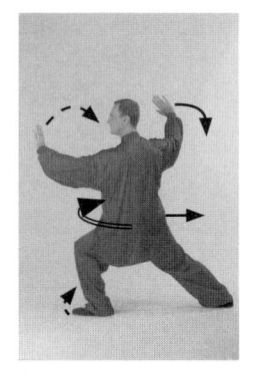

SECTION 8 (4 MOVEMENTS)

21. TURN, DEFLECT DOWNWARDS, PARRY AND PUNCH

转身搬拦捶 (Zhuǎnshēn Bānlánchuí)

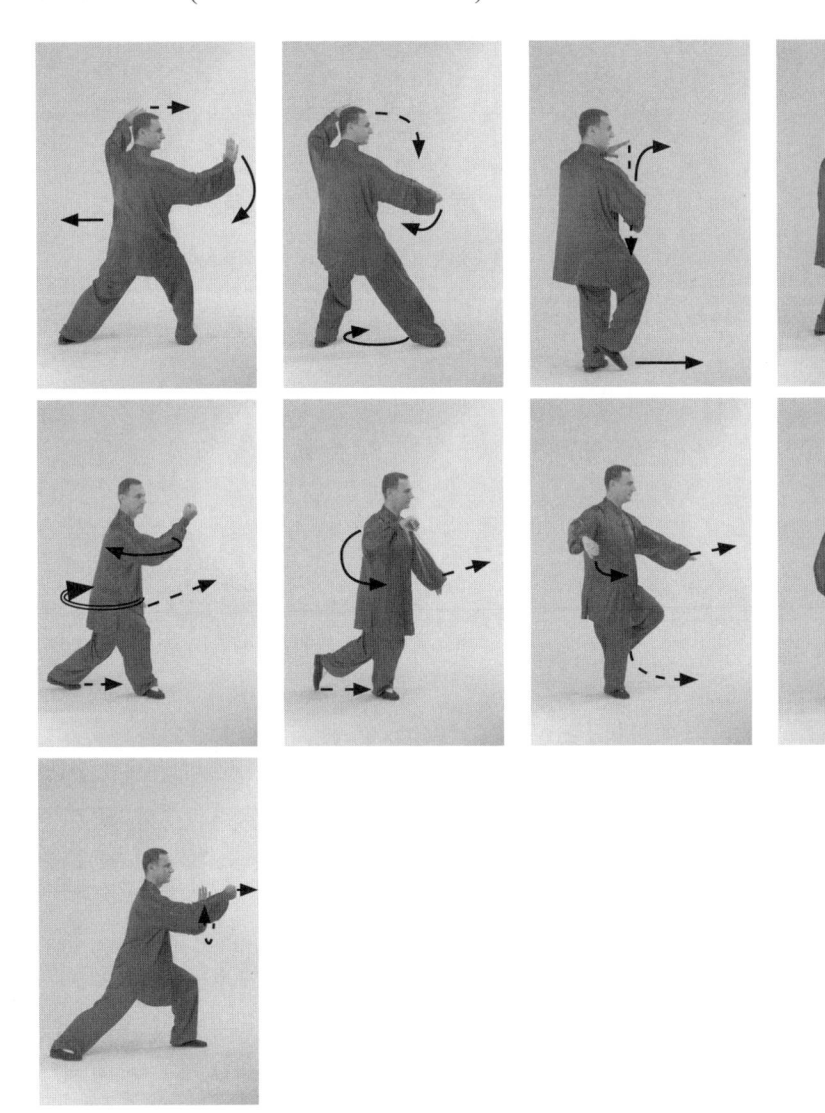

THE YANG TÀIJÍ 24-STEP SHORT FORM

22. APPARENT CLOSE-UP
如封似闭 (Rúfēng Sìbì)

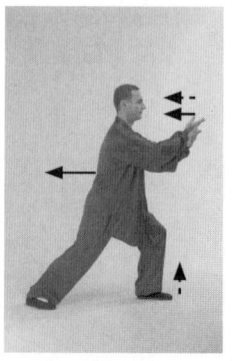

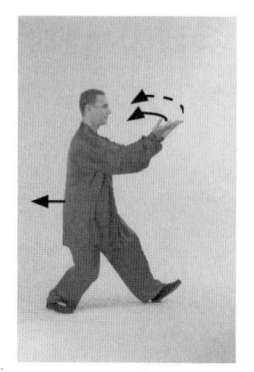

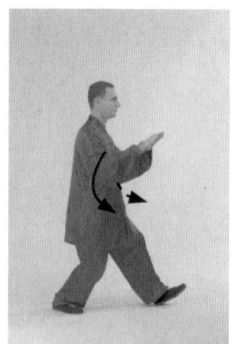

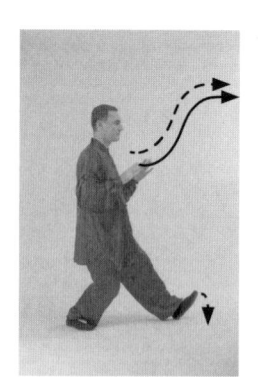

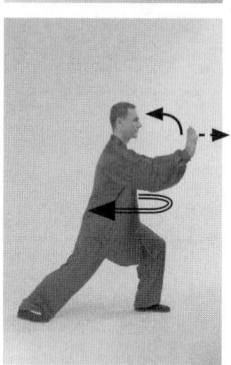

23. CROSS HANDS
十字手 (Shízìshǒu)

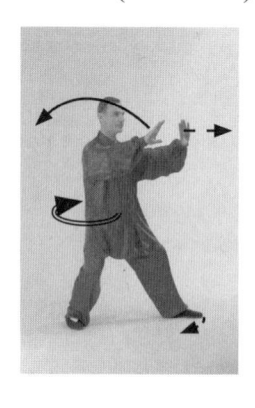

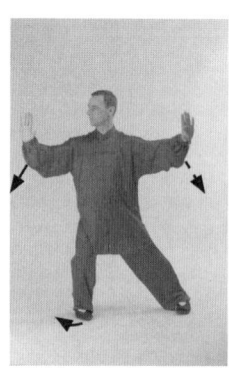

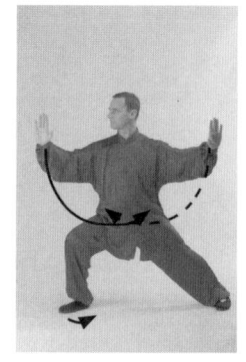

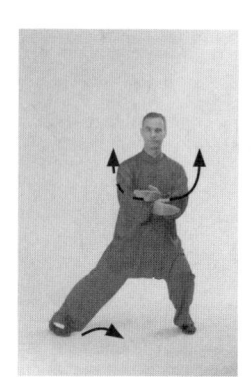

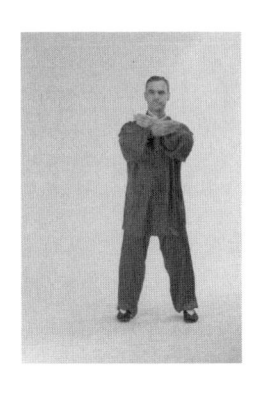

24. CLOSING FORM

收势 (Shōushì)

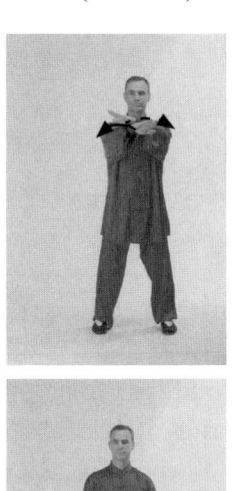

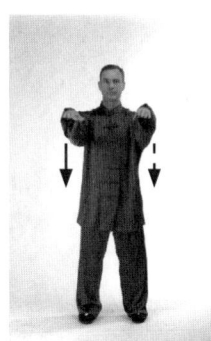

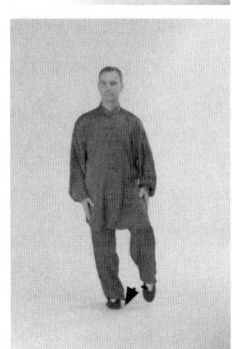

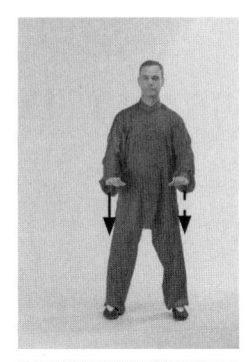

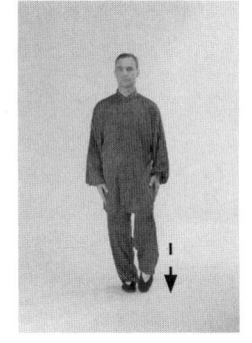

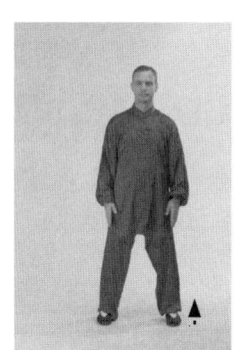

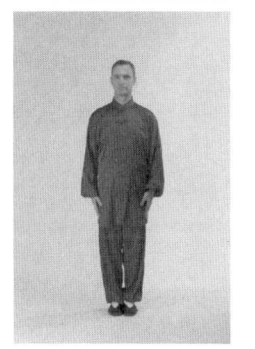

17

Beyond the Basics

GENERAL POINTS ON THE FORM

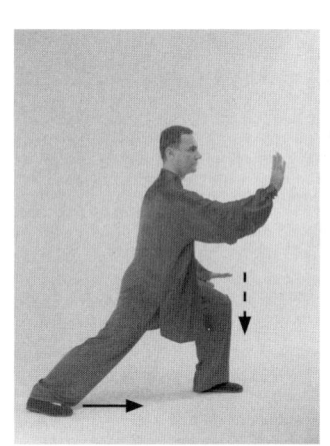

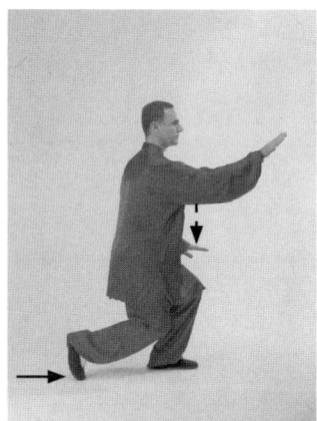

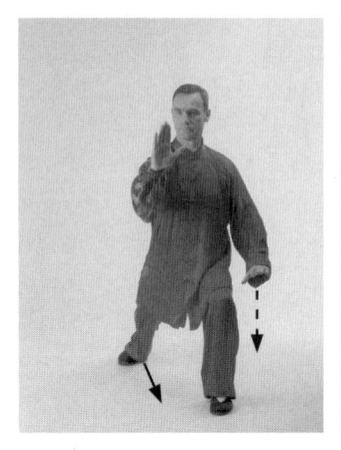

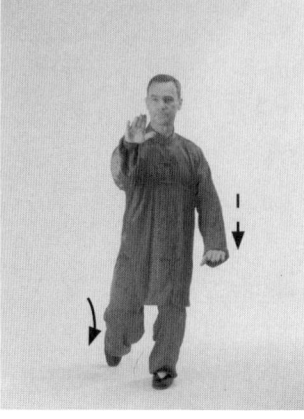

Bringing the rear leg forwards

If you are in (for example) a Bow Stance and want to lift your rear leg and bring it forwards, push downwards with the lower hand (if there is one). The pushing down of the hand helps to bring the weight into your front foot and makes the release of the rear leg much easier.

In addition, as you push the hand down, be aware of the use of the hip to bring the back leg forwards. It is the centre that moves the leg, not the leg itself.

Lowering an arm towards the body (inwards lowering)

First relax the chest as this will make the shoulder relax (1). Follow this by sinking the elbow as though resting it in someone's turned up palm (2), and then sink the forearm, then the wrist (3), the palm and the fingertips (4). The arm should feel heavy.

There are many occasions when this principle of sinking the arm takes place in the Yang Tàijí 24-Step Short Form. The most obvious examples are: Form 1 (both hands), the start of Form 7 (the left hand moving out of Repulse Monkey), Form 8 (the right hand in the transition and turn to the right side), Forms 7 and 8 (the lowering left or right hand when moving into Lǚ in Grasp the Bird's Tail), Form 10 (both hands alternately in Cloud Hands), etc. (See also 'Silk Reeling in tàijí movement', p.318.)

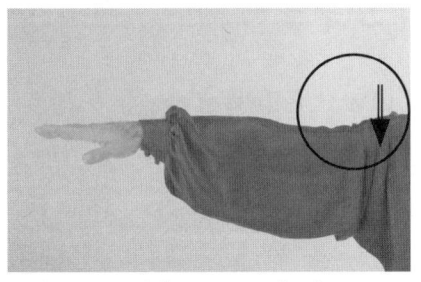

1. Arm out sideways and relax chest/shoulder

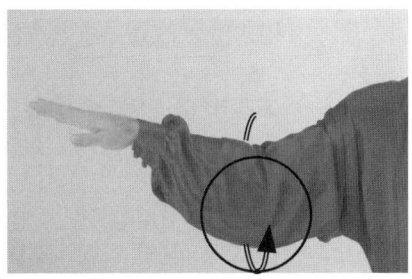

2. Sink elbow

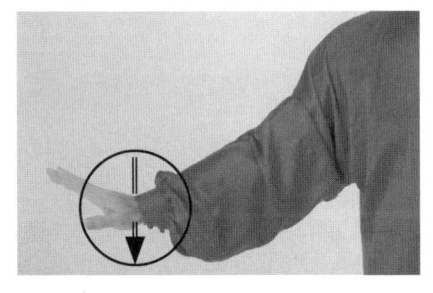

3. Sink wrist

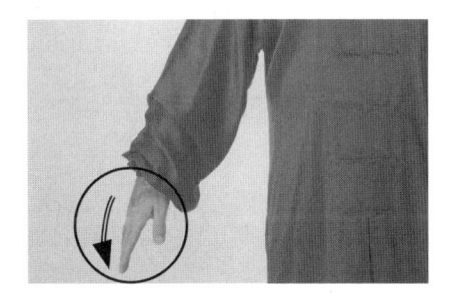

4. Fingers point at floor

Lifting an arm up the front of the body (inwards lifting)

If you want to continue the movement by lifting the arm up the centre of the body (as in e.g. Cloud Hands), lift the fingertips as though the arm is being hoisted upwards by someone pulling on your fingertips. The arms should be relaxed enough so that the elbow 'hangs' and feels heavy.

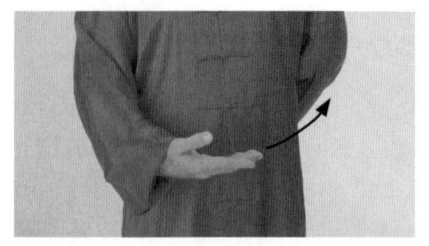

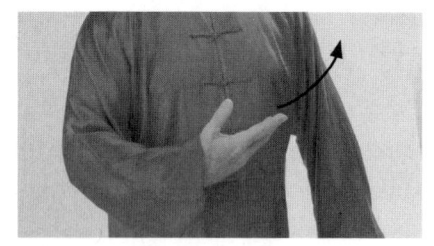

1. Right fingers starting to lift to left side; body turning left as in Cloud Hands

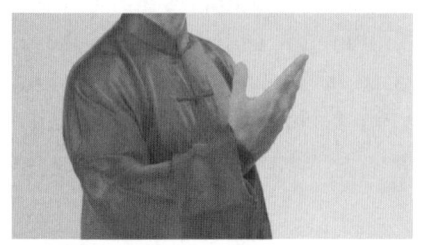

2. Lifted further to 45°

Lowering an arm down the centreline (outwards lowering)

This follows the same principles as in 'inwards lowering' above.

Irrespective of which way the palm is facing, relax the chest to soften the shoulder; by doing this you will feel the elbow sink (1). Then sink the back of the forearm (if the palm is turned upwards (2), otherwise sink the front of the forearm), then the back of the wrist, the back of the palm, and then the fingertips (3). The arm should feel heavy. The arrows in the photos below depict the direction of energy/relaxation.

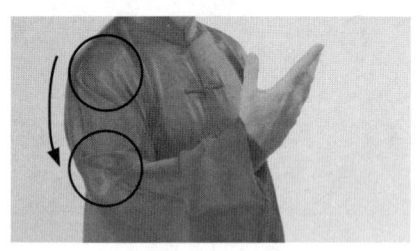

1. Right fingers in centre of body at throat height – palm upwards

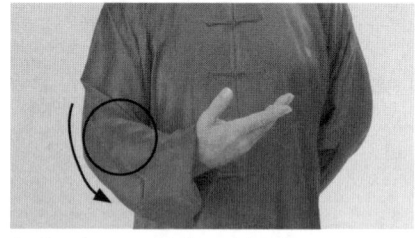

2. Sunk to middle of body

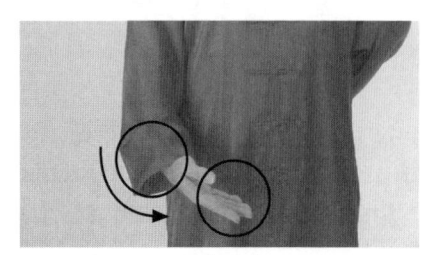

3. Sunk to waist-height

Lifting an arm away from the body with palm upwards (outwards lifting)

When an arm sinks to the leg (as in 'outwards lowering' above) and then lifts outwards and upwards to your side (e.g. in Repulse Monkey, and in Brush Knee and Twist Step), the forearm and palm should twist outwards *before* the arm lifts. There is a feeling of the hip and elbow forming a pivotal point, so that the elbow at no point feels as though it is moving *behind* the hip.

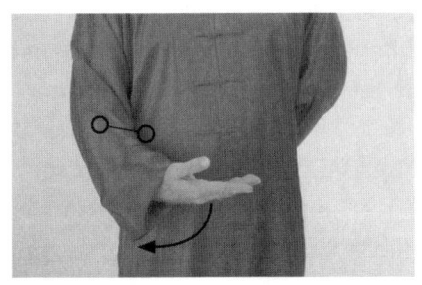

1. Right fingers in centre of body at waist-height – palm upwards

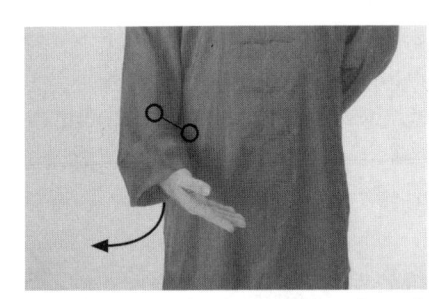

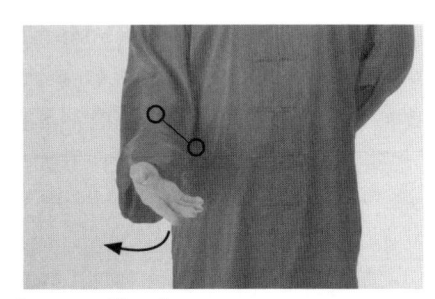

2. Half-pivoted out to right side – shown also with turn of body

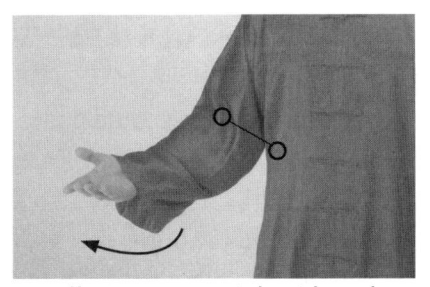

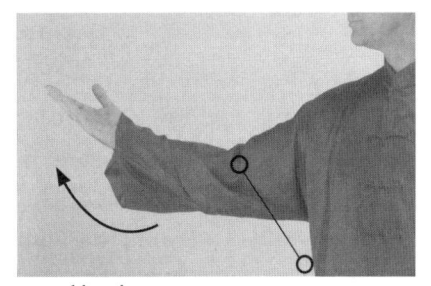

3. Full-pivot out to right side – shown also with turn of body

Silk Reeling in tàijí movement

All of the above 'inwards and outwards lifting and lowering' are simplified descriptions (upper limb only) of what the Chinese refer to as 'Silk Reeling Exercise' Chánsīgōng 纏絲功, sometimes also called 'Winding Silk Energy' Chánsījìng 纏絲勁.

In all movements, energy moves joint by joint through the limbs. The way to do this efficiently is to focus on and to relax/release the particular area of the body where you want the energy to move. You *can* do it by only thinking the energy to those specific points or areas, i.e. without the sense of relaxation and a tense body/limb, but the energy becomes more 'brittle', and the body becomes less integrated.

There is 'Silk Reeling' in every movement of tàijí. It can be seen in such movements as the vertical circling of Form 1 (Commencing Form), in the horizontal movements of Form 2 (Parting the Wild Horse's Mane), in the sideways circling of Form 10 (Cloud Hands), etc.

Silk Reeling is like pulling a weed carefully out of the ground; it is *feeling* the energetic connection of the plant right down to the smallest root and trying to draw it out without snapping it. It's the same when moving in tàijí – you have to feel the energetic connection from joint to joint in your body, so that, were someone to push (for example) your arm, there would be no moment of weakness, or disconnection from the centre, or disunity within the structure of the entire body. This is the body working in harmony.

The relationship between the upper and lower joints

There are a number of relationships within the body (and also, incidentally, in acupuncture); certain joints of the body work together in pairs, with the centre acting as the mainspring or fulcrum generating all actions.

The upper and lower joints should always work together, the shoulders/the hips, the elbows/the knees, and the wrists/the ankles. Usually the actions of one will be reflected in the other.

There is also a feeling of connection between the hips and the elbows (which doesn't mean that the elbow is 'glued' to the hip, but that the elbow will follow the movement of the hip).

This principle of connection underlies every tàijí movement; without it, the movements are just that – movements! But with it, the principle becomes the key to generating power/strength in the movements.

EXAMPLE OF HIP TO SHOULDER RELATIONSHIP

Moving from the end of Brush Knee and Twist Step 1 (right side) into the second Brush Knee: When you sit back on to the right foot, don't turn your hips or left foot to the left side; instead think of moving your right shoulder towards your left hip – whilst simultaneously tucking your pelvis under and gently pulling in your lower abdominal muscles.

Once you start to look for the relationships, you see them everywhere…just watch yourself walking!

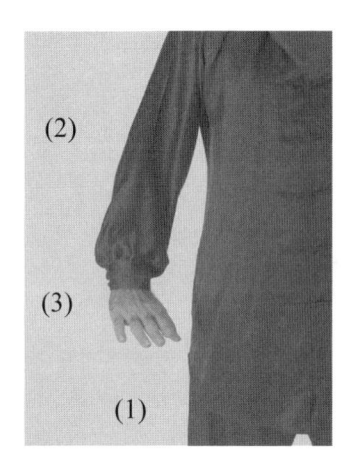

Pushing a hand downwards by the side of the body

There are many occasions where the hand is pushed downwards by the side of the body or leg (e.g. in the Yang Tàijí 24-Step Short Form, the final postures of the first five forms: Commencing Form, Parting the Wild Horse's Mane, Stork Spreads its Wings, Brush Knee and Twist Step, Play the Pipa, etc.).

When the arm pushes down, a feeling of 'Péng' should be retained in the arm; although the arm is mainly pushing downwards, the upper arm should retain Péng. This is achieved by a combination of 1) a definite downwards pressure with the heel of the palm, 2) a slight bowing of the elbow, and 3) a slight outwards 'pressure' with the hypothenar eminence.

The relationship between the shoulder joint and the hip joint

The shoulder/arm joint reflects the hip/leg joint.

THE SHOULDER JOINT

Because the humerus (the bone of the upper arm) is connected to, and articulates at, the lateral aspect of the scapula (it connects via a 'ball and socket' joint), beginners often lift the entire shoulder girdle (i.e. they lift and rotate the actual shoulder-blade) when raising the arm.

From a mechanical point of view, when lifting the arm to push, you should avoid lifting and rotating the shoulder-blade.

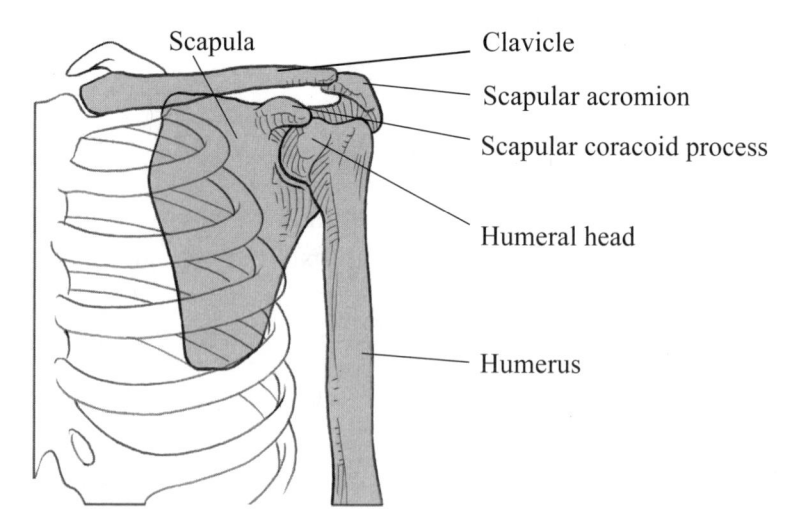

THE YANG TÀIJÍ 24-STEP SHORT FORM

Scapula
Clavicle
Scapular acromion
Scapular coracoid process
Humeral head
Humerus

Shoulder joint

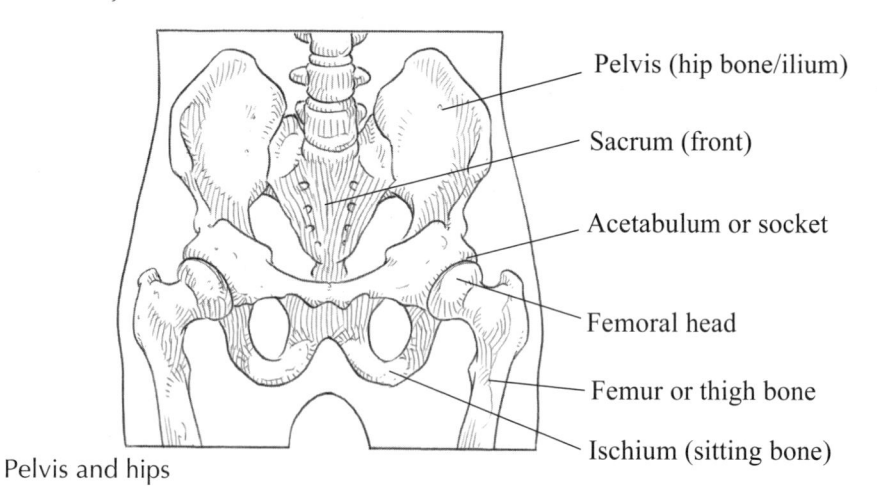

Pelvis (hip bone/ilium)
Sacrum (front)
Acetabulum or socket
Femoral head
Femur or thigh bone
Ischium (sitting bone)

Pelvis and hips

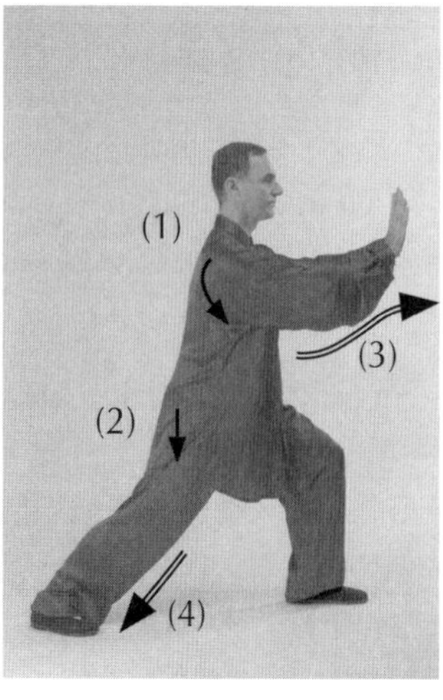

The same mechanical idea occurs with the hip joint; even more advanced practitioners have trouble connecting the hip joint correctly.

When going into Bow Stance, you shouldn't lift the femur (femoral head) out of the socket (acetabulum) – relax the hip of the outstretched rear leg.

When moving forwards into a Bow Stance and pushing with the arms, both the shoulder joint (1) and the hip joint (2) should connect correctly to the trunk. The power of the push with the arms (3) should work with the backwards push of the rear leg (4) (see also 'Yin and Yang in the Form', p.332).

The waist (Yāo 腰) and the pelvis (Gǔpén 骨盆)

Turning the waist (Yāo 腰) does not mean turning the pelvis (Gǔpén 骨盆; lit.: gǔ = 'bone/skeleton/frame/framework', and pén = 'basin/tub/pot/bowl') as well – the two are separate.

For example in Cloud Hands the pelvis/leg structure stays facing forwards whilst the upper body turns from the waist. Many people find this quite difficult, but it is just a matter of practice – the flexibility develops quite easily.

(See also 'Freeing the Waist' on p.323.)

Feeling comfortable in the postures

The general rule for any posture is that it should feel 'comfortable'. This idea is difficult for many beginners to grasp as most of the tàijí movements feel strange, particularly when the body weight is being taken on one leg, making the concept of 'comfortable' hard to understand. It means that there is a feeling of connection throughout the structure; the joints are aligned, and the body relaxed and soft.

CONNECTING THE BODY IN TÀIJÍ

There is an expression in tàijíquán: 'When one part of the body moves, everything moves.' This means that the geometrical relationship of the various parts of the body is so sensitive that the slightest alteration of one will affect the others, even down to a cellular level.

If my understanding is correct, this means that the person who originally made that statement had a grasp of quantum theory, and the statement is equally true for every minute event that you create in your life as it is for the use of the body.

At its most basic, this tàijí statement is saying that there is an interconnection amongst the parts of the body and that you cannot just move your arm independently – if you do, it's not tàijí.

When both learning and teaching tàijí, it is sometimes necessary to divide the body up, i.e. the body does this, the arms do that, and the legs do the other. There are advantages and disadvantages to this – it makes a movement much easier to learn, but makes the understanding of the *feel* of that movement much harder to grasp. In addition, the movements of all other parts of the body are often ignored – the hips, the back, the abdomen, the chest, etc.

It is important to understand that the waist (Yāo 腰) is the central pivot of the body and that the body splits above and below it – two limbs downwards plus hips, two limbs upwards plus shoulders, the shoulders and the hips both working in very similar ways and performing the same roles in their connection to the limbs.

The waist therefore acts as the coordinator; if it's too tense, messages between the upper and lower halves of the body can't get through; if it's too soft (lacking internal 'tone') the messages also don't get through or at least are slowed down.

Getting the right *feel* in the waist is like sailing in a dinghy; if you pull the mainsail in too tightly, not only is it tiring but the boat doesn't function so efficiently; if you leave the mainsail so slack that it flaps, the boat again doesn't function so well. You need to *feel* the wind and work with it.

If you want other examples, think of any of the elements and how, when using them, you work *with* them.

The same is true for the waist – if you don't relax it, you cannot *feel* through it, the pipeline becomes too restricted or too floppy!

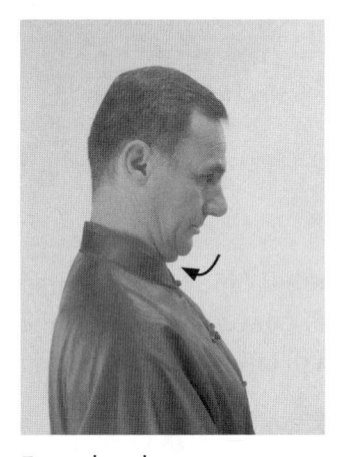

1. Straightening the head

There is plenty written about 'raising the crown as if supported by a silk thread'. When I was learning tàijí with one teacher we were always told to 'tuck the chin under'. I did this on a regular basis and often ended up with a headache.

Yes, it's true, you *do* tuck the chin under, but... you don't. The chin tucking under happens *as a result* of the releasing of muscles at the back of the neck and to the base of the skull, it is *not* the initiator. (See 'Freeing the neck' on p.31).

Once you have the feeling of the neck releasing, then the crown can be 'raised as if supported by a silk thread'.

N.B. If you try this out and then find that your shoulders have risen also, you haven't *released* the neck, you have *stretched* it.

Forced under

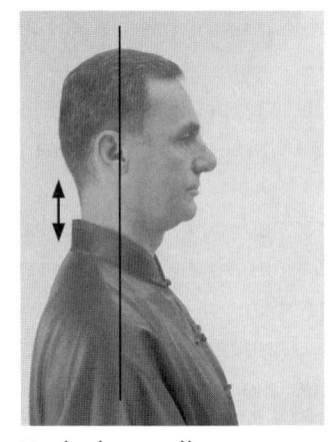

Tucked naturally

2. The chest and back

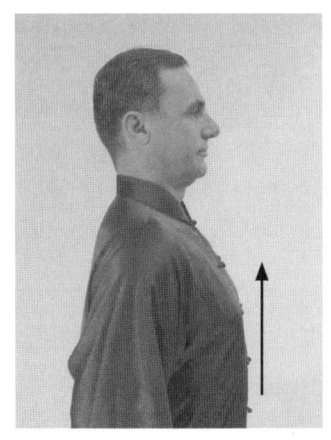

Hollowing the chest slightly allows the qì to sink to the dāntián, and softens the upper part of the body. Avoid the military posture – the shoulders pulled back, the chest protruding.

'Hollowing' means that there is a slight 'sinking' of the sternum/breast bone – try breathing out, and you will feel the sternum move inwards and slightly downwards.

Continue to breathe from the abdomen and you will no longer be lifting and lowering the ribcage in the same way that you were before.

Sink your shoulders and shoulder blades as you hollow the chest.

The hollowing of the chest and sinking of the shoulders produces a connection from one hand to the other around the back – this has been referred to as the 'Bow of the Arms' (see pp.347–8).

Over-lifted at the front

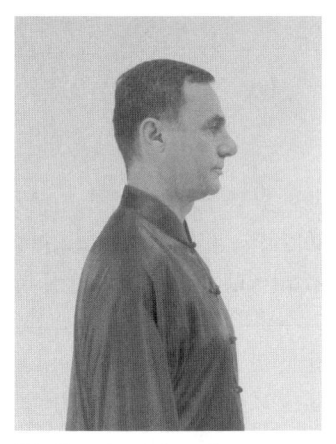

'Hollowing' the chest, and sinking the shoulders

3. Freeing the waist (Yāo 腰)

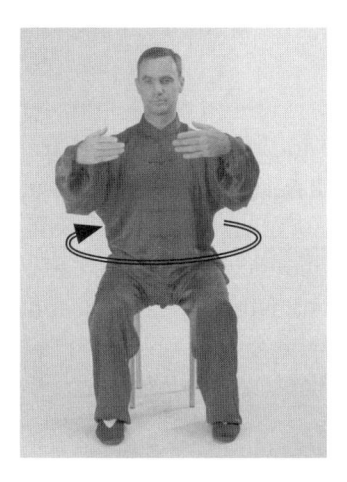

The waist is the body's main pivot, and is the key to connecting the upper body to the lower part of the body. In order for the body to move freely, we need flexibility in the waist – to see an example of non-flexibility in the waist, you only have to watch an old black and white film of Frankenstein's monster...the entire torso is locked into one unit.

When you relax and free the waist, the lower part of the body is no longer under the control of the upper part of the body. The pelvis starts to work independently without locking the legs, and the Kuà 胯 (inguinal grooves where the hips meet the legs) can begin to function correctly.

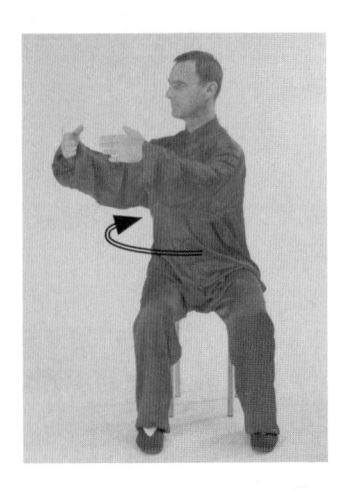

The third warm-up exercise above works on the freeing of the waist, but you can also loosen it by sitting on a chair with your arms held out ahead of you, or even folded across your chest, and then turn the upper body to left and right.

4. Full (solid) (Shí 实) and Empty (Xū 虚) Stance; transferring the weight

When there is more weight on one foot than the other, that leg is referred to as being 'full/solid' (Shí 实), and the other leg, with less weight on the foot, is referred to as being 'empty' or (Xū 虚).

The movements of tàijí involve a continuous process of the body weight transferring from one foot to the other; for example, when you move the body weight from the back foot in an Empty Stance, to the front foot (thereby turning it into a Bow Stance).

This is often likened to the structure of the legs being like an inverted 'U' that is half-filled with water. When the weight is on one leg (as in the photo below), that leg is filled with water; as the weight shifts to the other leg, the water 'pours' over the juncture of the legs (the pelvis) into the other leg, and, being water, it always sinks to the lowest part of the leg (the foot). Therefore if the hips aren't relaxed, it's as though you have 'left some water behind'.

When making such a move, there should be an awareness of the back foot pressing into the ground (to move you forwards), causing the shift of weight, and 'tipping' the weight into the other foot.

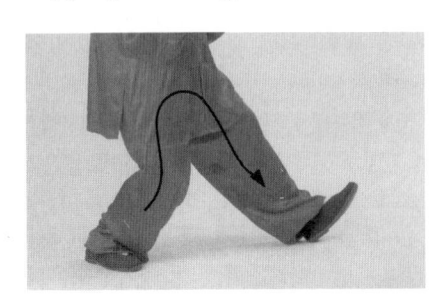

At all times when doing a weight transfer as above, there should be a feeling that you are connected to the earth – sinking into it; therefore as you push the weight forwards, your back foot is connecting to the earth, and as the weight transfers, your front foot simultaneously connects and sinks into it.

This helps to stop the body from rising and falling with the weight transfer, keeping it on a level plane.

The concept of 'full' and 'empty' is an extremely important one in tàijí, as many of the problems that beginners encounter in moving from one posture to another originate from the misunderstanding of how to transfer the weight.

The most common error when transferring the weight from front leg to back leg is the lifting of the pelvis/hips/buttocks as a result of not bending the back knee and sinking into the rear foot enough. The hips therefore make an upwards and downwards arc during the sitting back process – i.e. the hips and therefore the body rise and fall. The same is also true when moving forwards into a Bow Stance – the hips are not relaxed throughout the process, particularly at the end of the movement.

A useful way of looking at the weight transfer issue that might help beginners is thinking about the 'angles' formed by the knee joints:

Assume that you are in a Bow Stance, and you are going to sit back into an Empty Stance.

Your front leg in Bow Stance will be bent at an angle of (for example) 100°, and the back leg is almost straight. Start to move your weight on to the back foot, and for every degree that the front leg opens out and straightens as you move backwards, you think of bending the rear knee by the equivalent amount.

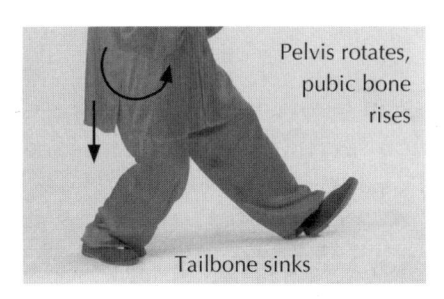

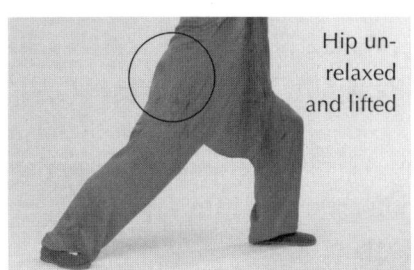

As you transfer the weight from front to back, allow the pelvis to relax and there should be a feeling of the tip of the tailbone dropping into the rear heel as the pelvis and tailbone tuck under, the pubic bone rising.

When moving from the back foot to the front foot, there is still the same sense of relaxation of the tailbone/sacrum, but the tucking under doesn't take place to the same degree. Nevertheless, there must be a dropping of the tailbone/sacrum.

This refers back to the freeing of the waist (above); in both cases – moving the weight forwards or backwards – the waist needs to be free so that the pelvis can alter angle, and tilt or not as necessary.

DOUBLE-WEIGHTEDNESS

The other expression that often crops up in tàijí is being 'double-weighted', and is argued as being something that should be avoided at all costs.

The usual description of double-weightedness is of a 50/50 weight distribution between the feet. In this position the 'full' and 'empty' are unclear and it is therefore inefficient for movement as it causes the body to become 'frozen', and there is a temporary loss of mobility.

This is easily demonstrated by standing in a wide shoulder-width stance and then trying to step sideways with either foot. You will find that, in order to step in one direction, you have to 'lock' the body and move in the other direction first; whereas if the weight is already on one foot you can alter direction immediately.

Although this might be partly correct, it doesn't allow for what you might call a 'vertical full and empty'. In other words, when in a wide shoulder-width stance and whilst the legs form a solid base, the upper body remains relaxed and soft, allowing for horizontal rotation of the body. The body is therefore not locked and the balance of 'full' and 'empty' within the body is retained, or to put it another way, there is still Yin and Yang in the body.

If this were otherwise, the start of almost every tàijí Form (for example in the Yang Tàijí 24-Step Short Form this would be Form 1: Commencing Form) and many Zhan Zhuang qìgōng positions would be double-weighted.

5. Sinking the shoulders and elbows

For most people who start tàijí, the shoulders seem to give the most trouble. At first, it's noticing that they are lifted like a pair of gigantic shoulder-pads, and then it's learning how to release them, then it's remembering to release them, and then it's feeling their connection to the hips and feet.

Lifting them will cause your energy to rise, will weaken the body, and will undermine your balance. It also causes both a muscular and an energetic disconnection in the shoulder joint and in the neck.

They should always be soft and relaxed, although for most beginners this is not as simple as it sounds.

When the shoulder is 'lifted', in fact it is the clavicle and the acromion (which are connected at the acromioclavicular joint) that are lifting, and because the acromion is part of the scapula, the scapula therefore rotates which lifts up the humerus (upper arm bone).

How *do* you relax the shoulders?

Clavicle
Acromioclavicular joint
Scapular acromion
Scapular
Humerus

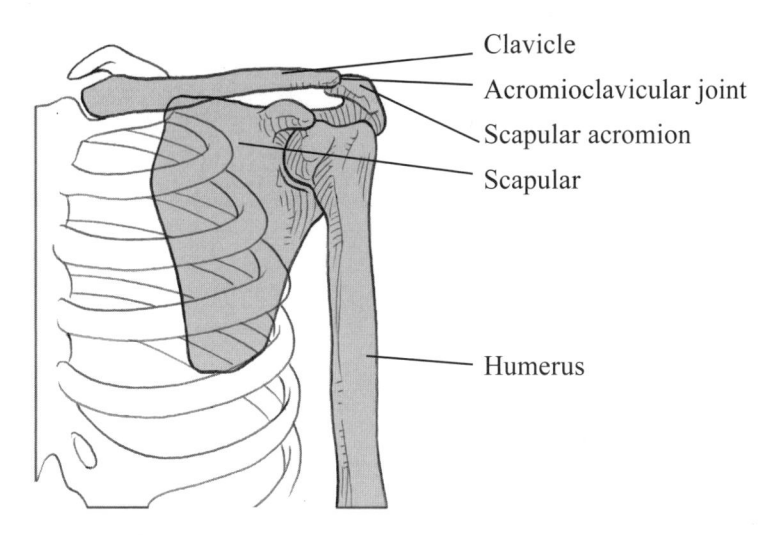

Shoulder joint

First of all it helps to think of sinking your chest. It is almost impossible to lift the shoulders if you breathe out and relax the chest.

It also helps to think of relaxing the shoulder blades, as this makes the entire shoulder girdle sink.

So you therefore think of both the chest and the shoulder-blades relaxing; this not only settles the shoulders, but also, because you are also relaxing your back, makes the shoulders 'widen'.

The problem mostly occurs when the arm or hand is lifted. When this happens, you have done what is known as 'recruiting' muscles, in other words you have borrowed muscles unnecessarily from other muscle-groups to do the job, i.e. lifting the arm. In the case of the arm this will often be the trapezius, as discussed previously.

The other way of thinking that helps when lifting your arm or hand is to think of dropping or sinking your elbow.

Sinking your elbow is like hanging up your shirt sleeve on the washing line; if you peg up the shoulder of the shirt and the sleeve, the arm just 'hangs'.

To teach the concept, I take hold the student's wrist or fingertips with one hand and lift it/them to about shoulder-height (without his providing any help to raise his arm). With the other hand I then try to push his elbow, which should be loose and should 'dangle'. If it doesn't, you know that he's still holding on to the muscles.

(See also 'The shoulders' on p.30.)

6. 'Mind' versus 'Force'

It is possible to align the body in such a way that it uses the minimum of its resources.
This has two results:

1. the body becomes very efficient, and

2. there is, in effect, an overflow of energy.

An analogy of the latter might be that of a dam: If the water in the dam is neither being used nor being lost (due to a poor structure), there is a build up of water, and it has to be drained off to avoid overflowing the dam.

The 'efficient' body requires some definition.

1. When in the condition of being efficient, the body is in a state of what you might call 'educated relaxation'; in other words the muscles are neither soft and flaccid, nor are they stretched – they are somewhere between the two. The Alexander Technique would refer to this condition as 'lengthened'; by relaxing the muscles, and by giving them a direction, they reach their natural length, and yet they are not stretched. (See 'Educated relaxation' on p.354.)

2. Because the muscles are in their most positive state – i.e. there is no tension within the body, the meridians or channels or Jīngluó within the body can transfer energy around the body in a very efficient manner – all the pipelines are open – there are no tension blocks. (This is assuming that there are no other physical problems, either chronic or acute.) The channels connect the body, completely integrating it.

3. It is also worth mentioning at this point that the practitioner can also become aware of the 'stabilizers' – the red muscle tissue which, in effect, holds the core structure of his/her body together. (For more details of this, see 'Skeletal connection – Stabilizer muscles' on p.346.) However, it is not essential to understand this in order to feel the energy building within the body, although certain exercises related to the stabilizers can help to enhance the awareness of them, and their importance in the structure of the body.

The overflow of energy manifests in the following way:

When perfectly aligned, a feeling of power or strength arises in the body. The body not only feels immensely strong and powerful, but it also feels remarkably calm and comfortable. There is a sensation of fullness both in the body and in the extremities; this can manifest as a feeling of warmth circulating around it. The Chinese say that this is the qì 气 moving in the body and that both acute and chronic problems can be cured using it. In the West we can only say that both qì and its curative potential are possibilities – no one has proved them!

With this kind of strength, there is no force, no tensed muscle, and therefore the strength is long lasting as there is no muscle to tire. This strength is wherever the mind is, not where the muscle is tensed; so the energy (strength) is directed by the mind – the yĭ 意.

Tàijí practitioners are aiming to perfect the production of and the use of energy so that it can be produced and directed at will.

7. Coordinating the upper and lower parts

This explains the use of the above energy in motion. It is said that in movement, 'Energy is rooted in the feet, is launched through the legs, controlled (ie. directed) by the waist, and manifested or expressed in the hands and fingers.'

The lower part of the body – the feet, legs and waist – work as one harmonious unit; they are the mobile foundation upon which the rest of the structure functions. Without a firm foundation the building is unsound.

When moving the body in any direction the energy should move seamlessly joint by joint through the body creating a 'connection'. It is a little like adding links to a chain, so that by the time you've added the last link the chain is complete.

For example, when pushing, you should feel the sensation of the push first at the ankle, then the knee, then the hip; it then moves up through the spine, to the shoulder, to the elbow and then to the wrist. In tàijí it will then usually be expressed through the fingertips.

The eyes, more often than not, follow the intention of the legs, body and hands, as they provide focus to the intention.

This is a chain-reaction in the sense of perpetuated motion, but also in the sense of a connective event in that the failure of one link in the chain means that the whole connection fails.

The back plays the main role in the coordination of the upper and lower body. There are no 'joints' in the back in the same way that there are in the legs and arms but, as osteopaths will tell you, there are certain key points in the spine that act as pivotal points or fulcra.

In order for the trunk to connect effectively to the legs, the pelvis needs to move into the 'correct' position. This involves an alteration to the way that it sits on the legs that also affects the middle and upper spine.

1. By gently lifting the pubic bone upwards towards the navel (contract the lower abdominal muscles) (1), and by releasing the small of the back so that it sinks, the pelvis pivots around the central point of the body (2) (sometimes referred to as the 'Wújí' point); not only does this connect the legs to the lower trunk, but it has an effect on the rest of the spine that automatically starts to alter the spine's shape.

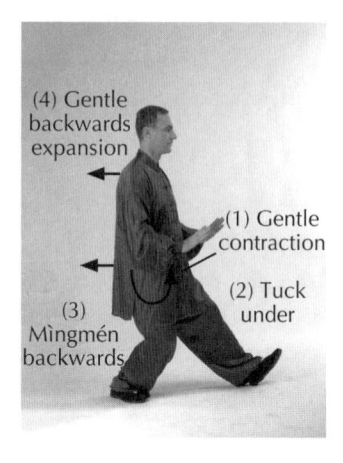

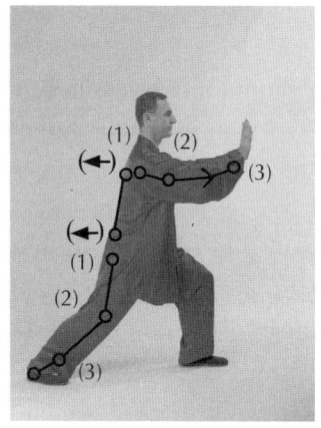

(4) Gentle backwards expansion
(1) Gentle contraction
(2) Tuck under
(3) Mìngmén backwards

2. In order for the lower spine to connect to the middle and upper spine, a wave-like or ripple-like movement needs to take place in the spine.

    As the pelvis tilts/tucks under and the lower abdominal muscles are gently contracted, push the point on your spine that is opposite your navel slightly backwards (if you don't tilt the pelvis this is virtually impossible); this point is Du 4 (Mìngmén 命門) (3).

3. Then push out the area between your shoulder-blades (approximately T4/T5/T6) (4). You'll feel the shoulders hyper-extend forwards slightly, thereby making the connection from the spine to the arms.

This is easiest to feel with either a slow push against a partner or against a wall.

It is then just a matter of thinking the push down the arms from shoulders (1) to elbows (2) to wrists (3), and down the legs from hips (1) to knees (2) to ankles (3).

Be very careful to relax the neck, bearing in mind that the tip of the spine (the coccyx) and the cervical vertebrae have a balancing act to play.

(See also 'The relationships between the upper and lower joints' on p.318.)

8. Harmony between the internal and external parts

If your mind is tense (stressed, worried, anxious), this will be reflected in your body; your movements will be uneven, heavy, or stiff. If your mind is calm and peaceful, your movements will be soft, gentle, smooth, and light.

In tàijí, where the structure of both the body (the way in which you use the body) and of the movements is concerned, there are only four important aspects: Empty (Xū 虚) or Full (Shí 实), Open (Kāi 开) or Closed (Hé 合). The concept of 'Kāi' and 'Hé' is discussed more fully later on (see Chapter 18), but in the context of the point being discussed here they mean not only the opening and closing of the four limbs, but also of the mind as well.

In tàijí, we are focusing on the mind (intention – yǐ 意) and awareness; the body follows, but the two need to work together.

9. Continuity in movement

The movements are continuous, without break. Yang Chengfu referred to this as being 'like a river which flows on and on without end' or 'like reeling silk thread from cocoons'. This refers not only to the external movement, but also to the internal. As the body moves forwards and backwards, it is important to maintain an unbroken flow of focus/concentration, and to keep the unbroken thread of energy within the body, which means that there are no uneven movements, and in particular that the movements originate from the dāntián/centre.

THE 'FLOW' OF MOVEMENT

The 'flow' of movement or energy is broken when the direction of movement of a limb suddenly reverses or dramatically alters, causing an angle rather than a curve.

When changing from (for example) a forwards movement to a backwards movement (from solid to empty) or vice versa, *feel* the movement of your energy in that particular direction and *even as you change direction, retain that feeling in that original direction – even though you have started a new direction.* If you do this with every movement, you will feel how the changes from empty to solid to empty are created, and you will feel the circles forming.

Then you can start to make the circles smaller.

This can also be done with the shifting of weight in the feet – as you finish sitting backwards or forwards, press the foot more firmly into the ground to reverse the direction as though driving the foot deep into the earth.

(See also 'Silk Reeling in tàijí movement' on p.318.)

10. Tranquil movement

The movements in tàijí are performed slowly because by so doing, the qì can be sunk to the dāntián (see 'The centre' on p.62), and the body and mind are calmed; this allows the body systems to function more efficiently, and the energy to flow unimpeded within the body. In my opinion, and speaking from my own experience, this can also allow the body to repair certain problems.

The movements should be practised as though trying not to disturb the surface of a lake – with great softness, slowness, smoothness, and sensitivity.

(See also 'Feeling comfortable in the postures' on p.321.)

YIN AND YANG IN THE FORM

All the moves in the Form fall into either a Yin move or a Yang move.

Yang moves expand, and Yin moves contract.

Yang moves also tend to rise, and Yin moves to sink.

Yang moves tend to move forwards, and Yin moves tend to move backwards.

The above are general rules for Yin and Yang, but it is important to realize that they are relative concepts. In other words a fire is Yang compared to, for example, water, but it is Yin compared to the sun! So this way of thinking in tàijí depends very much on what has preceded it.

In addition to this, as you make a tàijí move, overall a movement might be defined as 'Yang', for example a push – you might say that this is an 'assertive' or even 'aggressive' movement – very outwards going – and therefore is Yang. However, even when you do a push, internally it is a combination of both Yin and Yang, i.e. although the body is moving forwards (Yang), the chest is closing (Yin), and whilst the elbows are sinking and the arms closing (Yin), the legs are opening (Yang), etc.

The world is a clever system of 'opposites' that are never fixed as certainties. You only have to have a superficial look to see that life is like a sine wave that swings between these opposites to varying degrees – day to night, hot to cold, the waves that rise and fall, the governments that are popular and unpopular, the civilizations that come and go, the planets that grow and die, and so on, and so on...

In tàijí, the Yin and Yang theory is a method of making us aware of how the opposites are playing out in the microcosm of our bodies. To do this we use movement, but whilst seeing those opposites playing out, we are not just casual observers; we are aiming to become conscious of balancing these opposites within ourselves.

When they are balanced correctly, we become stronger, more flexible, more resilient, better focused, calmer and, to a very great extent, more in control of our lives in the way that we function both in ourselves, in society and in the world as a whole.

Once again we are back to the concept of the body being a microcosm; we are carrying around our very own practical test-kit for learning how to live efficiently and effectively in the world, because you can be absolutely certain that, whatever we discover about the way that our bodies work, it is just a reflection of how *everything* out there works.

To use a small example, if you put the back of your wrist against the back of someone else's wrist, and push directly against that person (who is doing exactly the same to you – Yang versus Yang), it becomes a simple matter of strength. Whoever has the greater strength will push the other person backwards. This is a little bit like whoever shouts the loudest is more likely to sell something, or whoever has the most money is going to make the biggest splash.

But tàijí is about 'moving a force of 1000 lbs with a force of 4 lbs'; it is about altering a situation or bringing about change with little or no effort.

So to return to the Yang versus Yang example above, you simply stay rooted (in other words, you retain your integrity) and by moving your arm sideways you deflect the other person's push, possibly even upsetting his balance in the process. Very little effort has brought about a change from Yang to Yin.

If the concept of Yin and Yang is a sine wave, the uphill Yang expansion cannot continue indefinitely, it has to change to its opposite.

Therefore one aspect of tàijí is learning the art of Yin and Yang: how to bring about that change.

Yin and Yang become apparent when you start to observe the body doing even the smallest of movements; it is impossible for you to move in any direction without pushing energy in the opposite direction.

Newton's third law of motion states that the force resulting from the interaction of two bodies acts with equal magnitude on both of them and in opposite directions. In other words: 'For every action, there is an equal and opposite reaction.'

THE YANG TÀIJÍ 24-STEP SHORT FORM

From a practical point of view, imagine that you are trying to push an object. If you put your feet *together* and push, it will be *your* body that is projected backwards. But if you put one foot forwards and the other further back (i.e. in a Bow Stance) you are able to push the object, because you are pushing an equivalent amount of energy backwards simultaneously. In other words, your body is expanding outwards from its centre.

As above, Yin and Yang are both relative concepts. Looked at from one perspective, you could say that one limb pushing backwards is Yin and one forwards is Yang. Looked at from the perspective of energy moving outwards from the dāntián, you could say that both are outwards movements from the centre and therefore Yang.

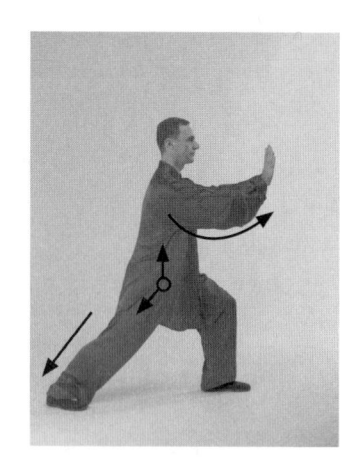

From the idea of 'equal and opposite reactions' we can learn about the way in which we manage the shoulder and hip joints: The '*above*-the-centre' shoulder/arm joint is the equivalent of the '*below*-the-centre' hip/leg joint; we *should* operate them in the same way, but we usually don't.

A push with the upper limbs is the equivalent of the rear leg extending into Bow Stance, i.e. the rear leg is pushing backwards (a push with the lower limb). When you push the hands forwards you don't lift the shoulder out of the socket so, when going into Bow Stance, you shouldn't lift the femoral head (the head of the femur (leg bone)) out of the acetabulum (the socket), but most people do – they lift it and destabilize the pelvis.

THE CENTRE

When I originally completed learning the basic moves of the Long Form (the 108-Step Form as it is also known), I then learned the aspect of what was termed 'Centre-Move' in the Form. This was the way in which your centre controls the movement of the limbs, in particular the arms; the arms themselves never have a 'life of their own', i.e. they never work independently of the body.

Location

First, the 'centre' is not the pelvis (Gǔpén 骨盆), nor is it the waist (Yāo 腰).

The 'dāntián' (丹田) is not really an actual part or place in the body; it is the concept of a core area around which other parts of the body are centred. Therefore, because the entire body ultimately works from the centre, the entire body really becomes the dāntián.

So the elbow can be a dāntián when the forearm is rotated (consciously using the elbow as a pivotal point), and in the same way the area of the chest can be rotated by, for example, turning the shoulders and consciously using the area of the breast bone as a dāntián.

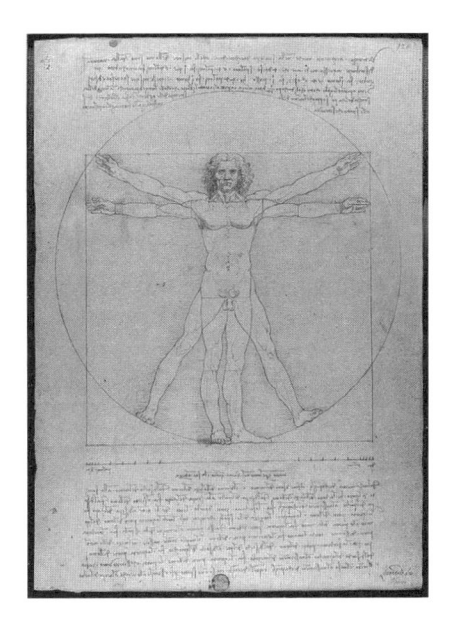

Da Vinci Vitruve Luc Viatour

These individual joint rotations are rather like the individual lives of planets in a solar system; they have their own orbits and rotations, but are ultimately controlled by the core of the solar system – the sun. The system works as one unit, the balance of the whole being dependent upon the interplay of the individual parts.

So the dāntián is really an integrated co-dependent system involving the entire body.

However, in tàijí, although these rotational points (and many others) come into play continuously, when we refer to the dāntián we are almost always referring to the *lower* dāntián.

The word 'dāntián' is often translated as the 'cinnabar field' or 'red field' or 'elixir field'. Dān 丹 translates as 'cinnabar' – mercuric sulphide, HgS, occurring in red crystals – the principal ore of mercury used as a pigment; or can translate as 'vermilion' (bright red) – artificial HgS used as pigment. Tián 田 translates as 'field', but also as 'arable land' or 'cultivate'. It therefore implies an area that can be cultivated.

Descriptions vary as to its location. It is sometimes described as three fingers in width below the navel and two fingers in width behind the navel. It is also described as being approximately 1–2 inches (2.5–5 cm) below the navel, and approximately one-third inwards towards the centre of the body. It is an 'area' rather than a specific acupuncture point, although some would argue that *Qìhǎi*

(Ren 6) or *Guānyuán* (Ren 4) is the dāntián. I have even come across a reference to its being '1.78 inches below the navel', and another reference to its being the *Huìyīn* (Ren 1 会阴 'Meeting of Yin') acupuncture point that lies between the thighs at the juncture of the two thighs between the genitals and the anus. I think that this latter desciption is incorrect!

The best description of the dāntián that I have come across is that it covers an area from the navel *Shénquè* (Ren 8 神闕 'Spirit Gate') down to *Qìhǎi* (Ren 6 气海 'Sea of Qi') which is 1.5 inches (4 cm) below the navel, and then down a further 1.5 inches to *Guānyuán* (Ren 4 关元 'Gate to the Original Qi'). The area has also been described as extending sideways of the centreline of the body to the two St.25 points *Tiānshū* (天枢 or 'Celestial Pivot/Hinge') and to the back point *Mìngmén* (Du 4 命門 'Gate of Life'). See the diagram below. I have also come across a reference to the area extending sideways of the centreline of the body to two extra acupuncture points called 'Xuanyu', although I am unable to find any reference to these extra points.

This circular area is 3-dimensional within the body.

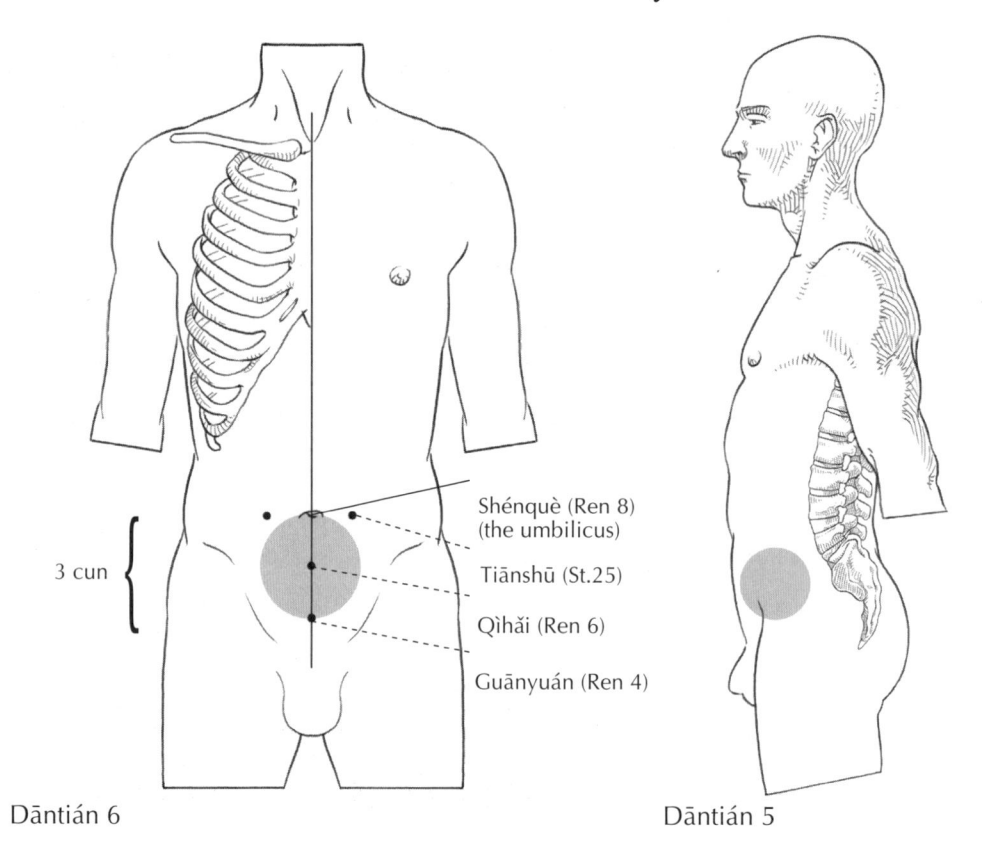

Dāntián 6   Dāntián 5

It is generally considered that there are three dāntiáns in the body: The *lower* dāntián has already been described; it is often called 'the lower cauldron'.

The area of the heart is often referred to as the *middle* dāntián (sometimes associated with the thymus gland).

The area in the brain slightly above the midpoint between the eyebrows and inwards towards the centre of the head is often referred to as the *upper* dāntián (sometimes called the 'third eye' and associated with the pituitary gland).

For the moment, our main interest is with the *lower* dāntián.

There are two points about this area that concern us as tàijí practitioners:

1. It is thought to be the place in the body in which the body's energy is stored.

2. It is considered to be the central control unit of body movement around which the tàijí movements rotate.

Feeling the centre

There are some simple exercises that can be done with a partner that go some way to feeling the centre, and feeling how to use it.

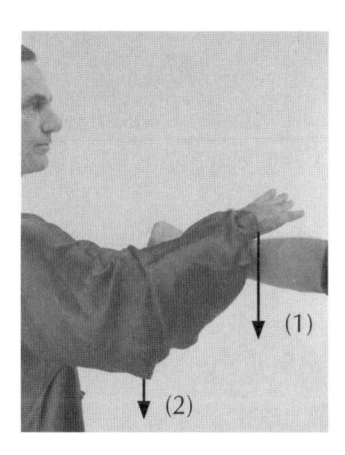

EXERCISE 1: PUSHING DOWNWARDS

Fold your left or right arm in front of your chest with the forearm parallel to the ground, and the palm facing the floor. Your partner then supports your wrist from underneath with his hand.

You now do a comparative test – (1) *not* using the centre, and (2) *using* the centre:

1. **Not using the centre:** Push your hand downwards whilst your partner tries to stop you. It is important that you try to push down with your *wrist*.

2. **Using the centre:** Then as a comparison, prepare the exercise in exactly the same way.

    This time when you push down, feel as though you are leading the downwards push of your hand with your elbow; also feel as though you are sinking your elbow into your abdomen.

In (1) you might find that you are tensing your shoulder and arm to push.

In (2) you should have a feeling of firmness in the abdominal muscles, as though you are also using them to do the movement.

The second part should feel more powerful, and should also feel as though you are combining the musculature of the body instead of using one limb to do the push.

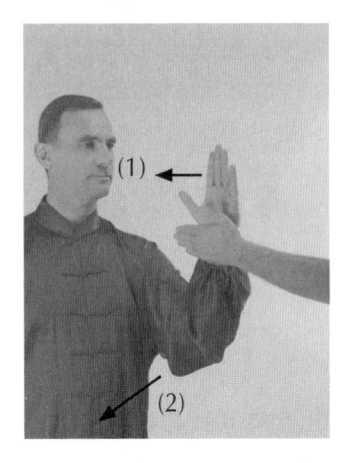

EXERCISE 2: PUSHING SIDEWAYS

This is similar in concept to the previous exercise but with a sideways instead of downwards movement.

Hold your arm in front of you with the fingers pointing upwards, your forearm therefore vertical. Your partner places a hand on your wrist.

1. Using your hand/wrist, try to push your partner's hand sideways.

2. Then to compare, prepare exactly as before and then move the hand sideways by feeling as though you are compressing your elbow and your abdomen together – moving them towards each other. However, note that you don't literally have to touch them together – this is a *feeling*, and anyone watching might not even notice that this is what you are doing.

Once again you should have a feeling of firmness in the abdominal muscles in the *second* part of the test, which means that you are using them to do the movement. The second part should feel more powerful, and again it should feel as though you are combining the musculature of the body instead of using one limb to do the push.

Moving the centre and centre-turn

The centre, dāntián, or core of your body plays a key role in tàijíquán. Every movement of the body is initiated by it, including the bending of both elbows and knees, and the turning of the body from left to right. It is like the mainspring in an analogue clock without which none of the cogs will rotate, or the hub of the bicycle wheel without which none of the spokes will move.

When you move the centre, it might, for example, make an arm move; it is important to feel the centre's involvement in creating the action of the arm as this unifies the body's actions. Furthermore, in the action of 'centre-move creating arm movement', every other relationship in the body has also changed simultaneously.

To repeat the Martial Arts expression (p.329) 'Energy is rooted in the foot, launched through the legs, controlled by the waist, and manifested in the hands', it might be better if this expression read: 'Energy is initiated in the dāntián, rooted in the feet, launched through the legs, controlled (directed) by the waist, and manifested or expressed in the hands and fingers.'

I am going to restrict 'centre-turn' to refer to the way in which you move the centre on a *horizontal* plane, rather than a vertical one. If I stand with my feet a shoulder's width apart and turn the centreline of my body towards my left knee, this will be called a 'centre-turn left'. Therefore a 'centre-turn right' would be for when turning towards the right knee.

An everyday example of this is the act of walking. In this, your centre will turn towards the leg that you place in front of you; if you don't, and you turn it the other way, you will walk like Frankenstein's monster! Therefore, when walking, if you place your left foot in front of you and move on to it, this would be called 'centre left' – you can call it left and forwards, but it isn't strictly speaking quite true, because 'forwards' is slightly different – there is no turn of the body.

The forwards and backwards movement of the centre would appear to be obvious, and in its most basic state, it is. For example if you look at the movements at the end of Grasp the Bird's Tail – *An* 按 followed by the push forwards – *Tuī* 推 (see pp.155–6), you can see that this is a straight push forwards – the centreline faces the direction in which you are pushing throughout.

If you're performing Brush Knee and Twist Step, you move the body forwards for the push – that is therefore 'centre-forwards', but, if you start to look closer at the movement you see that actually it isn't a pure 'centre-forwards', it's really 'centre-left-forwards' or 'centre-right-forwards'. But, for the sake of simplicity, this can still be referred to as 'centre-forwards'.

The same applies to the 'centre-backwards' movements, examples of which would be Play the Pipa (p.122), Stork Spreads its Wings (p.99), Repulse Monkey (p.129), and High Pat on Horse (p.195).

However, there are a couple of forwards/backwards centre movements that are less self-evident.

In the first move of the Form, you raise your hands away from and ahead of you to shoulder-height (1), and if your centre doesn't move backwards at the same time (2), you will fall forwards. This therefore would be what might be called a 'centre-back' move. The same goes for the next move that follows; your hands lower (moving closer to the body) and if you do not move your centre forwards again to compensate, you will fall backwards (a 'centre-forwards' move).

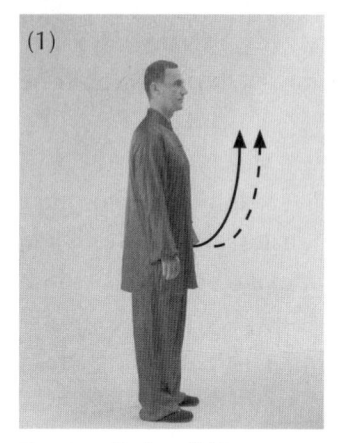

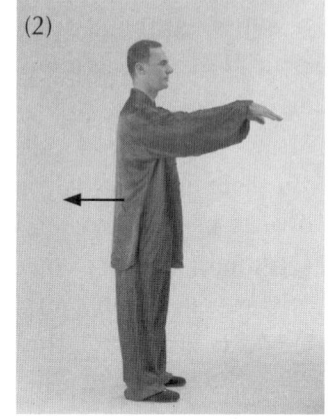

Form 1: Before lifting arms   After lifting arms

18

Open (Kāi 开) and Close (Hé 合)

Kāi 开 (lit. to open, start, turn on)

Hé 合 (lit. to combine, join, unite, gather)

The body undergoes a continuous process of what is known as 'opening' and 'closing' of both torso and limbs. This is more complicated than I am about to describe, but the basic idea is as follows: Opening and closing is the result of the centre's actions. It's not unlike the actions of a squid as it propels itself through the sea; by contracting its centre it compresses itself, and by altering its relationship to the surrounding water it produces movement. In compressing it 'closes'; in releasing the compression it 'opens'. The squid is a good example because you can visualize every cell of the creature working together as it compresses.

It's the same with the movements of tàijí; in its simplest format we compress the centre and then release it (or vice versa) thereby producing the 'posture' or movement. Every cell of the body should be involved in the movement; you don't compress one bit of the body, and leave the rest out.

For example, before opening the arms out in Parting the Wild Horse's Mane, we 'close' the body first – this generates the power for the movement. Moving into Repulse Monkey, from the arms open position we move to a closed position.

It is like producing power from a spring; there's no power if you don't first of all either stretch or compress the spring. It comes back to Yin and Yang again – you cannot have Yang (open – Kāi 开) unless you first of all have Yin (closed – Hé 合) or vice versa.

HOW TO CLOSE THE CENTRE

I have a particular memory of one tàijí class many years ago where the Chinese teacher was explaining the idea behind closing the centre. He gathered us around him, and having checked that there were no women present in the class (there weren't) said, in a very quiet voice, 'It's like having sex.'

It's the use of the hips/pelvis rather like a whip – a pelvic tilt.

The simplest description of the body closing is when you sit down on your heels in a squat; the centre of the body has compressed or 'closed', and the Kuà 胯 (see p.66) has folded – if you think that it doesn't, then try to squat with your backside sticking out, i.e. without tucking your backside under.

So in certain tàijí movements, you physically pull your lower abdomen inwards – gently tightening or firming the lower stomach muscles (it should feel a little as though you are pulling your navel inwards towards your spine) and you 'compress' the centre.

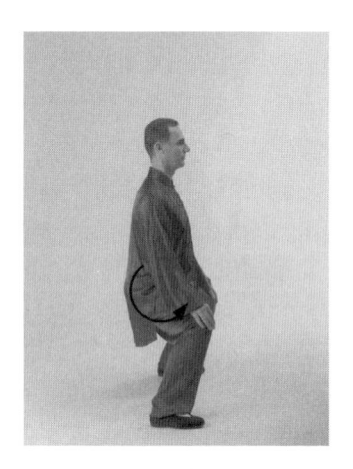

This pelvic movement recreates exactly the same action that you make when you sit down on a chair, except that you usually don't think about it when you go to sit down. We're all familiar with the jarring of the spine when sitting down on a chair that was higher than we expected; the lower spine wasn't in the right position – it hadn't curled under and formed a 'spring'.

So to 'close' the lower dāntián, you tuck the tip of your tailbone (the coccyx) under; you do a pelvic tilt.

Gently pulling your lower abdominal muscles inwards helps the front of the pelvis to tilt upwards, or to lift the pubic bone, but it is particularly important simultaneously to soften or release the area of the sacrum and the lumbar vertebrae, which will therefore allow the rotation to take place.

An analogy of this is to hold a football between your hands and rotate it. If you roll the ball, you might, for example, lift your right hand, but to keep the ball in the same place in space, you will need simultaneously to lower your left hand. You cannot leave the left hand stationary, otherwise the ball will move upwards to a different place in space.

You need to achieve the same effect with the body – leaving the centre at the same point in space; therefore the release of the back at the same moment as lifting the front is essential.

EXERCISE IN 'OPENING' AND 'CLOSING' THE ARMS

The feeling should come from the centre of the body.

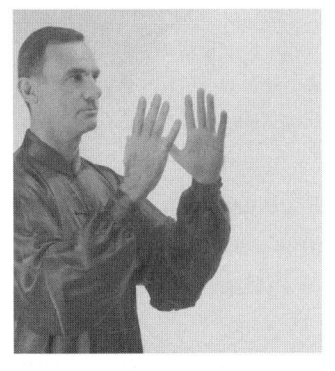

Starting position: To get the feeling of this, working with a partner, hold both of your arms in front of your chest so that they are bent at the elbows with the forearms vertical. Make fists if you like.

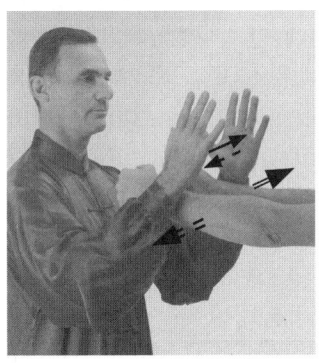

'Closing': Your partner puts his arms between your arms so that they press against the insides of the forearms.

As your partner begins to try to open his arms sideways, press your forearms together.

If he tries with medium strength, you'll find that, in order to close his arms you have to involve the chest to help you – using just the arms isn't enough. If he tries with maximum strength, you find that you have to involve your abdominal muscles also. This is the feeling for using the centre of the body and coordinating it with the arms.

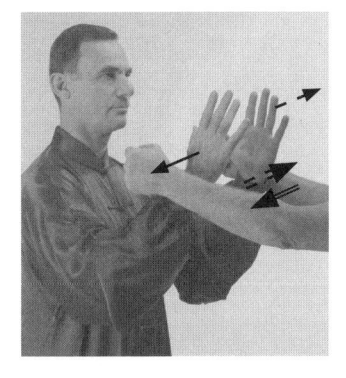

'Opening': Your partner places his arms so that they press against the outsides of your forearms.

As he applies pressure inwards, slowly open your arms.

FUNCTION OF CLOSING THE CENTRE

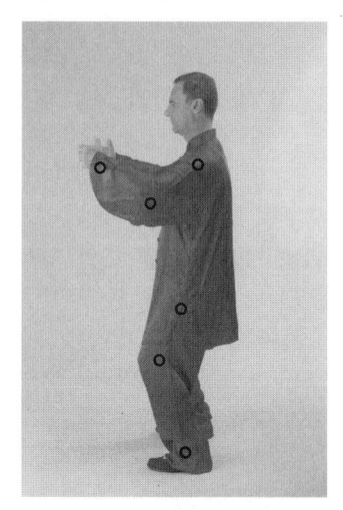

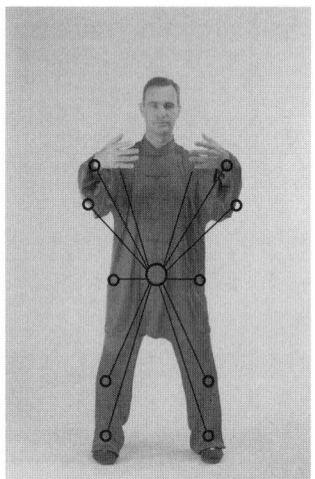

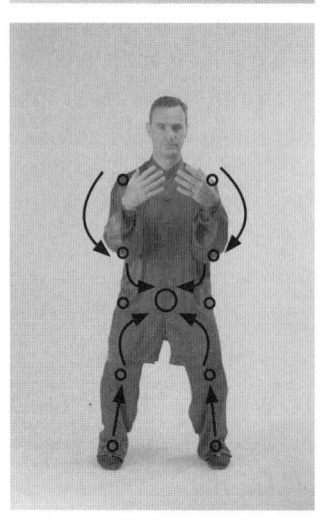

This rotational movement has a number of effects on the body, the most important of which is that it draws everything inwards – in particular your elbows and knees. It is as though the body is a loading spring, ready to expand outwards again – a tiger/leopard/puma, etc. about to pounce. It is also the body protecting its centre/core, and can be seen in many animals and insects – a woodlouse, an armadillo, a pangolin, or a hedgehog, as they roll themselves up.

The feeling should be a little like using the draw-string around the neck of a large canvas bag. When you pull on the draw-string, the eye-holes around the neck of the bag are drawn together. In the analogy, the draw-string is your dāntián, and closing it pulls the eye-holes (your shoulders and hips, elbows and knees, ankles and wrists) inwards.

'Closing' is not the body compressing into the centre, it should be thought of as the reverse – the centre drawing the body into itself. 'Opening' therefore becomes obvious: move out of the posture and the centre undoes and 'opens'.

Unlike 'centre-turn' mentioned above, 'opening' and 'closing' is a 3-dimensional action involving not only the horizontal plane but also the vertical – as well as the front and back of the body. The centre is also 3-dimensional, as discussed on p.336, and its actions will have an effect on every area of the body.

OPENING AND CLOSING THE LIMBS

Sometimes opening and closing are very clear-cut.
   For example:

Moving into Play the Pipa, the arms close, the body closes, and the legs close.

Moving out of Play the Pipa into Repulse Monkey, the arms open, the body opens, and the legs (by spiralling outwards) open (it's fractionally more complex than this in the action of the arms, but as an example it will do!).

But it isn't always so clear-cut; there are times when the arms open, but the legs close, or vice versa, or the body closes, but the legs don't, etc.
   For example:

In Cloud Hands, although the body stays closed throughout, sometimes the arms are open whilst the legs are closed, and vice versa.

However, as an overall concept, we can say that some movements are 'open' and some are 'closed' – possibly a case of taking a consensus of whether there are more 'opens' or 'closes' is any particular movement!

PÉNG ENERGY

In every posture in tàijí there should be Péng energy.
   Péng is often translated as 'ward off' which in English implies an action. However, 'ward off' in this case should be thought of as a descriptive adjective having a quality more like 'resilient' energy, or perhaps 'elastic' energy in the sense of having a bouncy, almost pliable quality to it. Although 'ward off' implies a deflection or a block, Péng energy is not only protective, but can also be an offensive/attacking energy as well as a sensing energy, a listening energy. For the person who comes into contact with it, there is a feeling of pushing against a soft, yet firm rubber ball – there is give, but there is also solidity and strength.
   Péng energy at heart is created by good skeletal connection, i.e. a good balance of Yin and Yang within the structure, calm focus/concentration, awareness, and what might be called 'educated' relaxation (see p.354).
   For Péng energy to exist, the body must be in a state where no joint is locked or rigid. As soon as there is rigidity, Péng is lost.

The body needs to be relaxed in such a way that any incoming force passing through it meets no resistance; it's almost as though the joints become like flexible tubes where the vibration of the opponent's incoming force can just pass through the middle of the tube, whilst the outside of the tube still supports the body.

The body therefore needs to become like a receptacle where the opponent's energy passes through it and then bounces back from the ground...a little like pouring your milk from a great height into one side of the cereal bowl; the milk goes down one side of the bowl, and then shoots up the other side and out of the bowl. If there's cereal in the bowl, the milk meets it like a dam (you've given it something to get hold of, i.e. your tension), builds up pressure and settles into the bowl.

I'm reminded of physics at school where you would send a vibration through a long spring; if something touches the spring, the vibration is compromised – tension is the something that gets in the way and compromises the vibration.

So the softening of the joints and sinking of your qì is of paramount importance.

Péng relies upon a good skeletal connection.

Skeletal connection – Stabilizer muscles

The body is 'held together' by the deep red muscle-tissue of the body, the 'stabilizers'. In theory these red fibres are not able to tire as they use oxygen to burn glucose and fat for energy and give off carbon dioxide. These muscle fibres, or 'slow-twitch' muscles as they are also known, are ideal for maintaining the upright posture, and the sustained contractions that are involved, without fatigue.

The skill of good connection therefore is to employ the stabilizers, without resorting to the white muscle tissue, or the 'mobilizers' – the 'fast-twitch' muscles. This latter group of muscles, although larger and stronger, *can* become fatigued; their energy stores become burned up and they produce lactic acid.

If you try too hard to connect the skeleton, the muscles may freeze up; in the Alexander Technique this result is known as 'end gaining', and you may end up in a worse position than before. Your breathing will often indicate 'end gaining' and stiffness; the stiffer you are, the shallower the breathing becomes.

The skill of good connection is to relax the muscles *but*, as stated earlier, to relax them *with direction*.

THE BOWS OF THE ARMS, LEGS AND BACK

The two arms, two legs and the spine work together as three interconnected 'hoops' around which the rest of the skeletal structure sits.

The way in which you hold and use these 'hoops' or 'bows' determines the efficiency of the body in performing an action (focused energy efficiency – no wastage).

The Bow of the Arms

This can easily be experienced as follows:

1. Standing upright, lift your arms up in front of you so that the wrists are at the same height as your shoulders, and with the palms facing away from you.

2. Move your arms out slightly sideways at the same height – a little less than 45° to each side is best.

3. Softening your shoulders completely, sink your elbows without moving the hands closer to the body.

4. Very slightly hyper-extend your shoulders forwards, *without lifting them*, and without tensing your neck; simultaneously be aware of gently hollowing the chest.

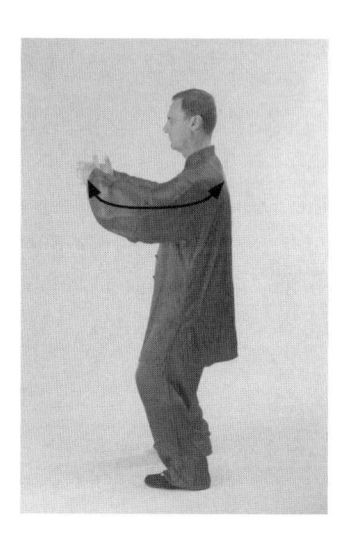

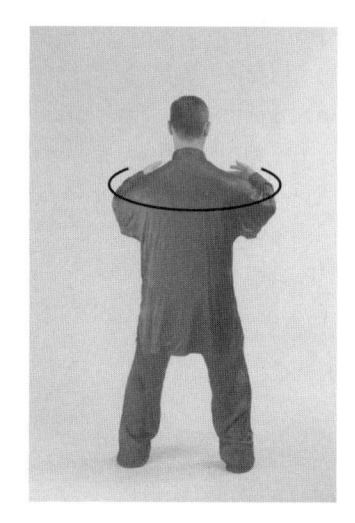

The arms are now what one might call 'connected', and you should now be able to feel a gentle stretch up the arms and around the back.

There is a very good 'test' for this Bow of the Arms that uses two partners. It is best to do it in two parts again, because it makes it *very* clear that enormous strength is derived from the correct way of doing it.

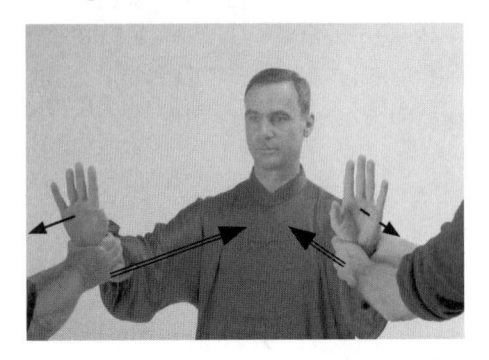

1. **The wrong method:** Stand in a Bow Stance, and hold your arms out as above, but without any hyper-extension. Sink the shoulders, but don't hollow the chest.

    Your two partners stand in front of where your arms are pointing and each takes hold of a wrist.

    Both partners then push towards you making sure that the pressure that they exert is equally balanced between the two of them.

    As they push, notice how much effort is involved, how the arms take all the strain, and how the muscles quickly tire.

2. **The right method:** Use exactly the same set-up as before, but this time, before your partners begin to push, use the gentle hyper-extension and hollowing of the chest as described above.

    You should find that you are considerably stronger; the arms are no longer tired, and you can hold the partners from you easily.

All we have done is to connect the arms and the back so that you are no longer using the arm muscles independently.

In (1) you are only using the muscles of the arms to resist the push, but in (2) you are using the entire structure of the body for the push – the push travels up the arms, connects to the spine, runs down the spine, and then down the back leg. When you are pushed, it feels as though your rear leg is being pushed into the ground, and the leg – being a very strong limb, simply has to push downwards into the floor to hold the push. In effect, the person pushing you is pushing the floor!

The Bow of the Legs

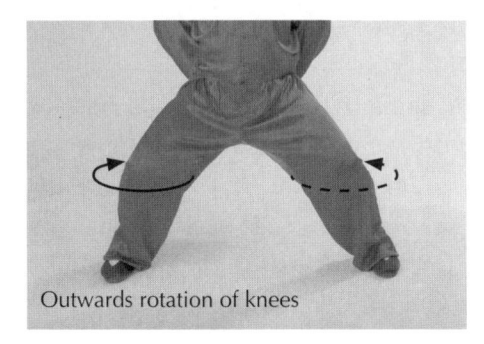

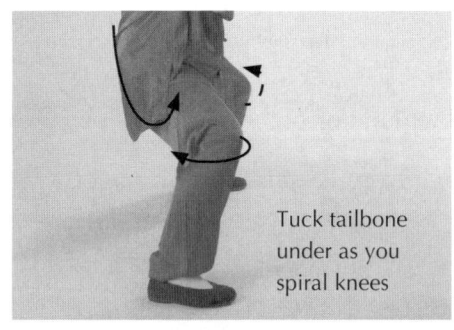

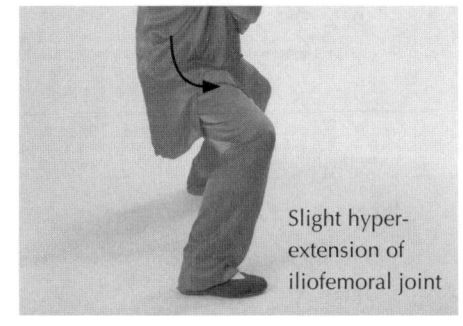

Outwards rotation of knees

Tuck tailbone under as you spiral knees

Slight hyper-extension of iliofemoral joint

The basic posture: Stand in a Horse Stance – both feet should point towards 12.00; the knees should be considerably bent.

Form the connection by allowing the knees to open outwards slightly. As you do so, pull your lower abdominal muscles in, soften the small of your back, and allow your tailbone to tuck under – i.e. do a pelvic tilt. To put it another way, using only your hips/pelvis, flick your tail between your legs.

Feeling the connection is almost like the leg equivalent of the Bow of the Arms – 'The right method' on p.348. Very gently hyper-extend the iliofemoral joint forwards – or, at least, *feel* as though you are.

It can help to imagine a strong elastic cord between your knees as you make the slight opening.

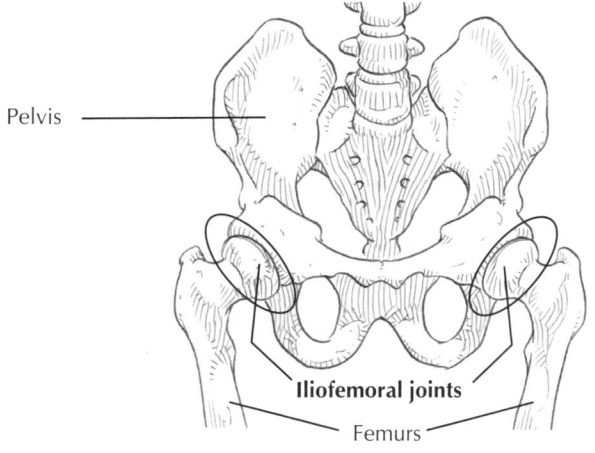

Pelvis

Iliofemoral joints

Femurs

The iliofemoral joints

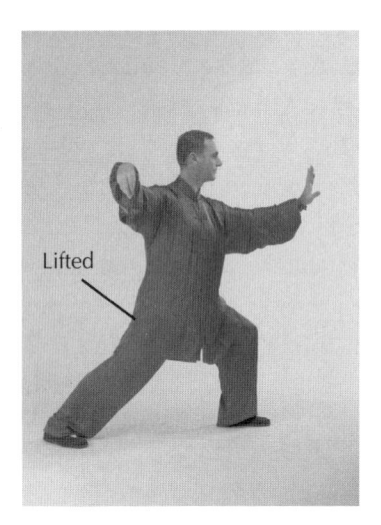

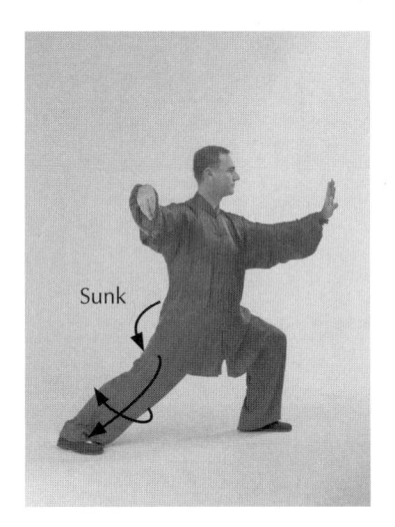

The 'Bow of the Legs' in a Bow Stance: When in a Bow Stance, many practitioners lift the hip of the rear leg. Stand in a left Bow Stance with approximately 70 per cent of weight on the front foot.

For the moment, straighten your rear right leg.

Now sink your right hip (it might help to think of sinking the right buttock or the tailbone/sacrum). The right leg will now want to bent slightly; however, this bend is achieved not by intentionally bending the knee but by sinking the tailbone or pelvic tilt. This provides the bow-like quality of the back leg, and you should feel a stretch in the anterior muscles (the quadriceps) of the right thigh.

There should be a feeling of rotating the knees outwards slightly.

Retain the same feeling that you had in the hips/pelvis/legs that you had in the Horse Stance above, including the elastic sensation between the knees – in particular in the right leg.

The posture should be comfortable, and without effort.

The Bow of the Back

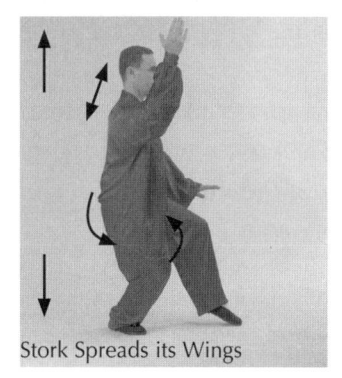

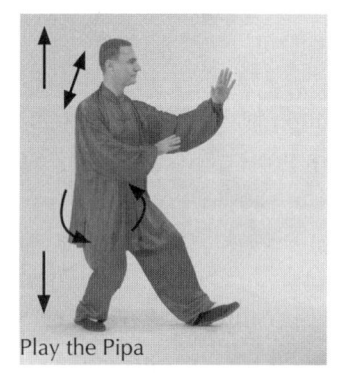

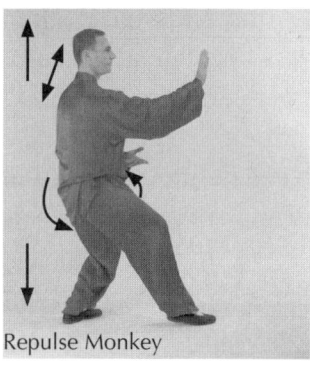

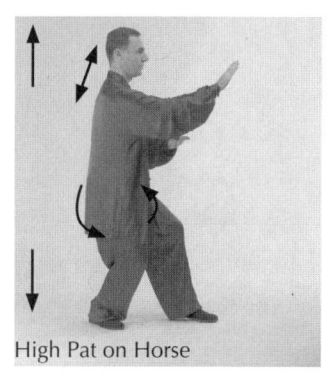

Stork Spreads its Wings

Play the Pipa

Repulse Monkey

High Pat on Horse

In order to feel this bow, the spine needs to be opened at the neck and in the small of the back; this has the effect of straightening out the spine. It can be forced, but it is far better if the result is achieved through relaxation.

Basic posture: It is easiest to feel the vertical connection in an Empty Stance, i.e. with the weight on the rear leg. The front foot can be flat, or with toes or heel raised.

Forming the connection: You need to perform three actions simultaneously: 1) the releasing or freeing of the neck, 2) the 'tucking under' of the tailbone (a pelvic tilt), and 3) the connection of the spine from shoulders to tailbone (thoracics, lumbars, sacrum and coccyx).

The first has been discussed earlier on in some detail, and in the classics is referred to as 'raising the crown'; I prefer the descriptions 'allowing the crown to rise' or 'freeing the neck' as these expressions imply no forcing or stretching. It is a releasing (in a vertical direction) of the muscles at the back of (and inside) the neck, in particular the muscles at the top of the neck, where the neck meets the skull.

The second can be achieved by forcing the tailbone under, but this can cause tension in the lumbar region; it is better to relax the waist, gently pull the pubic bone upwards towards the navel, and imagine that you are about to sit down on a stool which is directly below you.

The third is to gently flex the spine slightly pushing the vertebrae backwards one by one from bottom to top. (See also 'Coordinating the upper and lower parts', on p.329.)

As you do so, soften and sink the shoulders.

To feel the connection, the relaxation of the neck and the tucking under of the tailbone need to be simultaneous. If done correctly, you will feel the entire spine opening; it is a sensation of the spine stretching and bowing slightly, like a piece of thick elastic creating a natural tension.

This is the ends of the spine working in conjunction – rather like a seesaw; if you move one end of the seesaw, the other end reacts. The body works in exactly the same way – whatever you do to one part of the body should be balanced at the other end – Yin and Yang again.

Note: The pelvic bones should remain at the same level; otherwise the spine will take on a sideways twist in the lumbar region.

TESTING MOVES

In tàijí, 'testing' a move is usually done with a partner, and means that when your partner pushes you from a pre-arranged angle and in a pre-arranged direction, you try to absorb and withstand his push without being uprooted.

When being tested, you are aiming to feel not only comfortable but also strong as you are pushed. When your body is working in a connected or integrated way, when there is no tension in the joints (the bones are resting in their correct position so that they are not being pulled out of alignment by tension) and you have Péng energy within the posture with the Bows of Arms, Legs and Back in place (see also 'Péng Energy', p.345), it will feel effortless to withhold the push.

There is also a sense of borrowing the energy that your partner is expending in trying to push you, and using it to maintain your position.

Any tàijí posture can be used including the intermediate movements, but testing requires that you understand the direction and intention of the movements – which is why I use the term 'pre-arranged' above. If you do not understand the function of a movement, it is difficult to test it correctly as you will not understand the focus of the energy direction within the movement.

Testing is useful in that it makes clear certain aspects of tàijí that you are trying to apply when doing the Form alone.

The method of testing

To test your partner's posture, it is very important to go slowly with the push (or pull). Sudden movements are not helpful to either party when the posture is being tested because you are both looking to feel disconnections or breaks in the alignment of the body, and a sudden movement means that there isn't time to *sense*. In addition, you are more likely to tense up, which defeats the object.

Both parties are learning from the experience, because both of you are trying to feel when the posture is weak or strong.

The angle and direction of the test is very important.

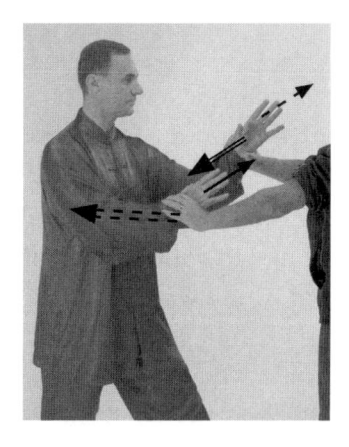

For example, if you are in the final posture of Play the Pipa – weight on your back foot, arms extended ahead of you, etc. (see p.127) – your partner takes hold of your wrists and pushes down the lines of your arms towards the midline of your body.

If your partner tries to lift your hands up, or pushes your arms sideways, this is not testing the movement for the purpose for which it was designed; the movement has a specific function; to test it incorrectly is a little like testing a designer car for its ability to plough a field, or a cricket or baseball bat for its potential as a spoon.

Having the posture tested is not just a case of getting into the posture and merely being a 'recipient', i.e. seeing if you are able to hold it without 'doing' anything, without engaging your own energy. The part of *being* tested requires that you use your own energy, and also make use of your partner's energy to help you hold the posture.

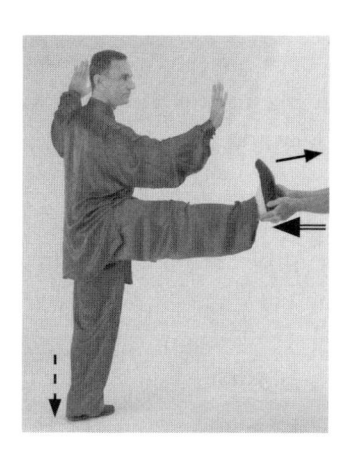

For example, you can test a kick by having your partner take hold of your ankle or foot (of the kicking leg) and push the foot directly towards your pelvis.

As the energy of the push comes towards you, feel as though you are not only pushing with the foot that your partner is holding, but also with the foot that is on the floor – so you are therefore simultaneously 'kicking' downwards.

EDUCATED RELAXATION

This is clearest in two-person exercises. It is the application of the principles of relaxation, and is the ability to 'listen' to a force and respond to it equally as it either comes towards you or moves away from you – it is the ability to 'stick'.

'Listening' is the main ingredient of 'sticking'.

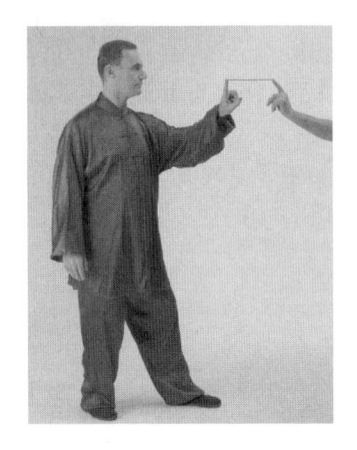

If you and a partner hold an unsharpened pencil (or similar thin stick) between your (for example) left hand index fingertips, and one of you moves the stick (forwards, backwards, up, down, sideways, etc.) whilst the other only has to follow without letting the stick fall, the one following is doing what is known as 'listening' or 'following'.

It is what you might term 'aware relaxation' or 'educated relaxation'; in other words your arm is still in the air ahead of you, so couldn't be said to be completely relaxed, and yet it is certainly not tense because you are sensing every slight movement of your partner and his intentions. The arm therefore works like an antenna.

This exercise is initially easier with the eyes closed.

When you perform the tàijí movements, this quality should still be present in the way that you hold your torso and limbs.

INTENTION (Yĭ) 意

In tàijí, as in everything, there is your inner experience and there is your outwards expression. Your intention or 'yĭ' 意 acts as the bridge between the two.

Your experience is the key to how you act outwardly, i.e. to how you express your experience. It is the sum of all that you have understood that has become part of who you are.

In tàijí that 'experience' is not just a matter of the number of times that you have performed a particular movement, nor is it only the understanding of a movement (although both of these can be contributory); the experience is a feeling that becomes a part of *you* – you become an expression of the tàijí movement, and the tàijí movement becomes as expression of you.

When you first begin to learn the tàijí movements this isn't possible; it takes time and patience, and a lot of practice so that the movements become second nature.

Once you have reached this level, you move to a different 'level', as only then can you begin to appreciate the purpose of the movement, the correct way to make it work for that purpose, and how the body integrates whilst doing the movement.

This is where your 'yǐ' 意 (intention) comes in.

Intention is a creative tool; in tàijí it *creates* the movement, bringing it into being and giving it life. It is the carrier of the sum of your understanding about that movement.

Tàijíquán is often referred to as 'shadow boxing'. The shadows that you are 'boxing' are your understanding of the purpose of the movements within the Form – so, as you perform the movements, you have an imaginary opponent or opponents.

So for example, if you are pushing, you feel as though you are actually pushing someone. Not only do you *visualize* him as being there, you *feel* what you would feel if he really were there – the slightest pressure on leg, body, arm or hand, and how your body would need to react, hold, and position itself in such an eventuality.

Your energy follows your intention – if you think of your finger, the energy will go to your finger. Thought is energy, so wherever you place that thought, that is where you will direct your energy.

This is very easy to experience, just think of the tip of your index finger; without touching it, try to feel the nail of the index finger, feel the sides of the finger, feel under the nail, feel the 'pad' of the finger... You will find that it possibly gets hotter, feels like it's swelling, starts to tingle and possibly even feels slightly uncomfortable.

All you've done is to increase the blood and energy supply to that finger; your intention has made it happen.

The most important point about intention is that you *feel*, and it certainly isn't necessary to do the movements faster; speed has nothing to do with it.

FĀ JÌN 发

This can be translated loosely as 'explosive energy', '...power', or '...force', although in the West we tend to use the word 'force' to mean muscular power.

Fā jìn is the art of releasing power in a split second; it is the art of moving 1) from a relaxed state, 2) to a state of effort, or energy expulsion, and 3) back to a state of relaxation – all in a split second.

The energy for this movement is always produced from the centre of the body, the dāntián and, when executed, feels internally something like a very brief physical whirlwind with minimal movement at its centre, but a lot at its perimeter.

Fā jìn is:

1. the sensing of your partner's/opponent's energy

2. moving with and following it

3. dissolving it

4. the perfect coordination and timing of your energy release based upon the sensing of the dissolved energy

5. finally followed by your total relaxation.

(1) and (2) need no explanation.

'Dissolving' your partner's energy (3) means that you both divert his energy (in effect making it lose its point), and (as a result) force him to withdraw it.

This 'diversion' of energy is like the batsman who allows the ball from the bowler (known as a 'pitcher' in baseball) to glance off his bat and go past him.

The 'withdrawal of energy' means that, in the case of your partner's energy, if he doesn't withdraw it, he is going to fall forwards as there is now nothing supporting him – he will feel as though his balance has been upset and he will want to regain it.

In tàijí from the Fā jìn practitioner's point of view, this usually involves the use of a circle, because the circle is the diversion. The circle doesn't have to be big, it can be tiny.

(4) is fairly self-evident.

(5) isn't so evident. Tension is a 'holding in' of energy; so if you push and then remain tense, you are keeping your own energy back. Nearly everyone who has played a ball game, golf, tennis, squash, cricket, baseball, etc. knows this; it's the follow-through, a release of energy that you can only do if you relax and use your 'intention' (yǐ 意) to direct the ball. It's no different in Fā jìn.

From a mechanical perspective, in the moment of the push and energy release (the precise moment of tension or explosion), it is the perfect unification of all parts of the body:

...the correct connection of centre to hip to knee to foot

...the correct connection of centre to shoulder to elbow to hand

...the correct connection of centre to both ends of the spine

...the correct use of the flexion of the spine, and the drawing up of the energy to between the shoulder-blades

...the simultaneous integrated employment of the ankle/wrist, knee/elbow, hip/shoulder connections

...the correct connection of centre to the earth.

But at the heart of it all is the correct 'sensing' of your partner's/opponent's energy, its dissolution, and the angle of redirection.

Fā jìn is also the extreme application of 'close' (Hé 合) and 'open' (Kāi 开).

Fā jìn exercises

The feeling of Fā jìn can be practised as a solo exercise, although it is preferable to practise with a partner.

CONNECTING THE LEGS AND THE CENTRE

Stand in an Empty Stance (with your weight therefore on the back leg); leave your arms hanging loosely by your sides.

Without moving too slowly, push your weight forwards *slightly* on to the front leg (maybe so the weight distribution is 50/50, maybe not even as much as that – less is better).

As the weight arrives on the front foot, push that foot firmly into the ground, applying in effect a 'brake' to the forwards movement; if you have left your hands hanging loosely by your sides, you should find that they continue to move forwards after you've 'braked'.

This exercise works on the same principle as getting the sauce out of a tight-necked bottle – pointing the bottle where you want the sauce to land, you throw the bottle forwards and then in effect pull it backwards suddenly. The sauce inside however, being 'relaxed', doesn't brake but carries on; the thicker it is (i.e. the tenser or more 'unrelaxed' it is), the shorter distance it travels out of the neck of the bottle.

To use another analogy, if your shopping is lying loose on the back seat of your car and you suddenly brake or hit, say, a wall with the car, everything will move from the back seat towards the front of the vehicle.

In Fā jìn it is the *instant* relaxation after braking that is so very important, because this is the moment that the power is released. In Fā jìn, you *want* the sauce to be propelled from the bottle; you *want* the shopping to land on the dashboard.

So two important factors are:

1. the ability to 'apply the brake' correctly, and

2. relaxation immediately after the Fā jìn.

However, in order to produce power, we first have to generate it. The sitting back procedure prior to the production of power is very important; as you sit back, tuck your hips/coccyx/sacrum under as much as you can – coiling the abdomen, hips and waist like a spring. Simultaneously, hollow the chest, dropping the elbows...which brings us to the arms...

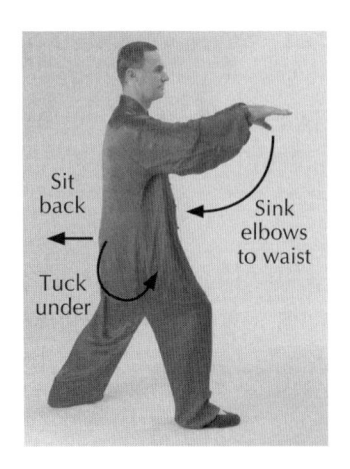

CONNECTING THE ARMS AND THE CENTRE

The arm movement of the solo exercise is circular. To get the feel of it, put 60–70 per cent of weight on to the front foot (you will not usually do this, but it helps to describe the shape that the arms create in the movement) and leave the arms outstretched (with palms down) ahead of you.

OPEN (KĀI 开) AND CLOSE (HÉ 合)

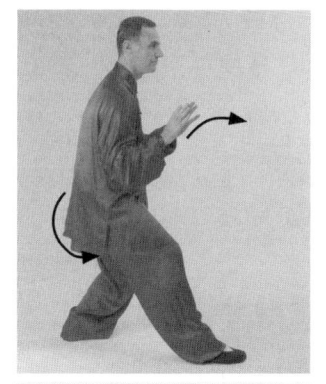

As you sit back on to your rear foot, push the palms towards the floor drawing them back towards your hips/waist.

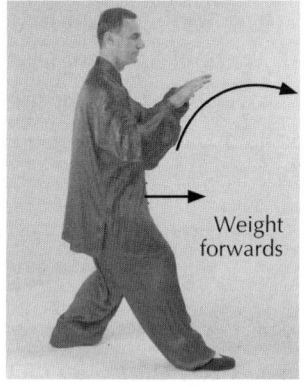

As you arrive on the back foot, the hands rise up the body in front of your chest, which brings us back to where we were before…
'Simultaneously, hollow the chest, dropping the elbows…'

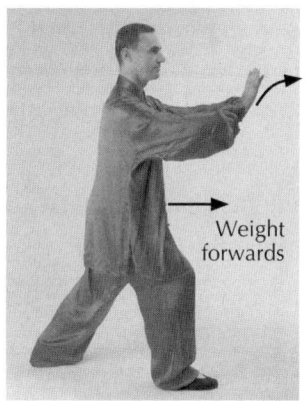

You then push the weight rapidly forwards, and…

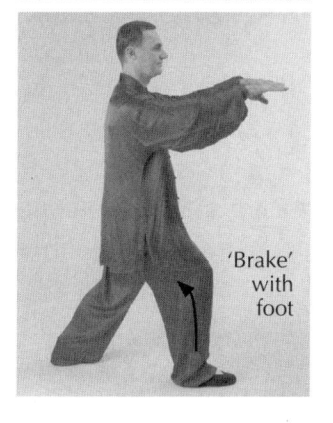

…as you apply the brake, the arms (the 'sauce' – the 'shopping on the rear seat') are ejected forwards as the spring uncoils, and the body immediately sinks back into the rear foot again.

This is the 'basic' solo exercise.

THE YANG TÀIJÍ 24-STEP SHORT FORM

WORKING WITH A PARTNER

The differences when working with a partner are:

- Your partner should grasp his own elbows, with his arms approximately parallel to the ground; it helps if he is a little tense. You place your hands on his arms.

- Because your partner's arms are there, you will not be able to lower your arms to the extent that you did in the solo exercise.

- When you push down with your palms as you sit back, feel the 'spring' of his arms. You are going to use this 'spring' to uproot him. Without any forwards or backwards movement, practise only pushing his arms down and feeling them spring back upwards again; when they do, don't lose contact, follow them.

- When gently pulling him forwards towards you as you sit backwards, feel his reluctance to move forwards. This means that his energy is already going backwards, and you will be able to use this when you push him.

- You are trying to connect his energy (his centre/core) to your energy, so that you are able to control it. Don't hurry, *feel* what is going on in his body; if you don't, you will lose half of the result. (This is what 'adhering' or 'sticking' in tàijí means – you are 'reading' someone, feeling his balance, his strengths, his weaknesses, his position, etc.)

- Generally, when working with a partner, the movements that you need to make will be much smaller than those when you work solo.

THE PUSH

When you make the Fā jìn push, you need to bring the energy up the spine.

When you've curled the pelvis under (done a pelvic tilt), the energy is in the lower dāntián.

To feel the next part, put your hands on your partner's arms (you are sitting back ready to push). Sink the elbows and slightly hyper-extend the shoulders forwards, hollowing the chest, whilst feeling the palms completely connected to your partner's arms. You will have a sensation first of the lumbar spine pushing backwards, and then of the thoracic vertebrae (somewhere between thoracics 4 and 8) expanding slightly, almost as though the spine is curving back in those areas. Simultaneously, release your neck – don't let it compress – and, more to the point, don't let your chin jut forwards.

Push…and instantly release.

… And then try putting that concept into the solo Form, but so subtly that it is almost invisible.

THE TIMING

As you practise this, you will find that by far the most difficult part of this is the timing of the push. There are exercises to teach this, but they are beyond the scope of this book.

THE YANG TÀIJÍ 24-STEP SHORT FORM MUSIC: BREAKDOWN OF BEATS PER MOVEMENT

Musical introduction

The 'official' music can be purchased from most retailers that supply taijiquan DVDs, and taiji equipment such as weapons and clothing.

The music is approximately six and a half minutes long, and begins with an introduction, giving the practitioner time to prepare.

Usually there are two versions; one with the names of the various forms spoken over the music (in Chinese) so that you know where you should be in the form at any given point, and the other with only the music.

The description that follows is to help with the unspoken version.

This is the Ready Position 预备势 (Yùbèishì). It is 16 beats (4 bars) long (although there is a considerable amount of 'rubato' in the playing, i.e. the timing is slowed and lengthened).

Before the main theme begins, there are four bass notes, and it is during the last *two* of these that you step to the left with the left foot (see 'Commencing Form 起势 (Qǐshì)' in the table on the following page).

Form no.	No. of beats	Related postures
Commencing Form 起势 (Qǐshì)	4	**Beginning:** Step out with left foot
1	8 (4 + 4)	**Raise and lower hands**
2	8 + 8 + 8	**Parting the Wild Horse's Mane** (1–3)
3	8	**Stork Spreads its Wings**
4	10 + 8 + 8	**Brush Knee and Twist Step** (1–3)
5	8	**Play the Pipa**
6	8 + 8 + 8+ 8	**Repulse Monkey** (1–4)
7	8	**Grasp the Bird's Tail (L):** Hold the ball and Péng (R)…
	8	…from Péng to the point where you connect heel of palm to heel of palm still sitting back; this is to just before Jǐ. (*On count 5, the arms are approximately out to the right side*)…
	10	…from Jǐ to Àn (R)
8	2	**Grasp the Bird's Tail (R):** Sit back and connection to right side
	8	Turn, hold the ball and Péng (L)…
	8	…from Péng to the point where you connect heel of palm to heel of palm still sitting back; this is to just before Jǐ. (*On count 5, the arms are approximately out to the left side*)…
	10	…from Jǐ to Àn (L)
9	8 (4 + 4)	**Push left** (4) and **Push right** to Crane's Beak (4)
	4	**Single Whip**
10	8 + 8 + 8	**Wave Hands Like Clouds** (on first beat of the second '8', draw the right foot in; on the fifth beat of the second '8', step with the left foot. Repeat this pattern for the remainder of steps)

OPEN (KĀI 开) AND CLOSE (HÉ 合)

Form no.	No. of beats	Related postures
11	4	**Turn to the right corner** and into Crane's Beak (4)
	4	**Single Whip**
12	8	**High Pat on Horse** (arms open by count 4)
13	10	**Kick with Right Heel** (separate the arms for the first time on approximately beat 5)
14	8 (4 + 4)	**Strike (Opponent's) Ears with Both Fists** (count 4 is sitting back)
15	10	**Turn and Kick with Left Heel**
16	2 (slow feel)	Preparatory to Snake Creeps Down (1)…
	8 (6 + 2)	…**Snake Creeps Down (L)** (count 6 is left hand by knee/leg; then 2 counts to body upright – not on 1 leg yet)…
	4	**Golden Cockerel on One Leg (R)**
17	4 (slow feel)	Preparatory to Snake Creeps Down (2)…
	8 (6 + 2)	…**Snake Creeps Down (R)** (count 6 is right hand by knee/leg; then 2 counts to body upright – not on 1 leg yet)…
	4	**Golden Cockerel on One Leg (L)**
18	8 + 8	**Jade Lady Weaves Shuttles** (1 and 2)
19	8	**Needle at Sea Bottom**
20	6	**Flash Arms**
21	8	**Turn, Deflect Downwards** (to Bān)…
	8	…through **Parry** (Lán) to **Punch** (Chuí)
22	8	**Apparent Close-Up to Àn**
23	8	**Cross Hands**
24	8	**Closing Form**: Separate and lower hands and feet together
		Depending on the orchestral version of the music, there are two notes that could be interpreted as: 1. weight shift to right foot 2. left foot in and hands by sides

THE YANG TÀIJÍ 24-STEP SHORT FORM IN COMPETITION

General principles of evaluation

In traditional routine competition, the contestant is appraised on overall technical ability as displayed in performance. The following evaluation guidelines are taken from the BCCMA Competition Manual with the kind permission of the BCCMA.

Each contestant commences the evaluation with a maximum score of 10 points; this represents the highest level of achievement. Whenever errors in the performance occur, points will be deducted according to various criteria.

No additional points may be awarded for any spectacular techniques displayed by the contestant.

In tàijíquán, slow and smooth movement are displayed to give the impression of softness with firmness of the yĭ (focus one's intention or subconscious).

The evaluation consists of three parts:

1. the quality of movements (6 points)

2. a) power and coordination (2 points)

    b) style and spirit (2 points)

3. The deduction criteria for other errors.

1. The **quality** of the movements in the 24-Step Form refers to:

    - the correct method of *forming* the *hand(s)*
    - the correct method of demonstrating the *stances*
    - the correct method of holding the *body*

    and to the **technique** of the movements which refers to:

    - the correct methods of *using* the *hand(s)*
    - the correct methods of executing the *leg* techniques, for example the kicks
    - the correct methods of using the *body* in movements
    - the correct methods of using the *feet*, for example in stepping, and balance.

2. The **overall** skills refer to the power and coordination, and the style and spirit of the performance.

   - **Power** refers to the techniques being executed smoothly, the appropriate force being applied accurately in unison with all other movements.

   - **Coordination** refers to the body integration when executing a technique (the potential for producing power so that the technique will be effective).

   - **Style** refers to the Form not being performed in the manner of a different style of tàijí (e.g. Chen or Sun).

   - **Spirit** refers to the yĭ which shows through the facial expression and eyes, but also in the clarity in performance of the movements.

3. The **deduction criteria** are an incomplete routine and/or forgetfulness of the routine, and 'errors', which fall into three categories: 1) slight errors, 2) apparent errors, and 3) severe errors.

A few examples of these are:

Movement	Slight error	Apparent error	Severe error
	Deduct 0.1 point	Deduct 0.2 point	Deduct 0.3 point
Stork Spreads its Wings	1. Fingers bunched together or too loose and soft. 2. Body leaning forwards and buttocks protruding. 3. Transition is not distinguishable from one stance to another. 4. Shoulders too rigid and as a result movement is restricted. 5. Eyes looking to the floor.	Repeating the same error twice.	Repeating the same error more than three times. (This is the maximum points that can be deducted for the same error occurring throughout the whole routine.)

And again:

Movement	Slight error	Apparent error	Severe error
	Deduct 0.1 point	**Deduct 0.2 point**	**Deduct 0.3 point**
Play the Pipa	1. Transition is clumsy from one stance to another in execution. 2. The front heel is not placed gently on the floor. 3. The right hand is too far apart from the left elbow, and the fingers point at the floor. 4. The shoulders are too rigid. 5. The body leans forwards and the buttocks protrude.	Repeating the same error twice.	Repeating the same error more than three times. (This is the maximum points that can be deducted for the same error occurring throughout the whole routine.)

Some examples of deduction criteria for **power** and **coordination** are:

Type of expression	Minor error	Apparent error	Severe error
	Deduct 0.1–0.5 points	**Deduct 0.6–1.0 points**	**Deduct 1.1–2.0 points**
Power	1. Force is applied rigidly or loosely. 2. Inaccurate focus. 3. Insipid force is applied and there is no clear distinction between emptiness and firmness. 4. Lack of lightness and agility.	1. Reckless and tense movements restrict the delivery of intended force. 2. Repeat the same error twice.	1. Movements too abrupt and weak to deliver the intended force to designated target. 2. Repeating the same error more than three times.

| **Coordination** | 1. Inconsistent coordination of movements.
2. Transition from one stance to another is not agile.
3. Eyes do not coincide with the hand movements. | 1. Hand and waist movements are poorly coordinated.
2. Perception irregular and dispersed.
3. Lack of continuity between various movements. | 1. Hand and foot movements not coordinated, and obstruct each other.
2. No evidence of coordination of movements.
3. Execution of routine is mechanical, devoid of tàijí characteristics. |
|---|---|---|---|

GENERAL GUIDELINES

1. Poor performance: 7.9 points
2. Average performance: 8.0–8.5 points
3. Good performance: 8.6–9.0 points
4. Excellent performance: 9.1–10 points

Key points to observe

In evaluation, it is essential that judges pay attention to the main points of the routine with the entire performance in mind.

1. Tàijíquán should be performed slowly, calmly, and with agility to give the appearance of softness yet firmness.

2. The way in which the body is used is the main factor in deciding whether the contestant's posture is correct or not.

    The body should be erect and relaxed, with its weight naturally distributed. The movements should be easy but not soft, stretching but not rigid.

3. Coordination is the key to the contestant's overall performance.

    Therefore, to achieve integrated performance, the waist must lead the arms and legs in order to generate the power to the hands.

4. The way in which the hand is held is important.

   The middle of the palm must be hollow with fingers slightly apart, relaxed and firm.

   The fist must be clenched firmly and softly, but not tightly and rigidly.

5. Transition from one stance to another must coincide with the hand movements.

6. The overall skill performance (power, hand techniques, coordination, spirit and style) shall be evaluated at the end of the contestant's performance.

19

Footprint of the Form

KEY TO FOOT PATTERNS

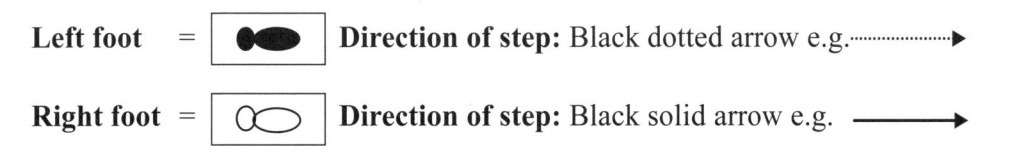

Left foot = 🯅 **Direction of step:** Black dotted arrow e.g. ┄┄┄►

Right foot = ⬭ **Direction of step:** Black solid arrow e.g. ──────►

The arrow, depending upon its positioning, refers either to the direction of the next step, or to where the foot has come from.

A double arrow ═══► signifies the rotation of the body.

▼▲ or ▽△ signifies toes *down* or toes *up*, and the colour again refers to left (black) or right (white).

▼⌒ (or e.g. ⌒▽) shows the angle of the foot when on the ball of the foot.

● or ○ signifies the foot raised off the ground – the colour again referring to left (grey) or right (white).

'Slipping the heel' is shown by a small arrow which starts from the heel, dotted for the left foot, and solid for the right foot. The previous foot position is shown in feint: or

'Turning the toes' is shown by a similar method:

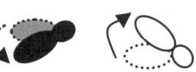

369

THE YANG TÀIJÍ 24-STEP SHORT FORM

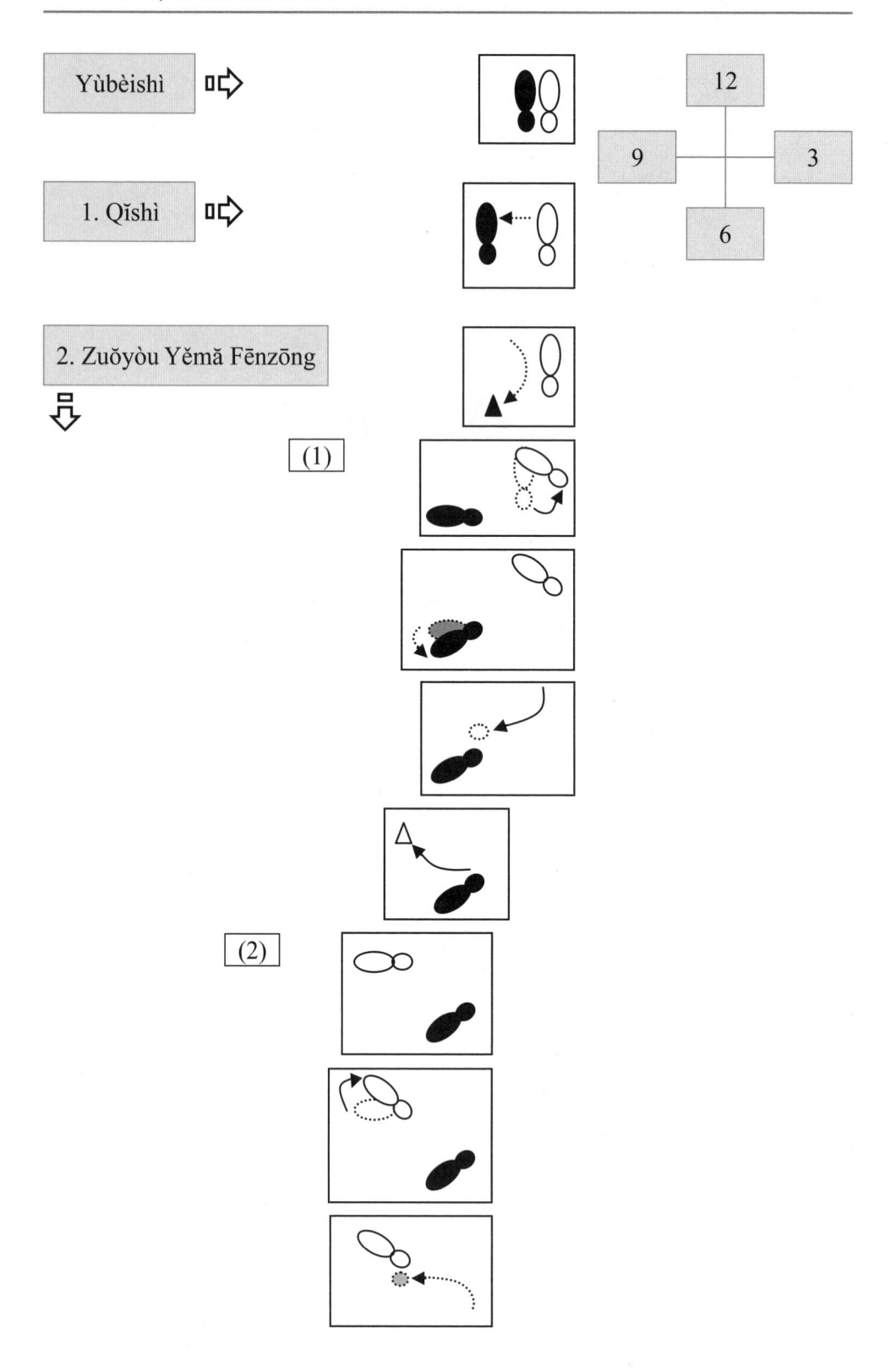

Yùbèishì ⇨

1. Qǐshì ⇨

2. Zuǒyòu Yěmǎ Fēnzōng ⇩

(1)

(2)

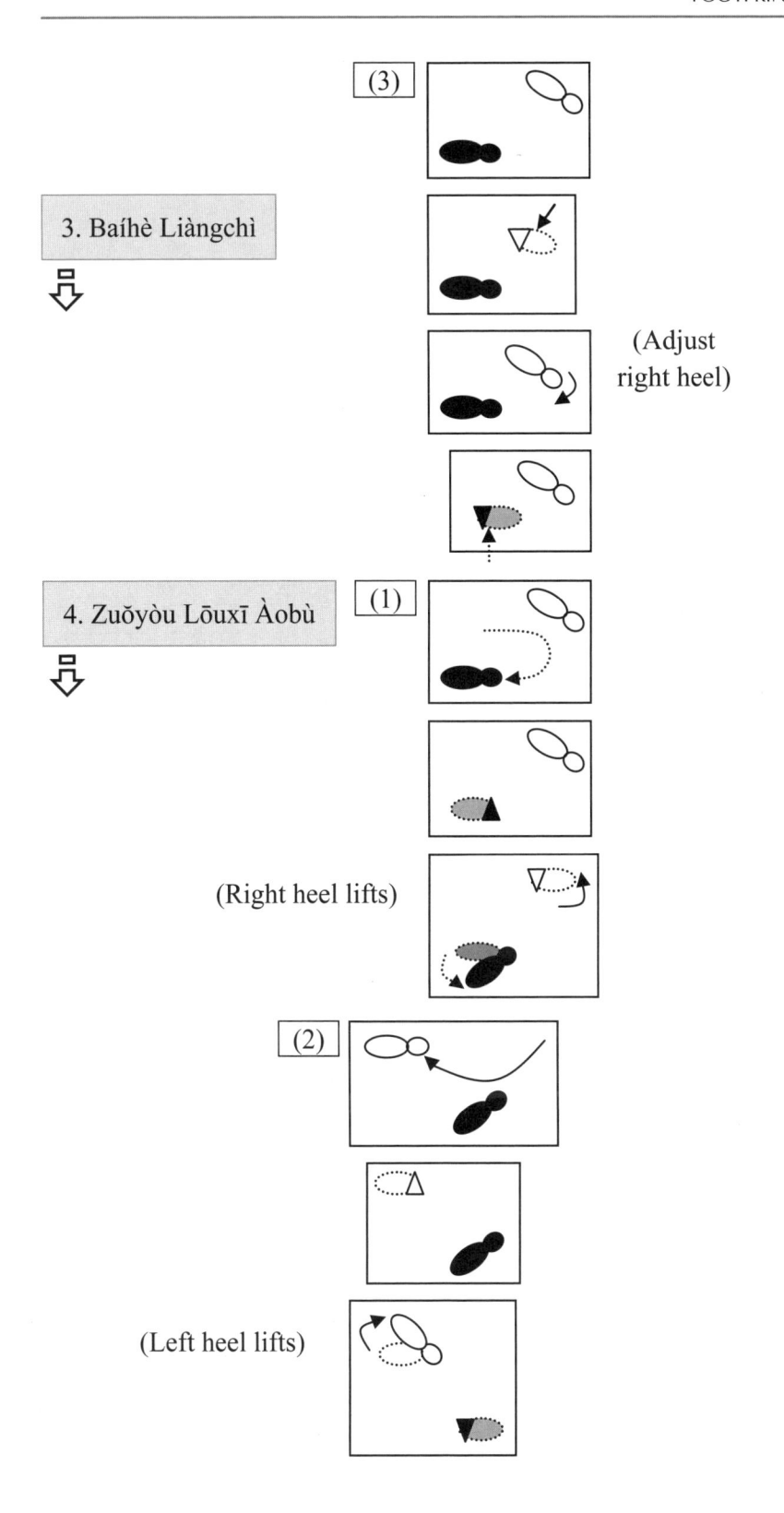

FOOTPRINT OF THE FORM

3. Baíhè Liàngchì

(3)

(Adjust right heel)

4. Zuǒyòu Lōuxī Àobù

(1)

(Right heel lifts)

(2)

(Left heel lifts)

THE YANG TÀIJÍ 24-STEP SHORT FORM

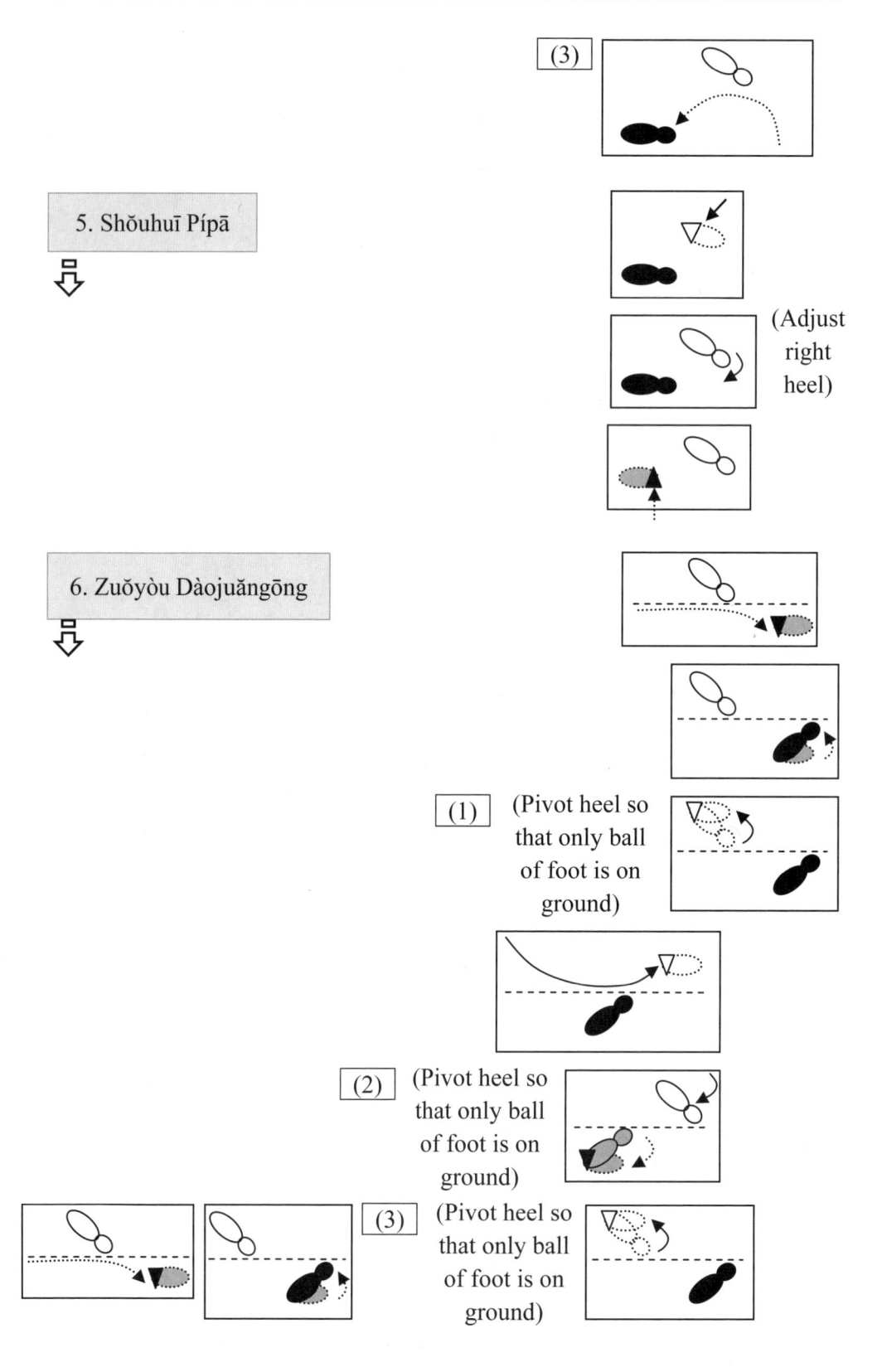

(3)

5. Shǒuhuī Pípā
⇩

(Adjust right heel)

6. Zuǒyòu Dàojuǎngōng
⇩

(1) (Pivot heel so that only ball of foot is on ground)

(2) (Pivot heel so that only ball of foot is on ground)

(3) (Pivot heel so that only ball of foot is on ground)

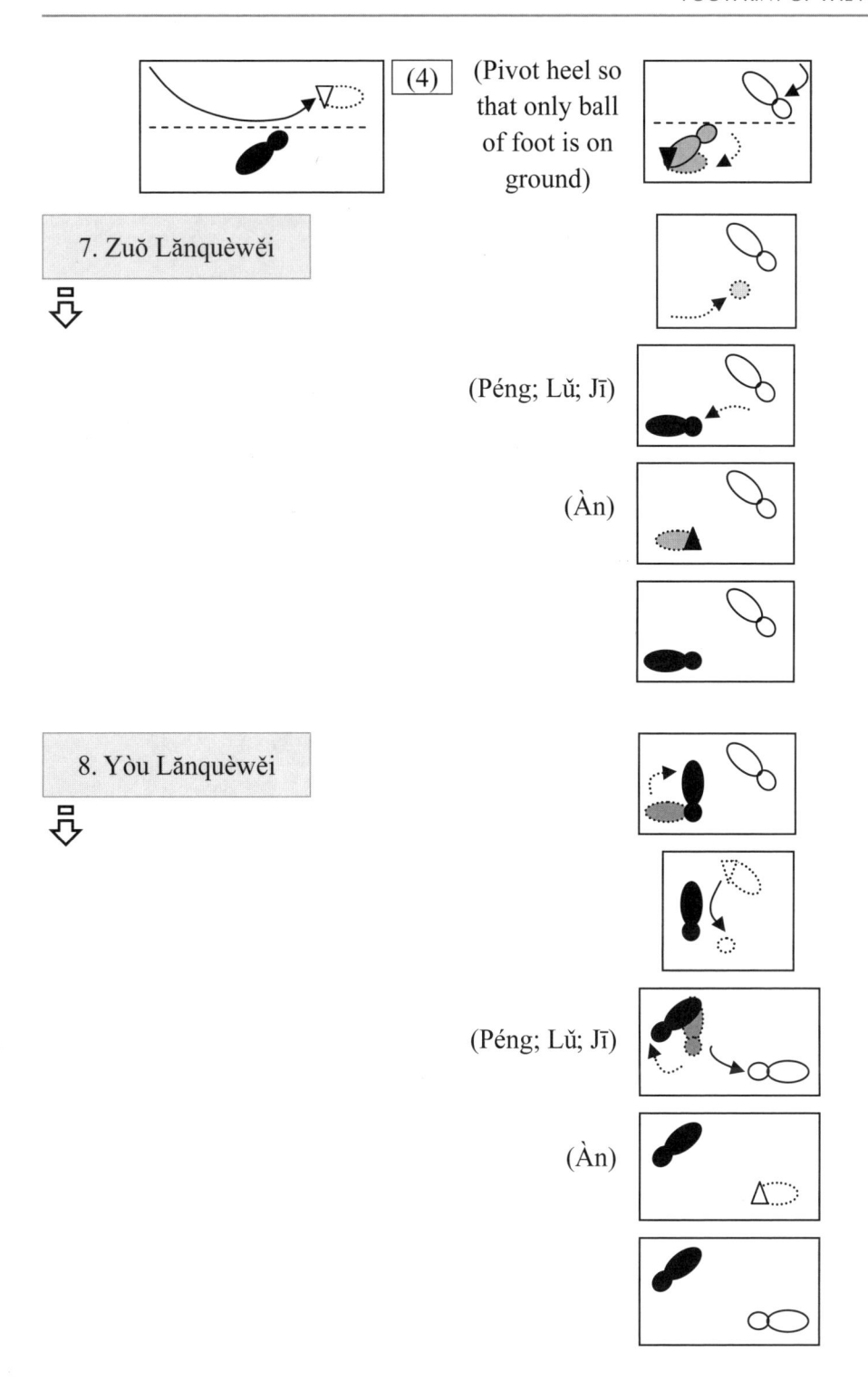

FOOTPRINT OF THE FORM

(4) (Pivot heel so that only ball of foot is on ground)

7. Zuǒ Lǎnquèwěi

(Péng; Lǔ; Jī)

(Àn)

8. Yòu Lǎnquèwěi

(Péng; Lǔ; Jī)

(Àn)

373

THE YANG TÀIJÍ 24-STEP SHORT FORM

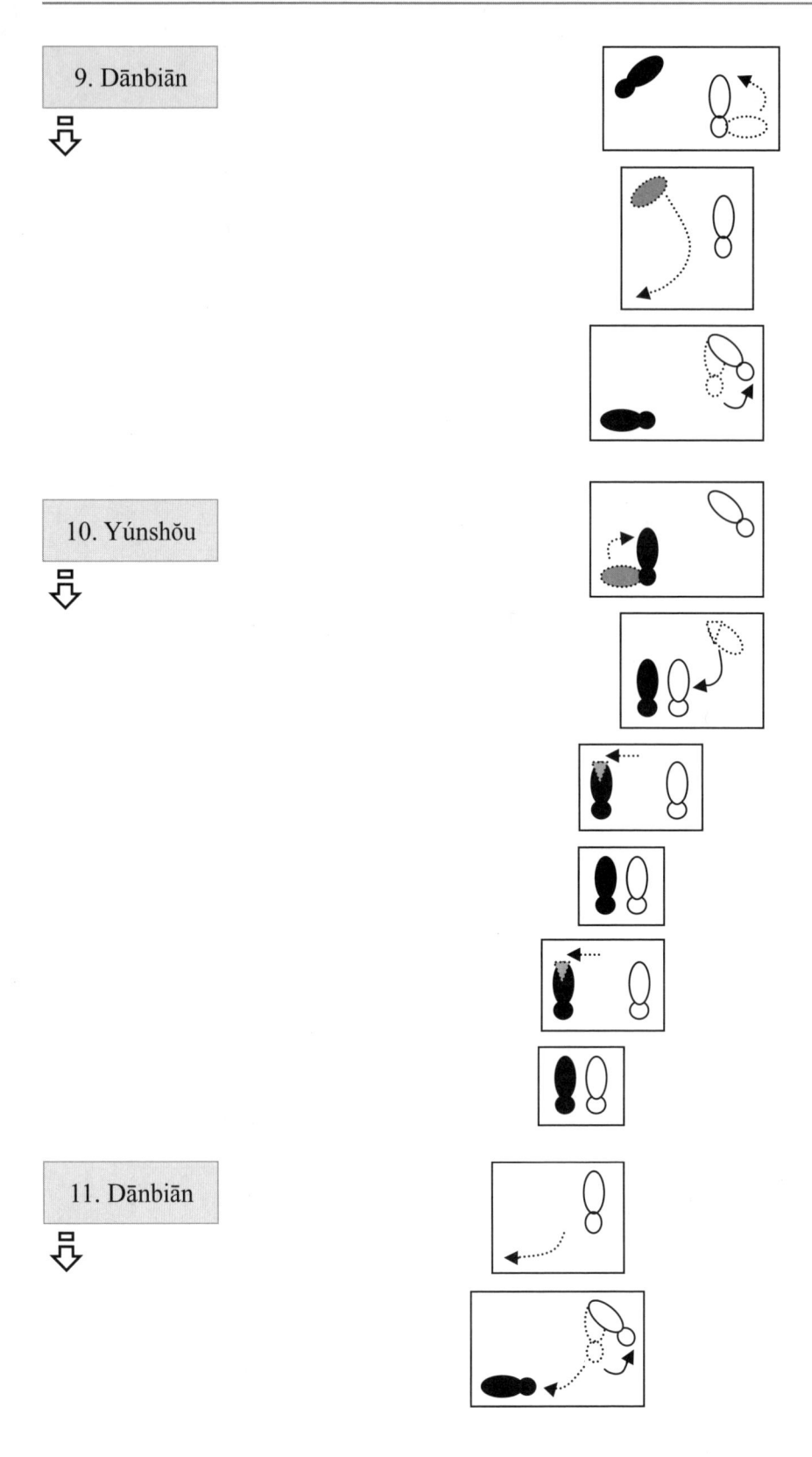

9. Dānbiān
⇩

10. Yúnshǒu
⇩

11. Dānbiān
⇩

374

FOOTPRINT OF THE FORM

12. Gāotànmǎ

(Adjust right heel)

(Optional adjustment of left toes inwards)

13. Yòu Dēngjiǎo

Variation
Angle of foot

Variation

Right foot kick

Variation

14. Shuāngfēng Guàn'ěr

Variation

Variation

THE YANG TÀIJÍ 24-STEP SHORT FORM

15. Zhuǎnshēn Zuǒ Dēngjiǎo
⇩

Variation

Left foot kick

16. Zuǒ Xiàshì Dúlì
⇩

17. Yòu Xiàshì Dúlì
⇩

376

FOOTPRINT OF THE FORM

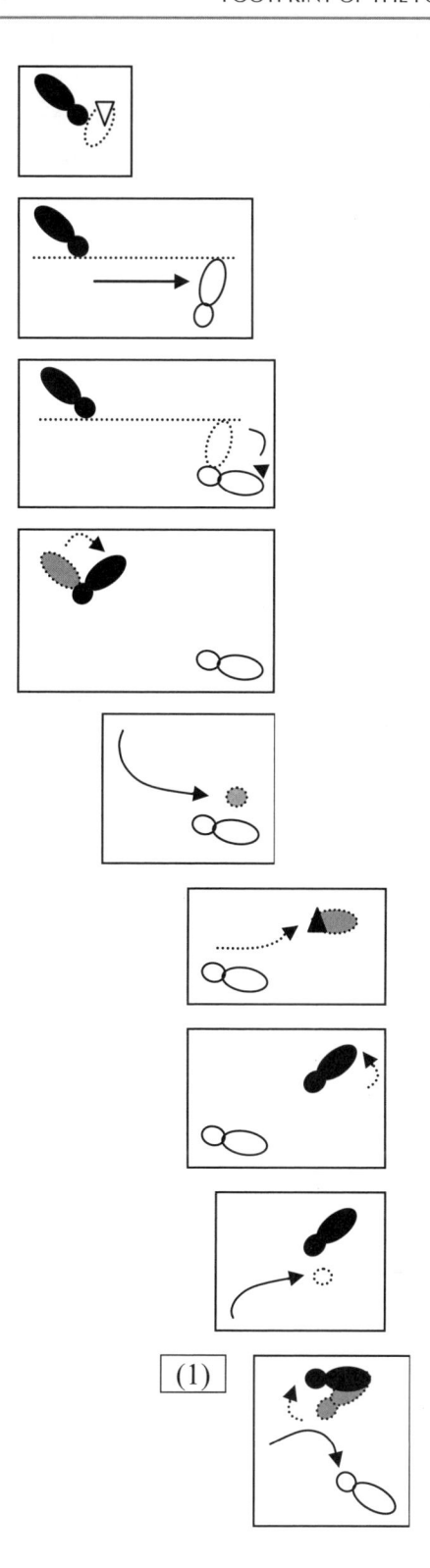

18. Zuǒyòu Chuānsuō

(1)

377

THE YANG TÀIJÍ 24-STEP SHORT FORM

(Optional sitting back between previous and following movements)

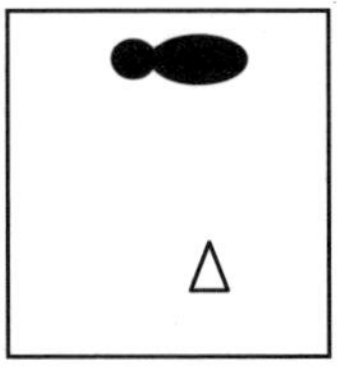

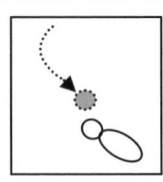

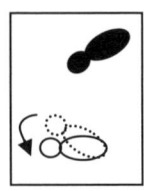

19. Hǎidǐzhēn

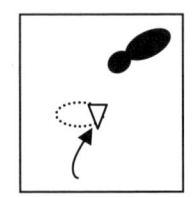

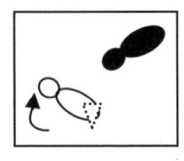

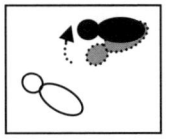

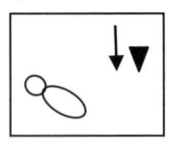

20. Shǎntōngbì

(Optional to bring the left foot in prior to re-stepping)

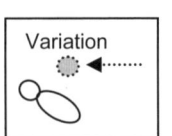

Variation

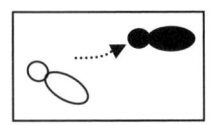

378

FOOTPRINT OF THE FORM

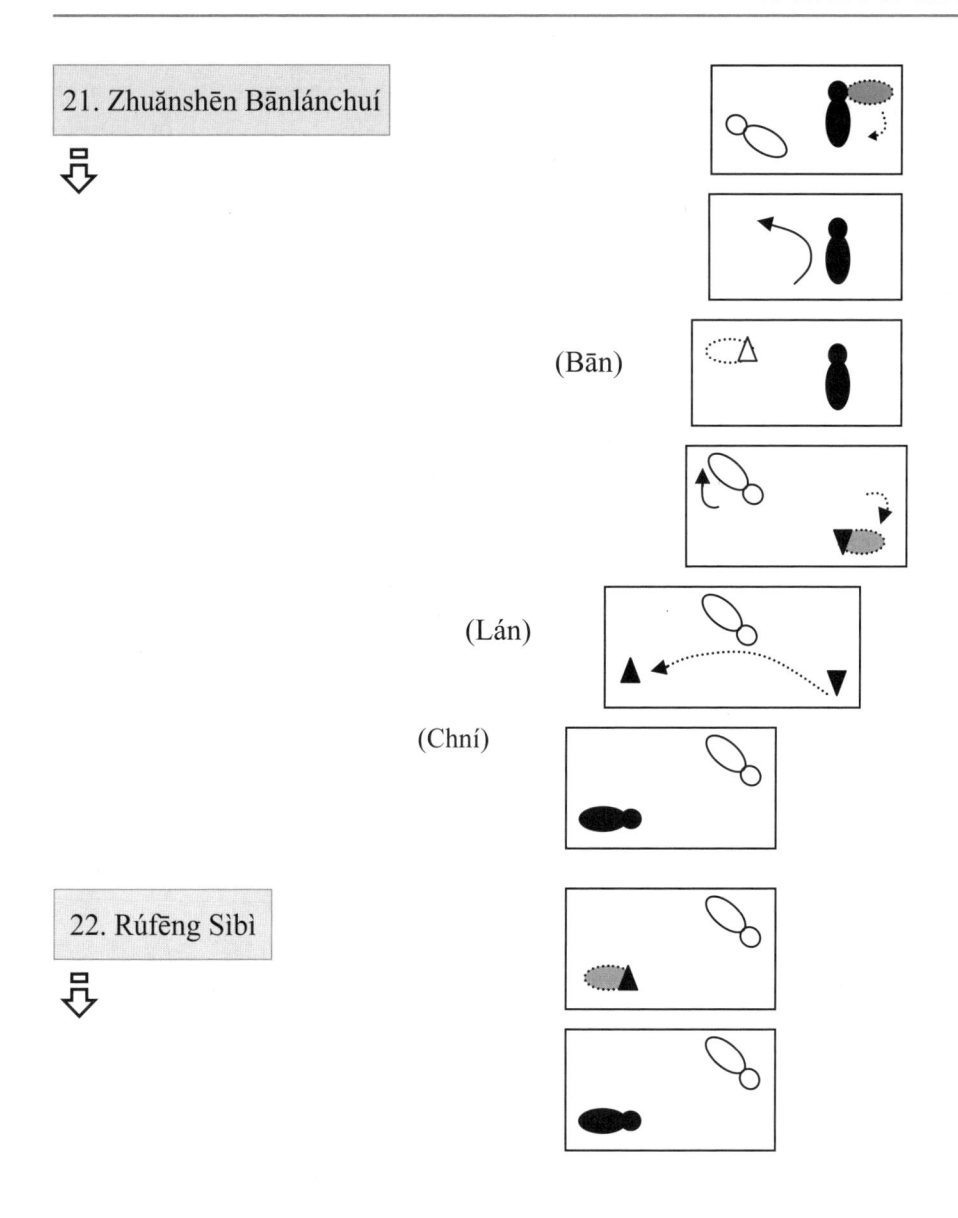

21. Zhuǎnshēn Bānlánchuí

(Bān)

(Lán)

(Chuí)

22. Rúfēng Sìbì

379

THE YANG TÀIJÍ 24-STEP SHORT FORM

23. Shízìshǒu

(Adjusting the right toes is optional)

24. Shōushì

(Some people treat *this* as the start of Form 24)

About the Author

James Drewe became involved in the Chinese Health Arts in 1975 when he began by studying Gongfu and Tàijíquán. He rapidly became interested in the philosophy behind these forms of exercise and also in both meditation and the use of diet to promote health. Since then he has taken an interest in a variety of other health arts and qualified as an acupuncturist.

In 1980 he began learning the Yang family style of Tàijíquán and Zhan Zhuang Qìgōng under Master Chu King Hung and has also studied Zhan Zhuang Qìgōng with Master Lam Kam Chuen.

He later broadened his tàijí training with Richard Watson, learning the core syllabus of both Hand and Sword Forms of the 'modern' Yang style. He has also studied many of these with both Professor Li Deyin and Master Wang Yanji.

He has studied the Chen 56-Step Competition Form, the Wudang Tàijí Sword Form, the Sun 97-Step Form, the Yang Broadsword, and the Fan Form with Professor Li Deyin; the Chen Broadsword with Simon Watson, and the Sun 73-Step Competition Form with both Simon Watson, and Master Huang Ping.

He currently teaches a wide variety of forms. These are taught alongside various two-person forms (both for barehand and sword), Pushing Hands, Da Lu, Applications of the Forms, and Fā jìn techniques.

In Qìgōng, apart from Zhan Zhuang Qìgōng, he has studied a therapeutic Qìgōng called Daoyin Yangsheng Gong, which consists of sets of exercises for the cardiovascular, digestive, respiratory and skeletal systems, as well as exercises for the five major organs with Richard Watson, Mark Atkinson, Hu Xiao Fei, and Professor Zhang Guande.

James is vice-chairman of the Longfei Taijiquan Association, and runs classes in both London and Kent.

Details of courses and classes can be found on the website at www.taiji.co.uk and www.qigonghealth.co.uk, and he can be emailed at james@taiji.co.uk.

Further Reading

Li Deyin (2008) *Tàijíquán* (Book and DVD). London: Jessica Kingsley Publishers.

Jan Diepersloot (1995) *Warriors of Stillness: Meditative Traditions in the Chinese Martial Arts, Vol 1*. London: Paul H. Crompton.

Dan Docherty (2009) *Tai Chi Chuan: Decoding the Classics for the Modern Martial Artist*. Wiltshire: The Crowood Press.

Neale Donald Walsch (2003) *The New Revelations: A Conversation with God (Conversations with God)*. London: Hodder Mobius.

Yang Zhenduo (1991) *Yang Style Tàijíquán*. Beijing: Morning Glory Publishers.